T-CELL LEUKEMIA

Edited by **Olga Babusikova, Sinisa Dovat**
and **Kimberly J. Payne**

T-Cell Leukemia
Edited by Olga Babusikova, Sinisa Dovat and Kimberly J. Payne

Published by InTech
Janeza Trdine 9, 51000 Rijeka, Croatia

Publishing Process Manager Martina Blecic

Technical Editor Teodora Smiljanic

Cover Designer InTech Design Team

Additional hard copies can be obtained from orders@intechopen.com

T-Cell Leukemia, Edited by Olga Babusikova, Sinisa Dovat and Kimberly J. Payne
p. cm.
ISBN 978-953-307-400-9

For EU product safety concerns:
IN TECH d.o.o., Prolaz Marije Krucifikse Kozulić 3, 51000 Rijeka, Croatia,
info@intechopen.com or visit our website at intechopen.com.

Contents

Preface

1. Introduction

T cell malignancies include a spectrum of diseases. The most common of them are: 1) Adult T-cell leukemia (ATLL); 2) Childhood T-cell Acute lymphoblastic leukemia (T-ALL); 3) Cutaneous T-cell lymphoma – that includes mycosis fungoides and Sezary syndrome; and 4) Anaplastic large cell lymphoma – anaplastic lymphoma kinase (ALK)-positive. Although these diseases are distinct clinical entities, they all pose challenging treatment problems for oncologists. Many of these illnesses carry a poor prognosis, and novel treatment modalities are essential to improve survival. Over the last 10 years, significant progress has been made in understanding the molecular pathogenesis of these diseases, which promises to lead to novel targeted chemotherapeutic agents. The purpose of this book is to provide a comprehensive review of the scientific advances in T-cell malignancies and to highlight the most relevant findings that will help the reader understand both basic mechanisms of the disease and future directions that are likely to lead to novel therapies. In order to assure a thorough approach to these problems, contributors include basic scientists, translational researchers and clinicians who are experts in this field. Thus, the target audience for this book includes both basic scientists who will use this book as a review of the advances in our fundamental knowledge of the molecular mechanisms of T-cell malignancies, as well as clinicians who will use this book as a tool to understand rationales for the development of novel treatments for these diseases.

2. Adult Human T-Cell Leukemia and Molecular Mechansims of HTLV-1

The first chapter, "Adult Human T cell Leukemia" by Herbeuval J-P., provides an overview of human ATLL. This chapter spans the role of HTLV-1 virus, including its genomic and epidemiological characteristics; the clinical picture and treatment of ATLL, and immune response to HTLV-1 with a brief overview of the role of specific types of immune cells. This chapter gives a comprehensive review of ATLL, with sufficient depth of knowledge for practical oncologists, without extensive molecular mechanistic details of the pathophysiology of the disease.

The subsequent three chapters are primarily concerned with the molecular mechanisms by which HTLV-1 causes ATLL. Chapter 2, "Human T-Cell

Lymphotropic Virus (HTLV-1) and Adult T-Cell Leukemia," by Abbaszadegan M.R. and Gholamin M., provides an overview of the structure, epidemiology, function and pathophysiological effects of HTLV-1 in A-TALL. This chapter provides up-to-date knowledge of the first discovered human retrovirus along with its primary molecular functions. In Chapter 3, "Roles of HTLV-1 Tax in Leukemogenesis of Human T-Cells," Nakamura M. focuses on detailed molecular mechanisms of the role of the Tax1 gene of HTLV-1 in malignant transformation and the development of ATLL. The author specifically addresses the role of Tax1 in promoting cell growth, deregulating cellular signaling, and in the modification of apoptosis and cellular immortalization. Chapter 4, "Host Imune System Abnormalities Among Patients with Human T-Lymphothropic Virus Type 1 (HTLV-1)-Associated Disorders" by Yagishita N., Araya N., and Sato T., centers on the immunological abnormalities of HTLV-1-positive patients. Specifically, functional changes in CD4+ T cells and abnormalities of the cytotoxic T lymphocyte (CTL) response, as well as abnormalities of innate immunity following HTLV-1 infection are described.

3. Signaling Pathways in T-Cell Malignancies

The next four chapters describe the role of specific genes or pathways in the pathogenesis of ATLL, T-ALL, and other T-cell malignancies. Chapter 5, "Constitutive Activation of the JAK/STAT and Toll-Like Receptor Signaling Pathways in Adult T-Cell Leukemia/Lymphoma" by Tsukada J., et al., focuses on the functional specificity of these pathways in HTLV-1 infected cells and their role in malignant transformation. In Chapter 6, "The Role of Ikaros in T-ALL," Dovat S. and Payne K.J. dissect the role of the Ikaros (Ikzf1) tumor suppressor gene and its regulatory signal transduction pathways in the control of proliferation in malignant cells. The novel findings that Casein Kinase 2 (CK2) and Protein Phosphatase 1 (PP1) control the ability of Ikaros to regulate tumor suppression in T-cell leukemia are summarized. Chapter 7, "p16^{INK4A} – Connecting Cell Cycle Control to Cell Death Regulation in Human Leukemia" by Ausserlechner M.J. et al., focuses on the role of the INK4 inhibitor protein p16INK4A in the regulation of cell cycle and cell survival in T-ALL. The role of the INK4A gene in the generation of induced pluripotent stem cells and in hematopoietic stem cells is discussed. Chapter 8, "Accumulation of Specific Epigenetic Abnormalities During Development and Progression of T cell Leukemia/Lymphoma" by Yoshino T. et al., describes recent findings on the role of epigenetic changes in the development of T cell leukemia and in cellular proliferation. This chapter summarizes the scientific advances in epigenetic regulation of gene expression related to T cell leukemia/lymphoma, and provides an overview of the role of DNA methylation and histone modifications in the regulation of gene expression. Chapter 9, "Roles of MicroRNA In T-Cell Leukemia" by Tomita M., centers on another emerging field of molecular biology – microRNA and its role in the regulation of gene activity. This chapter gives a nice overview of the mechanism of microRNA action that is easily understandable for both basic scientists and clinicians and describes the role of microRNA in different types of T-cell malignancies.

4. Complications of T-Cell Malignancies and Experimental Therapy

The last three chapters cover the mechanisms of a common complication of ATLL – hypercalcemia, as well as a novel therapeutic approach for this disease. Chapter 10, "Mechanisms of Humoral Hypercalcemia of Malignancy in Leukemia/Lymphoma" by Rosol T.J., et al. provides an overview of hypercalcemia of malignancy. The chapter emphasizes the roles of various factors in the pathogenesis of humoral hypercalcemia of malignancies (HHM), the clinical significance of HHM in various T-cell malignancies, and therapeutic approaches to HHM. Chapter 11, "The Role of T-Cell Leukemia Translocation-Associated Gene (TCTA) Protein in Human Osteoclastogenesis" by Nanke Y. et al. concentrates on the mechanism by which the TCTA protein regulates osteoclastogenesis. The role of the receptor activator NF-kB ligand (RANKL) in osteoclastogenesis, and recent discoveries about the role of TCTA as an inhibitor of RANKL-induced osteoclastogenesis is described in detail. Chapter 12, "Retrovirus Infection and Retinoid," Maeda Y et al. describe retinoids as a potential novel treatment agent for ATLL. The growth inhibition effect of All-Trans Retinoic Acid (ATRA), its downregulation of IL-2Rα/CD25, and its inhibition of NF-kB transcription activity by ATRA are described. The potential clinical use of retinoids for T-cell malignancies is discussed.

5. Summary

This book provides an up-to-date overview of advances in our understanding of the pathogenesis of T cell malignancies and will serve as a tool for both basic scientists and clinicians by providing a basis for further studies and an aid in the search for more effective therapies for these challenging diseases.

Sinisa Dovat
Pennsylvania State University College of Medicine
United States of America

Kimberly J. Payne
Loma Linda University
United States of America

1

Adult Human T Cell Leukemia

Jean-Philippe Herbeuval
CNRS UMR 8147, Université Paris Descartes
France

1. Introduction

Human T cell leukemia virus 1 (HTLV-1), the first characterized human retrovirus, has been identified as the causative agent for adult T-cell leukemia/lymphoma (ATLL). This aggressive lymphoid proliferation is associated with a bad prognosis due to the resistance of HTLV-1-infected cells to most classical chemotherapeutic agents.

HTLV-1 is transmitted intravenously, by sexual contact, or through breast-feeding from mother to child, and epidemiological evidence predicts that ATLL development occurs following childhood infection. ATLL exhibits diverse clinical features: the acute, the sub-acute or smoldering, the chronic forms and the ATL lymphoma. In the two most aggressive forms (acute leukemia and lymphoma), the tumor syndrome comprises massive lymphadenopathy, hepatosplenomegaly, lytic bone lesions and multiple visceral lesions with skin and lung infiltration.

HTLV-1 virions infect $CD4^+$ T cells, which represent the main target for HTLV-1 infection in peripheral blood. HTLV-1 associated diseases occur after long periods of virus latency. For years it has been thought that unlike other retroviruses, free virions were poorly infectious. However, a recent study reported that freshly isolated myeloid dendritic cells (mDC) and plasmacytoid dendritic cells (pDC) are efficiently and productively infected by cell-free HTLV-1. Furthermore, infected mDC and pDC were able to transfer virions to autologous $CD4^+$ T cells, clearly demonstrating that cell free HTLV-1 can be infectious and target dendritic cells. Innate immune response against HTLV-1 is poorly documented.

We describe here immune response against HTLV-1 and physiological consequences.

2. The Human T cell leukemia virus 1 (HTLV-1)

In 1980 the group of Robert C. Gallo characterized the first human retrovirus, the Human T cell leukemia virus 1 (HTLV-1) (Poiesz, Ruscetti et al., 1980). This virus was recovered from the peripheral blood cells of a patient suffering from adult T-cell-leukemia/lymphoma (ATLL). This form of leukemia is a severe T-cell lymphoma proliferation with bad prognostic due to the resistance of HTLV-1-infected cells to most classical chemotherapeutic agents.

We first describe here the epidemiology, the genomic of HTLV-1 virus and its receptor complex.

2.1 HTLV-1 genomic characteristics

HTLV-1 is classified as a complex retrovirus, in the genus delta-retrovirus of the subfamily Orthoretrovirinae. HTLV-1 retrovirus genetic material is composed by a

diploid single strain RNA (Figure 1). The length of the HTLV-1 genome is 9.032 basepair (bp). The group antigens are similar to other retroviruses-(gag), polymerase (pol), and envelope (env) genes are flanked by long terminal repeats (LTR). The LTR consists of U3, R and U5 regions. The U3 region of HTLV-1 controls the virus transcription. It contains essential elements such as the TATA box, which is necessary for viral transcription, a sequence that causes termination and polyadenylation of the RNA messenger and Tax responsive elements (TRE) involved in Tax protein transcription which regulates the transcription of the HTLV-1 provirus. The R region overlaps the 3′ of the U3 region and contains the majority of the Rex response element. The "gag" gene encodes the virus core protein, which is initially synthesized with approximatively molecular weight of 53 kD. During viral maturation this precursor is cleaved to form the matured matrix P19 (MA), the capsid P24 (CA) and the nucleocapsid P15 (NC).
HTLV-1 virions are enveloped into a lipidic membrane and a nucleocapsid that protect the genetic material, the ribonucleic acid (RNA). The lipidic membrane is derived from cellular plasma membrane. The envelope proteins are constituted by the glycoprotein (gp) 21 (Transmembrane subunit, TM) and gp46 (Surface subunit, SU), which are coded by env and are integrated to the lipidic membrane. Matrix protein p19 and p24 are coded by gag and constitute the intern core of viral envelope. The nucleocapsid p15 is also coded by gag and is enveloping the genetic material composed of a diploid single stranded RNA (Figure 1).

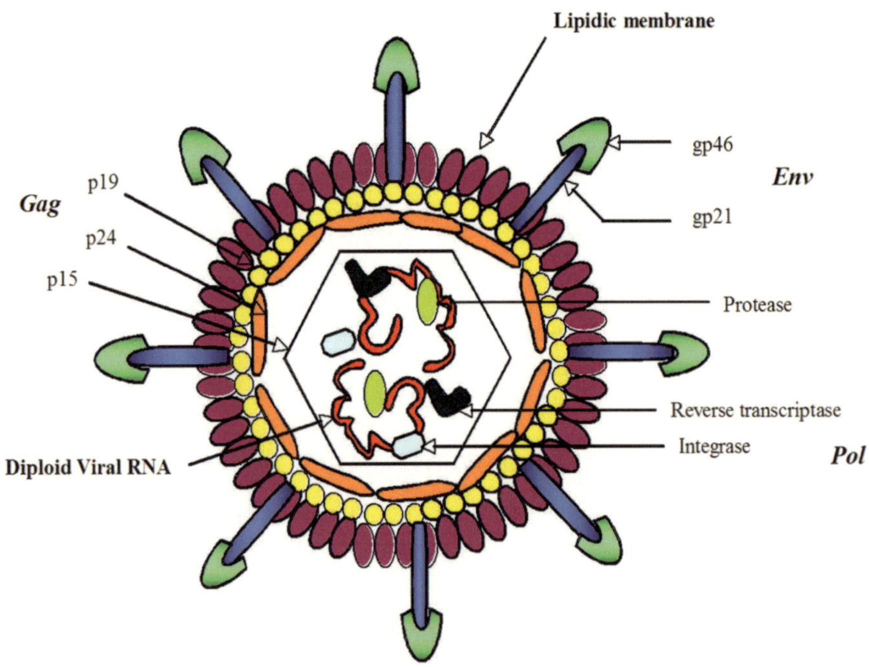

Fig. 1. Genomic and proteic structure of HTLV-1 virion.

2.2 HTLV-1 epidemiology

Over the course of more than 30 years, the epidemiology of HTLV-1 has matured. Epidemiologic studies are based on serologic diagnosis by detection of specific antibodies using enzyme-linked immunosorbent assay (ELISA) or by agglutination assay. Thus, the serologic is confirmed by immunoblot of specific antibodies and polymerase chain reaction (PCR) of genomic DNA from cells of infected patients.

The number of HTLV-1 infected people is elevated and the most recent studies estimated at 15-20 millions people infected worldwide (Verdonck, Gonzalez et al., 2007). Epidemiologic studies revealed that density of infected individuals were in Malaysia, Caribbean, Africa (Gabon, Cameroun), South America (Brazil, Guyana, Colombia) and South Japan (Figure 2). However, these numbers are only estimations and probably do not reflect the reality. Indeed, most of infected people are not diagnosed due to the complex and expensive methods of diagnosis. Thus, number of people really infected might be higher especially in developed countries.

Among the HTLV-1-infected population, around 3 to 6% develop the ATLL syndrome. HTLV-1 infection is highly concentrated in some regions especially in South Japan where the prevalence can reach as high as 37% in a selected population (Mueller, Okayama et al., 1996; Yamaguchi, 1994). The reasons for HTLV-1 clustering, the high ubiquity in southwestern Japan but low prevalence in neighboring regions of Korea, China and Eastern Russia are still unknown. For nonendemic geographic regions, HTLV-1 is mainly found in immigrants. The contamination is largely due to sexual contacts with sex workers. However, the prevalence in Europe and North America remains extremly low and does not exceed 0,01% (Proietti, Carneiro-Proietti et al., 2005).

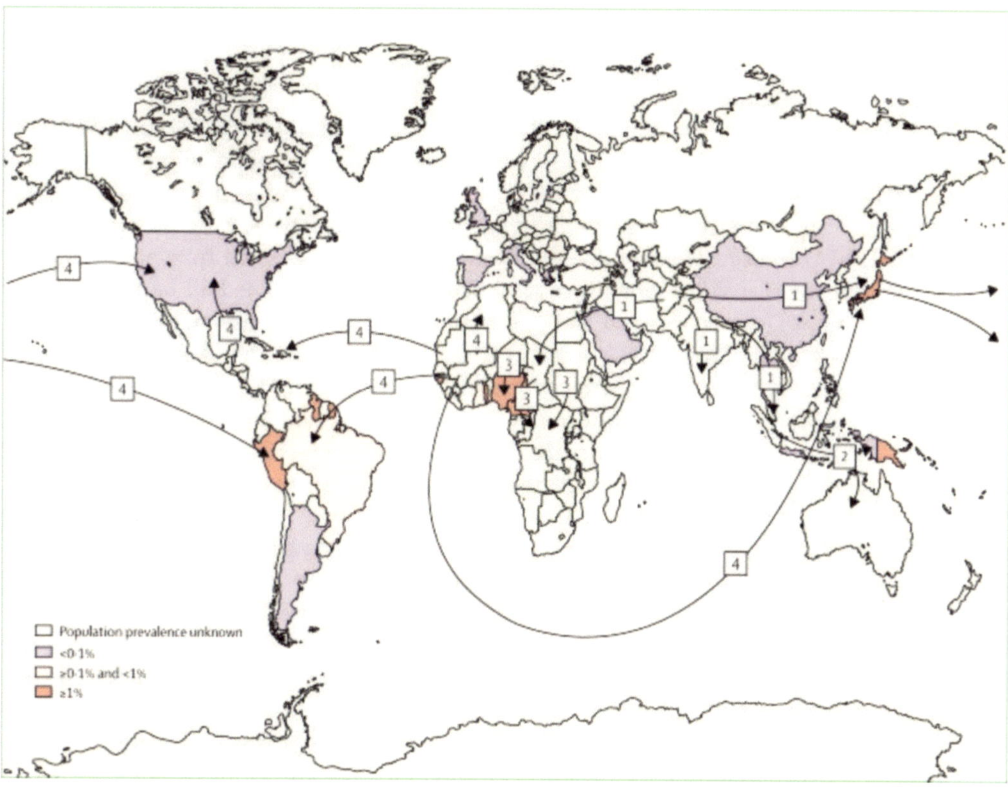

Fig. 2. Origin, spread, and prevalence of HTLV-1.

HTLV-1 is transmitted intravenously, by sexual contact, or through breast-feeding from mother to child, and epidemiological evidence predicts that ATLL development occurs following childhood infection. Mother to child transmission occurs very frequently (around 20%) and is related to mother viral load and prolonged breast-feeding. Indeed, it is now well accepted that HTLV-1 could be transmitted through mother's milk and is one of the major factor in vertical transmission. Thus, screening of HTLV-1 among blood donors had been extended and breast-feeding among HTLV-1-infected women had been refrained in Japan decreasing vertical transmission.

Finally, it is also possible that HTLV-1 could be transmitted by saliva, which contains HTLV-1 antibodies and proviral DNA. However, there is no clear study demonstrating this way of contamination (Fujino and Nagata, 2000).

Origin and spread hypothesis based on phylogenetic and anthropological data. HTLV-1 originated in African primates and migrated to Asia where it evolved into STLV-1. This early STLV-1 lineage spread to India, Japan, Indonesia, and back to Africa (arrows 1). It crossed the simian–human barrier in Indonesian human beings who migrated to Malesia, resulting in the HTLV-1c subtype (arrows 2). In Africa, STLV-1 evolved through several interspecies transmissions into HTLV-1a, HTLV-1b, and HTLV-1d, HTLV-1e, and HTLV-1f (arrows 3). Because of the slave trade and increased mobility, HTLV-1a was introduced in the New World, Japan, the Middle East, and North Africa (arrows 4). Colours indicate current prevalence estimates based on population surveys and on studies in pregnant women and blood donors. In some countries, HTLV-1 infection is limited to certain population groups or areas. (Verdonck, Gonzalez et al., 2007).

2.3 HTLV-1 receptor complex

For years the HTLV-1 receptor remained unknown and a real mystery. Serious evidences indicated that HTLV-1 entry requires the viral envelope glycoprotein (Env), the surface subunit gp46 and the transmembrane subunit gp21, generated from the clivage of a precursor gp61. Mutation in any of this proteins or use of blocking antibodies dramatically reduced HTLV-1 infection. Thus, one study demonstrated that glucose transporter GLUT1 was the receptor for HTLV-1 (Manel, Kim et al., 2003). GLUT1 matched all requirement for HTLV-1 entry. GLUT1 is overexpressed by activated T cells, which are targets of HTLV-1. Using small interfering RNA siRNA strategy they demonstrated that downregulation of GLUT1 in cell lines reduced HTLV-1 infection. Furthermore, GLUT1 transfection of GLUT1 negative cells restored HTLV-1 infection, demonstrating that GLUT1 is an essential component of HTLV-1 receptor. More recently, it has been suggested that two other molecules are involved in HTLV-1 infection of target cells: neuropilin 1 (NRP-1) and Heparan Sulfate Proteoglycans (HSPG) (Ghez, Lepelletier et al.).

The Neuropilin-1 was initially identified as a embryonic neurons guidance factor. NRP-1 is a glycoprotein receptor for Semaphorin 3a and VEGF (Vascular endothelial growth factor). It also has been showed that NRP-1 was a key molecule in angiogenesis and is also implicated in the regulation of immune response (Tordjman, Lepelletier et al., 2002). It has been showed that NRP-1 directly binds HTLV-1 virus. The interaction appeared functionnaly relevant since NRP-1 overexpression enhanced syncytium formation *in vitro*. Furthermore, confocal analysis revealed a strong polarisation of NRP-1 and viral glycoprotein Env at the interface of an infected cell and a target T cell (Ghez, Lepelletier et al., 2006).

HSPG family members are composed of a core protein associated with one or several sulphated polysaccharide side chains (i.e. sulfate glycosaminoglycans). Sulphated polysaccharide side chains confer to HSPG members electrostatic properties that allow binding to a very large range of proteins, including cytokines, receptors, hormones, chemokines and extracellular matrix proteins. HSPG enhances infection by facilitating the attachment of the particles on target cells and/or allowing their clustering at the cell surface before specific interactions between viral proteins and their receptors that lead to fusion. HSPG had been showed to bind the HIV-1 protein gp120, therefore facilitating HIV-1 infection. Studies demonstrated that inhibition of HSPG dramatically reduced syncitium formation and infection in CD4+ T cells (Lambert, Bouttier et al., 2009). Furthermore, inhibition of HSPG also reduced infection of dendritic cells. Thus, a model involving three partners had been proposed (Figure 3).

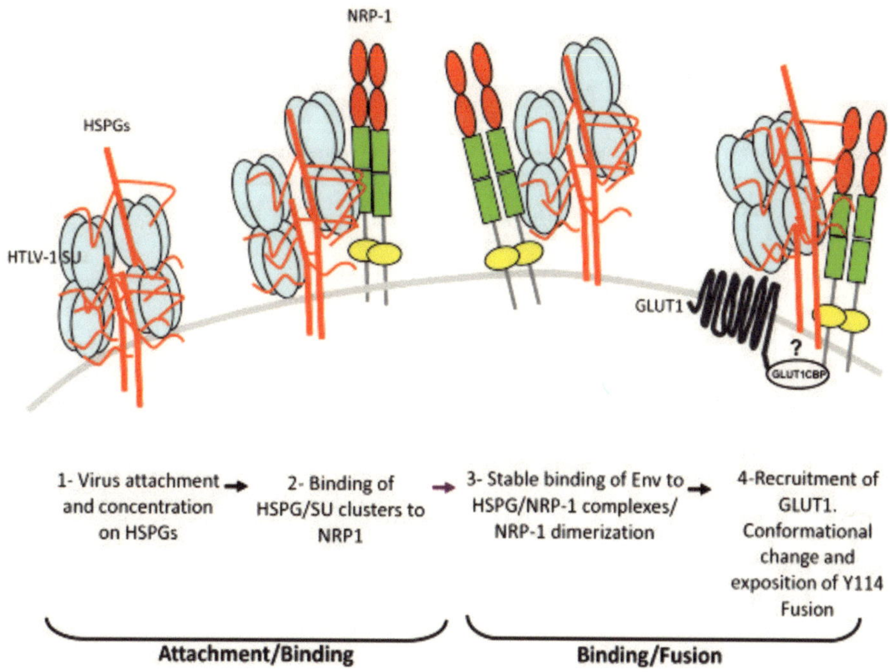

Fig. 3. Model for HTLV-1 receptor complex.
From Ghez, Lepelletier et al., 2006.

More recently, one study proposed another model for HTLV-1 entry into target cells (Pais-Correia, Sachse et al.). This model proposes that HTLV-1-infected T lymphocytes transiently store viral particles as carbohydrate-rich extracellular assemblies. These carbohydrate assemblies are attached to cell surface and held together by virally-induced extracellular matrix components. This extracellular matrix is made of protein such as collagen, agrin, galectin-3 and tetherin. It should be noted that HSPG is probably a protein of the HTLV-1 extracellular assemblies. This kind of structure was first discovered for bacteria and called "biofilm". Authors showed that extracellular HTLV-1 biofilms adhere to other cells facilitating viral binding and infection. This form of viral infection is extremely efficient due to high concentration of extracellular viruses on cell surface.
Thus, HTLV-1 may use several strategies to infect target cells. However, further studies are needed to clarify the entry of HTLV-1 in patients.

3. The adult T-cell leukemia/lymphoma (ATLL)

Adult T cell leukemia/lymphoma (ATLL) had been shown to be a consequence of HTLV-1 infection (Hinuma, Gotoh et al., 1982). HTLV-1 infection is also responsible for myelopathy/tropical spastic paraparesis (HAM/TSP) (de The, Gazzolo et al., 1985; Gessain, Barin et al., 1985), uveitis and infective dermatitis in children (Manns et al., 1999). We focus in this section on the complex T-cell leukemia/lymphoma induced by HTLV-1 infection.

3.1 HTLV-1 induces T cell leukemia

In the late seventies, a group of leukemia patients with characteristic clinical features and particular geographical distribution were identified. Uchiyama *et al* proposed adult T cell leukemia (ATL) as a new disease. In 1980 the group of Robert C. Gallo characterized the first human retrovirus responsible for ATL, the Human T cell leukemia virus 1 (HTLV-1) (Poiesz, Ruscetti et al., 1980).

Since then, HTLV-1 has been identified as the causative agent for two major syndromes: the adult T-cell leukemia (ATL) (Poiesz, Ruscetti et al., 1981; Robert-Guroff, Nakao et al., 1982) and the HTLV-1-associated myelopathy/tropical spastic paraparesis (HAM/TSP) (Jacobson, 1996). More recently, HTLV-1 also has been shown as the causative agent for uveitis and infective dermatitis in children (Manns, Miley et al., 1999). Among the HTLV-1-infected population, around 3 to 6% develop the ATL syndrome. At the present time, it is not known why some infected patients develop ATL and others do not.

3.2 ATL syndrome

The ATL exhibits diverse clinical features and outcome is directly correlated to ATL subtype. The malignancy ranges from a very indolent and slowly progressive lymphoma to a very aggressive and nearly uniformaly lethal proliferative lymphoma. The incidence of ATL is estimated to be 61/100,000 HTLV-1 carriers, and the crude lifetime risk for developing ATL is 7.3% for males and 3.8% for females. Four types of ATL had been described based on the number of abnormal T cells in peripheral blood, tumor lesions in organs, serum lactic acid dehydrogenase (LDH) level and clinical course: the sub-acute or smoldering (5%), the acute (55%), the chronic forms (20%) and the ATL lymphoma (20%).

Patients with smoldering ATL exhibit skin lesions, minimal lymph node enlargement and few leukemic cells in blood. Chronic ATL is characterized by mild symptoms and longer clinical course. In the two most aggressive forms (acute leukemia and lymphoma), the tumor syndrome comprises massive lymphadenopathy, hepatosplenomegaly, lytic bone lesions and multiple visceral lesions with skin and lung infiltration. Acute ATL is also characterized by general malaise, fever, cough, high lactate deshydrogenase (LDH) serum levels, and appearance of multilobulated nuclei leukemic cells. This aggressive lymphoid proliferation is associated with a bad prognosis due to the resistance of HTLV-1-infected cells to most classical chemotherapeutic agents. The cancer is thought to be due to the pro-oncogenic effect of viral DNA incorporated into host lymphocytes DNA, and chronic stimulation of the lymphocytes at the cytokine level may play a role in development of malignancy. The time between infection and onset of cancer also varies geographically. It is believed to be about sixty years in Japan, and less than forty years in the Caribbean.

3.3 The ATL cell

The ATL cell is easily characterized by histological and/or cytological infiltration by flower cells (Matsuoka, 2005) that are malignant activated lymphocytes with convoluted nuclei and basophilic cytoplasm, a multilobed nucleus with a flower shape (Figure 4). ATL cells express most of T cell markers (CD2, CD3, CD4, CD45RO) and more rarely CD8. However, ATL cells also express the alpha chain of IL-2 receptor, CD25, and T cell activation markers such as major histocompatibility complex HLA-DR and HLA-DQ. ATL is well known to infiltrate various organs and tissues, such as the skin, lungs, liver, gastrointestinal tract, central nervous system and bone. This infiltrative tendency of leukemic cells is possibly attributable to the expression of various surface molecules, such as chemokine receptors and adhesion molecules. Skin-homing memory T-cells uniformly express CCR4, and its ligands are thymus and activation-regulated chemokine (TARC) and macrophage-derived chemokine (MDC). CCR4 is expressed on most ATL cells. In addition, TARC and MDC are expressed in skin lesions in ATL patients. Thus, CCR4 expression should be implicated in the skin infiltration (Yoshie, 2005). On the other hand, CCR7 expression is associated with lymph node involvement (Kohno, Moriuchi et al., 2000). OX40 is a member of the tumor necrosis factor family and was reported to be expressed on ATL cells (Imura, Hori et al., 1997; Kunitomi, Hori et al., 2002).

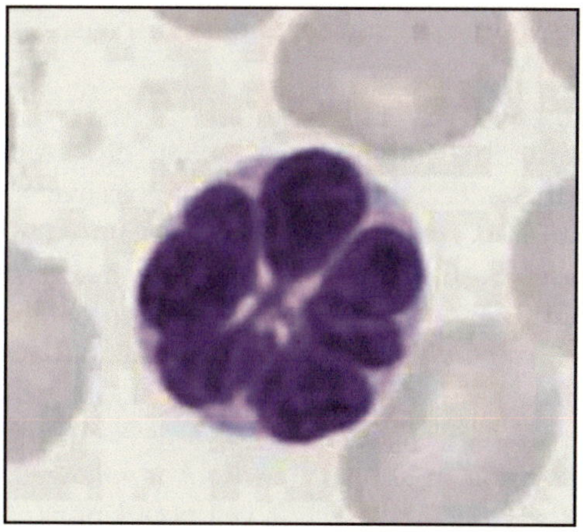

Fig. 4. Typical "flower cell" in the peripheral blood of an acute ATL patient observed on microscope. In the peripheral blood of an acute ATL patient, leukemic cells with multilobulated nuclei (Matsuoka, 2005).

3.4 Treatment of ATL

Adult T cell leukemia is an agressive malignant disease that results from HTLV-1 infection. The prognostic is directly correlated to the ATL subtype. Since ATL is a neoplasm of mature T cells, it has been treated with chemotherapies for non-Hodgkin's lymphoma. Conventional chemoterapy (LSG15) had only transcient effect and the prognostic remains poor. The median survival time (MST) never exceeded 10 month.

Therefore, new therapeutic strategies were tested to adapt treatment to ATL subtype reviewed by Kimiharu Uozumi (Uozumi). New strategies can be divided in 3 main groups: chemical anti-tumor agents, monoclonal antibodies and vaccination.

Among new chemical anti-tumor agents the combined use of anti-retroviral drug AZT and recombinant interferon alpha (IFN-α) showed promising results (Hermine, Bouscary et al., 1995). The MST was increased in most patients and this therapy constitutes one of the most efficient at the present time.

Similarly the combined use of arsenic trioxid and interferon alpha exhibits an anti-leukemia effect in very poor prognosis ATL patients despite a significant toxicity (Hermine, Dombret et al., 2004).
Treatment using monoclonal antibodies and recombinant cytokines are also very promising. We will describe later in section 4 the use of TNF-related Apoptosis Inducing Ligand (TRAIL), a Tumor Necrosis Factor (TNF) superfamily member (Wiley, Schooley et al., 1995), as a new therapeutical strategy to induce ATL cells apoptosis.

4. HTLV-1 and immune response

HTLV-1 is a retrovirus and therefore is recognised by the immune system as foreign agent. Immune system is activated after infection and produce specific anti-HTL-1 antibodies. Most of immune cells respond to HTLV-1 virions. However, because symptoms occur after a long period of latency it is extremely hard to study acute infection. Thus, most of immunologic studies are performed using samples from patients infected since several years. We review in this section the interactions between immune cells and HTLV-1 and provide some new features concerning innate immune response.

4.1 Immune cell activation by HTLV-1

HTLV-1 like HIV-1 is a retrovirus and induces a chronic disease. Although a large number of studies have indicated that initial virus infection involves majority viral invasion of $CD4^+$ T cells, which represent an important target for HTLV-1 infection in the peripheral blood, additional evidence has demonstrated that HTLV-1 can infect several additional cellular compartments *in vivo*, including $CD8^+$ T lymphocytes, monocytes, dendritic cells, B lymphocytes residing in the peripheral blood and lymphoid organs or resident central nervous system (CNS) astrocytes (Koyanagi, Itoyama et al., 1993; Macatonia, Cruickshank et al., 1992; Nagai, Kubota et al., 2001; Richardson, Edwards et al., 1990).
Transient phase of reverse transcription of viral RNA is followed by a persistent phase of clonal expansion within the $CD4^+$ and $CD8^+$ T cell populations (Mansky, 2000; Mortreux, Leclercq et al., 2001). Very little viral gene expression and low amounts of infectious virus production of HTLV-1 infected monocyte/macrophage lineage and dendritic cells are likely attributable to their postmitotic status and relatively short lifetime (Banchereau and Steinman, 1998; Valledor, Borras et al., 1998).
This differential viral gene expression between T and dendritic cells depending of viral clonal expansion and expression drives the HTLV-1 immune response. Although dendritic cells have a low level of viral gene expression, recent evidence has suggested that HTLV-1-infected dendritic cells exhibit an enhance capacity to stimulate antigen-specific T cell activation (Makino, Shimokubo et al., 1999). Furthermore, the Th1-type cytokines IL-1b, interferon-γ (IFN-γ), and TNF-α were overexpressed in asymptomatic carriers and patients with HAM/TSP, while the Th2/Th3-type cytokine transformin growth factor (TGF-β) was overexpressed in patients with ATL (Tendler, Greenberg et al., 1991). Several events may lead to stimulation of a Th1 or a Th2/Th3 T cell response besides the subset of dendritic cells (DC1 and DC2) that are first encountered antigen, or depending of the pathogen, recognition receptors and site of exposure (Pulendran, Palucka et al., 2001). Furthermore, the type of T cell response is dependent of both DC ontogeny, but also of the dendritic cell activating stimulus (Grabbe, Kampgen et al., 2000). Consequently, the initial route of

infection determines the preferential infection of dendritic cell subsets but these consequences of event remain unknown.

Furthermore, the proportion of blood and secondary lymphoid organs HTLV-1+ DC is proportional to the total proviral DNA load in the blood, providing a correlation of proviral DNA load and the frequency of effector/memory Tax- $CD8^+$ T cells (Nagai, Kubota et al., 2001).

HTLV Tax oncogene may be released and act as a cytokine on neighboring cells in the CNS inducing NF-kB nuclear localization and immunoglobulin κ light chain, IL-2Ra, IL-1b, IL-6, TNF-α, and TNF-β expression (Lindholm et al., 1990; Lindholm et al., 1992; Marriott et al., 1992; Dhib-Jalbut et al., 1994). The cytokine like effects of Tax may induce a signaling cascade by binding to a specific cell surface receptor (DC1 and/or DC2 NP-1).

Interestingly, one of the members of the interferon regulatory factor (IRF) family – IRF-4 – was shown to be highly expressed in cells derived from patients with ATL and in HTLV-1 infected cell lines (Imaizumi, Kohno et al., 2001; Mamane, Grandvaux et al., 2002; Mamane, Loignon et al., 2005; Sharma, Grandvaux et al., 2002; Sharma, Mamane et al., 2000; Yamagata et al., 1996). A detailed analysis of IRF-4 has implicated the viral Tax protein in mediating activation of the Sp1, NF-kB and NF-AT pathways leading to a feed back loop mediated by Tax (Grumont and Gerondakis, 2000; Sharma, Grandvaux et al., 2002; Sharma, Mamane et al., 2000).

4.2 ATL and TRAIL-induced apoptosis

Induction of tumor cell death by apoptotic molecules is one of strategy that could be used to selectively reduce cancer cell proliferation without damaging normal tissue. The tumor necrosis factor (TNF)-related apoptosis-inducing ligand (TRAIL), a TNF superfamily member, has been shown to induce apoptosis of the vast majority of tumor cell lines (Wiley, Schooley et al., 1995). TRAIL-induced apoptosis is finely regulated by the expression of two groups of receptors. Three receptors do not induce apoptosis (Decoy Receptors, DcR) and two activate apoptosis of target cells (Death Receptor 4 and 5, DR4, DR5) (Sheikh, Burns et al., 1998; Sheridan, Marsters et al., 1997; Wu, Burns et al., 1997). The two biologically active forms of TRAIL, membrane-bound (mTRAIL) and soluble TRAIL (sTRAIL), are regulated by type I interferon (interferon-alpha and beta: IFN-α and IFN-β)(Ehrlich, Infante-Duarte et al., 2003; Sato, Hida et al., 2001; Tecchio, Huber et al., 2004). TRAIL active form consist of a trimer stabilized by a zinc molecule. TRAIL is secreted by leukocytes, including T lymphocytes (Kayagaki, Yamaguchi et al., 1999), natural killer cells (Smyth, Cretney et al., 2001), dendritic cells (Vidalain, Azocar et al., 2000; Vidalain, Azocar et al., 2001), monocytes and macrophages (Herbeuval, Lambert et al., 2003). TRAIL can activate both intrinsic or extrinsic apoptosis pathway. DR4 and DR5 induced apoptosis through the formation of a death inducing signaling complex (DISC) containing the death receptor, adaptor proteins such as Fas-associated death domain (FADD), and initiator caspases such as pro-caspase-8 or pro-caspase-10 (Bellail, Tse et al., 2009; Jin, Kurakin et al., 2004; Walczak and Haas, 2008). Consequently, pro-caspase-8 or pro-caspase-10 are activated by autoproteolytic processing, which then cleave and activate downstream effector caspases (Gomez-Benito, Martinez-Lorenzo et al., 2007), such as caspase-3 (extrinsic pathway). Additionally, the Bcl-2-interacting protein Bid is also cleaved by caspase-8. Truncated-Bid causes the loss of mitochondrial membrane potential and caspase-9 cleavage, resulting in apoptosis. Very little is known concerning death and decoy receptors regulation. Among these receptors, death receptor is the most studied, and authors showed that DR5 transcription is regulated (at least partially) by the protooncogene p53 (Sheikh, Burns et al., 1998; Wu, Burns et al., 1997). It should be noticed that TRAIL death receptors 4 and 5 not only induce apoptosis but may also play a crucial role in inflammatory responses (Collison, Foster et al., 2009). Figure 5 illustrates TRAIL pathway and regulation.

TRAIL is a very promising candidate for cancer treatment due to its sophisticated way of inducing apoptosis. While the vast majority of normal cells express decoy receptors and are therefore protected from TRAIL-mediated apoptosis, tumor cells generally express death receptors. Indeed, TRAIL induces apoptosis in human tumor cell lines (Griffith, Chin et al., 1998) but not in normal cells (Gura, 1997). TRAIL also induces apoptosis of infected cells. For example, plasma TRAIL has been reported to be an early pathogenic marker in acute HIV-1 infection and is correlated to viral load in chronic disease (Gasper-Smith, Crossman et al., 2008; Herbeuval, Nilsson et al., 2009). HIV-1 upregulates DR5 expression on the membrane of $CD4^+$ T cells *in vitro* (Herbeuval, Boasso et al., 2005; Herbeuval, Grivel et al., 2005) making them prone to TRAIL-mediated apoptosis (Lichtner, Maranon et al., 2004). Furthermore, the percentage of CD4+ T cells co-expressing TRAIL and DR5 are elevated in the blood of viremic progressors (Herbeuval, Grivel et al., 2005). Thus, TRAIL does not exhibit cytotoxic effects on normal cells and tissues and is potentially efficient to eradicate a large panel of cancer cells. Several clinical trial are currently evaluating TRAIL anti tumor effect, alone or in combination with other chemotherapeutic drugs.

Thus, it remained pertinent to determine whether ATL cells were sensitive to TRAIL-mediated apoptosis. One study characterized the sensitivity of ATL cells to TRAIL cytotoxicity. Authors tested several cell lines and also primary cells from both chronic and acute ATL. Unfortunately, the vast majority of primary ATL cells or cell lines appears to be resistant to TRAIL induced cell death (Matsuda, Almasan et al., 2005). This resistance was due to multiple parameters, including the lack of DR4 and DR5 expression, abrogation of death signal upstream caspase-8, attenuation of both extrinsic and intrinsic apoptotic pathways. More recently, it has been shown that the resistance upstream caspase 8 was due to an over expression of the cellular caspase-8 (FLICE)-inhibitory protein (c-FLIP) that blocks caspase recruitment and apoptosis. However, other study show that ATL cells might be sensitive to TRAIL-induced apoptosis (Hasegawa, Yamada et al., 2005), therefore TRAIL effect in ATL should be clarified.

Surprisingly, most of ATL cells expressed TRAIL on their surface. This finding suggested that constitutive expression of TRAIL would participate in the development of TRAIL-resistant clones observed in patients. The natural resistance of ATL cells would have excluded the use of TRAIL as therapeutic agent. However, a recent study demonstrated that the herbal compound Rocaglamide restores TRAIL sensibility in ATL cells. Indeed, Rocaglamide induces suppression of c-FLIP expression in ATL cells that sensitizes these cells to TRAIL-mediated apoptosis. Authors suggest the use of Rocaglamide as an adjuvant to TRAIL as new therapeutic strategies against HTLV-1-mediated ATL (Bleumink, Kohler et al.). It has also been observed that the use of a combination of a p53 activator, Nutlin-3a, and TRAIL synergized to induce ATL cell apoptosis (Hasegawa, Yamada et al., 2009). This could be explained by the fact that p53 regulates TRAIL death receptor 5 on cell surface. Thus, Nutlin-3a treated ATL cells would express DR5 and then become sensitive to TRAIL-mediated apoptosis.

Therefore, the understanding of ATL sensitivity to TRAIL-mediated apoptosis appears to be crucial to develop new therapeutic options.

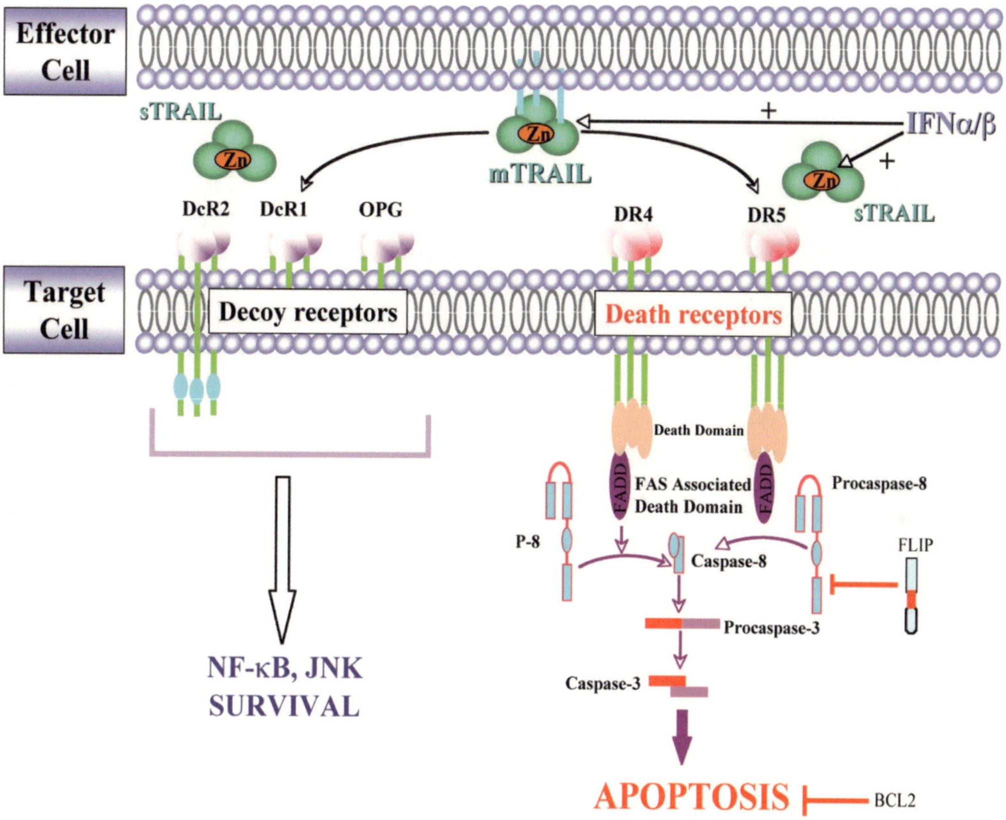

Fig. 5. TRAIL apoptotic pathway. Membrane (mTRAIL) or soluble TRAIL (sTRAIL) bind to 3 decoy receptors (DcR1, DcR2 and OPG) and 2 death receptors (DR4 and DR5) which activate the caspase pathway leading to apoptosis.

4.3 Myeloid dendritic cells and HTLV-1 infection

HTLV-1 targets CD4+ T cells which represent an important target for HTLV-1 infection in the peripheral blood. However, there are some additional evidence that showed that HTLV-1 can also infect including CD8+ T lymphocytes, monocytes, B lymphocytes, astrocytes (Richardson, Edwards et al., 1990) and dendritic cells (DC) *in vivo*. Myeloid dendritic cells do not exhibit high viral gene expression, but recent work suggested that HTLV-1-infected dendritic cells show better capacity to stimulate antigen-specific T cell activation (Makino, Shimokubo et al., 1999). Moreover, the proportion of lymphoid organs containing HTLV-1 positive dendritic cells is proportional to the total proviral DNA load in the blood, providing a correlation of proviral DNA load and the frequency of effector/memory Tax-CD8+ T cells (Nagai, Kubota et al., 2001).
More recently, findings demonstrated a central role to myeloid dendritic (mDC) and plasmacytoid dendritic cells (pDC) in HTLV-1 infection. For years it has been thought that unlike other retroviruses such as HIV-1, free virions were poorly infectious (Donegan, Lee et al., 1994). However, a recent study reported that freshly isolated mDC and pDC are efficiently and productively infected by cell-free HTLV-1 (Jones, Petrow-Sadowski et al.,

2008). Furthermore, infected mDC and pDC were able to transfer virions to autologous CD4+ T cells, clearly demonstrating that cell free HTLV-1 can be infectious and target dendritic cells (Jones, Petrow-Sadowski et al., 2008).

5. HTLV-1 and plasmacytoid dendritic cell response

Plasmacytoid dendritic cells were discovered in 1997 as professional IFN-alpha producers and innate immune cells (Grouard, Rissoan et al., 1997). These cells are rare but play a central role in host defense against viruses and bacteria by producing cytokines and antiviral factors. The role of pDC in HTLV-1 infection remained unknown until recent years probably because of the extreme difficulty of studying HTLV-1 acute infection. We describe here recent data providing some new features in the understanding of HTLV-1 innate immune response.

5.1 The Plasmacytoid dendritic cell (pDC)

PDC are cells of hemopoietic origin that are found at steady state in the blood, thymus and peripheral lymphoid tissues. Early studies described pDC as being oval-shaped with typical plasmacytoid morphology. The ability of plasmacytoid-derived DC (also named DC2) to induce a Th2 differentiation of naïve CD4 T cells formed the basis for the concept of type 1 and type 2 DC (Review Nat immunol, 2001). The role of these DC in mouse and human was studied in different models and is not completely elucidated (Liu, 2005). A little later, it was shown that pDC were specialized in the production of type I IFN (Siegal, Kadowaki et al., 1999). They are the principal source of type I IFN in human blood and very rapidly produce all type I IFN isoforms in response to microbial stimuli, such as virus (Cella, Jarrossay et al., 1999; Siegal, Kadowaki et al., 1999), CpG-containing oligonucleotides (Kadowaki, Antonenko et al., 2000), or the synthetic molecules imidazoquinolines (Gibson, Lindh et al., 2002). PDC-derived type I IFN has direct anti-viral activity against a variety of virus, including HIV, and has important adjuvant functions on other immune cell-types, such as NK cells, T cells, macrophages and DC. Thus, pDC activation triggers a dual type of response: type I IFN production and DC differentiation (Colonna, Trinchieri et al., 2004; Yang, Lian et al., 2005).

PDC and plasmacytoid-derived DC express the Toll-Like receptor TLR7 and TLR9 (Jarrossay, Napolitani et al., 2001; Kadowaki and Liu, 2002) and respond to their respective ligands, imidazoquinolines (Hemmi, Kaisho et al., 2002) and single strand RNA (Diebold, Kaisho et al., 2004; Heil, Hemmi et al., 2004; Lund, Alexopoulou et al., 2004) for TLR7, CpG-containing oligonucleotides (Hemmi, Takeuchi et al., 2000) and DNA viruses (Lund, Sato et al., 2003) for TLR9. They do not express TLR2, TLR3 and TLR4, and do not respond to such ligands as peptidoglycan, LPS (lipopolysaccharides) or double-stranded RNA (Jarrossay, Napolitani et al., 2001; Kadowaki and Liu, 2002). Activation of pDC through TLR7 and TLR9 can trigger both types of response, including large quantities of type I IFN production and/or DC differentiation (Liu, 2005). Synthetic CpG-containing oligonucleotides of the types A and B (CpG-A, CpG-B) selectively induce type I IFN production and DC differentiation, respectively (Duramad, Fearon et al., 2005) while some viral stimuli, such as *influenza* virus (Flu), herpes simplex virus (HSV) or CpG-C can induce simultaneously both responses (Liu, 2005). Two factors seem to be key for the induction of large quantities of type I IFN in pDC: 1) the ability of the TLR ligands to bind its receptor in the early endosomal compartments (Guiducci, Ott et al., 2006; Honda, Ohba et al., 2005); 2) the phosphorylation and nuclear translocation of the transcription factor IRF-7 (Honda, Yanai et al., 2005). This last step was shown to depend on the kinases IRAK-1 (Uematsu, Sato et al., 2005) and IkB kinase-a (IKK-a) (Hoshino, Sugiyama et al., 2006) in mouse pDC. It has been recently shown that the PI3-kinase pathway was critical to control the nuclear translocation of IRF-7 and the subsequent production of type I IFN (Guiducci, Ghirelli et al., 2008). At the present time, it is not known whether additional molecular pathways are involved and modulated HTLV-1 diseases.

PDC express a panel of surface receptors but their function remain largely unknown. The best characterized is the lectin BDCA-2 (Blood dendritic cell antigen-2) (Dzionek, Inagaki et al., 2002; Dzionek, Sohma et al., 2001). BDCA-2 mediates antigen uptake and inhibits pDC production of type 1 IFN induced by *influenza* virus (Dzionek, Sohma et al., 2001). This inhibition is mediated by the induction of a B cell receptor-like signaling cascade (Cao, Zhang et al., 2007). Neuropilin 1 (NRP1), also called BDCA-4, is another surface receptor constitutively expressed at high levels on human pDC. NRP1 is involved in the interaction between myeloid DC and T cells within the immune synapse (Tordjman, Lepelletier et al., 2002). However, its role in pDC function remains unknown. Recently, we have shown that NRP1 was a coreceptor for the HTLV-1 virus and might be involved in viral entry (Ghez, Lepelletier et al., 2006). Thus HTLV-1 could provide a link between the molecular pathways downstream of NRP1 and the physiopathology of pDC in HTLV-related diseases.

There is increasing evidence that pDC are involved in several disease settings. They were observed *in situ* in a variety of pathological conditions, such as HPV-related cervical cancer, skin melanoma (Salio, Cella et al., 2003), psoriasis (Nestle, Conrad et al., 2005) or allergic contact dermatitis (Bangert, Friedl et al., 2003) and in the nasal mucosa as early as 6 hours after allergen challenge, suggesting an active recruitment of blood pDC at the site of inflammation. Moreover, a dysregulated TLR-induced IFN response has been linked to autoimmune diseases (Colonna, 2006; Marshak-Rothstein, 2006), particularly lupus erythematosus and psoriasis (Nestle, Conrad et al., 2005).

5.2 pDC and HTLV-1 infection

Three molecules have been characterized for HTLV-1 entry into cells, heparin sulfate proteoglycans (HSPG) (Jones, Petrow-Sadowski et al., 2005) and NRP-1 (also called BDCA-4) for the initial virus binding to target cells (Ghez, Lepelletier et al., 2006), and glucose transporter 1 (GLUT-1) for the post-attachment and the viral fusion (Manel, Kim et al., 2003; Takenouchi, Jones et al., 2007). Interestingly, NRP-1 is expressed by mDC and T cells but cells expressing the highest level of BDCA-4 in blood are pDC (Grouard, Rissoan et al., 1997; Siegal, Kadowaki et al., 1999), strongly suggesting that HTLV-1 could interact with pDC. Nevertheless, HTLV-1-induced immune response by professional "sentinel" pDC has not been reported. Viral activation of pDC can be regulated by either of two Toll-like Receptors (TLR), TLR7 or TLR9, which are considered to be the receptors that human pDC use for recognition of RNA/retroviruses and DNA, respectively. HIV-activated pDC were recently reported to express the tumor necrosis factor (TNF)-related apoptosis-inducing ligand (TRAIL) (Chaperot, Blum et al., 2006; Hardy, Graham et al., 2007; Stary, Klein et al., 2009). TRAIL has been shown to induce apoptosis of cancer (Herbeuval, Lambert et al., 2003; Walczak, Miller et al., 1999) and infected cells expressing death receptor-4 or -5 (DR4, DR5). We recently demonstrated that HTLV-1 stimulated pDC expressed TRAIL and acquired cytotoxic activity, transforming them into a new subset of killer innate immune cells, which may play a central role in viral immunopathogenesis and tumor development (Hardy, Graham et al., 2007).

The role of pDC in HTLV-1 infection was unknown until Jones *et al* reported that freshly purified mDC and pDC could be productively infected by HTLV-1 free viruses (Jones, Petrow-Sadowski et al., 2008). Authors clearly demonstrated that infected pDC and mDC could also infect CD4$^+$ T cells *in vitro*. These findings were major discovery for two reasons: first, they showed that, unlike researcher thought for years, free particles of HTLV-1 could directly infect T cells, and secondly because it was the first demonstration of pDC-HTLV-1 interaction.

However, the infection of target cells by HTLV-1 is not totally understood and need to be clarified. HTLV-1 infection is a sequential process that potentially involves the recruitment of at least three molecules.

5.3 pDC activation by cell free HTLV-1 virions

Due to abvious evidences that pDC and HTLV-1 could interact, we decided to study pDC response against HTLV-1. The first parameter we tested was the IFN-α production, which is characteristic of the innate immune response. Our first results were disappointing. Using supernatants from chronically HTLV-1-infected cell lines we stimulated pDC *in vitro*. The IFN-α produced by pDC exposed to supernatants from MT-2 cell line remained very low compared to *Influenza* A (Flu) stimulation. The difference between the two stimulation was the purity of the viruses: Flu was a purified virus while HTLV-1 stimulation was made from supernatants. Thus, we decided to purify HTLV-1 by ultracentrifugation. Pelets were collected and the quantity of viruses was determined using p19 ELISA. Thus, we could calculate the concentration of purified HTLV-1 and use a large range of viral concentration to stimulate pDC. Therefore, we showed that purified cell free HTLV-1 particles could induce massive IFN-α by pDC, similarly to Influenza A virus (Flu) or HIV stimulation. For the first time, we clearly demonstrated that free HTLV-1 particles, as other retroviruses, could generate an IFN-α response by pDC (Colisson, Barblu et al, 2010). We also tested IL-10 and TNF-α production by HTLV-1-exposed pDC and found high levels of IL-10 and TNF-α production.

We and others reported that Flu or HIV-1 activation of pDC resulted in cytokine production but also activation markers (CD40, HLADR), maturation markers (CD80, CD86) and migration marker CCR7 (Beignon, McKenna et al., 2005; Chaperot, Blum et al., 2006; Fonteneau, Larsson et al., 2004). We found that HTLV-1, like other retroviruses, induced activation and maturation marker expression by pDC. However, it remained unclear whether the lymphoid migration marker CCR7 was expressed by pDC after HTLV-1 exposure. This might have essential consequences in immunopathogenesis. Indeed, HIV-1 induces migration of pDC from the blood to lymphoid organs by upregulating CCR7 expression on cell surface. Thus, activated pDC migrate to tonsils and other lymphoid organs and participate to CD4+ T cell depletion in tissues (Stary, Klein et al., 2009). We observed that CCR7 was not or weakly expressed by pDC after HTLV-1 exposure. Consequently, we could imagine that pDC do not migrate to lymphoid tissues in HTLV-1 infected patients, in contrast to HIV-1 patients. Further studies are needed to better characterized *in vitro* and *in vivo* CCR7 expression and pDC migration in patients.

We next wanted to better characterize pDC activation by HTLV-1. We previously reported that HIV-1 induced pDC transformation into TRAIL-expressing pDC, which were able to induce apoptosis of CD4$^+$ T cells expressing DR5 (Hardy, Graham et al., 2007). This new subset of killer cells was called Interferon-producing Killer pDC (ie IKpDC). Using cell free purified HTLV-1 particles, we stimulated isolated pDC from healthy donors and cells were analyzed using three dimensional (3D) microscopy. Microscopy revealed some surprising results. We found high levels of TRAIL in non activated pDC. This result was not expected as it has never been observed before. However, it was not clear whether TRAIL was located on membrane or in cytoplasm. Thus, using the ImageJ tool "3D interactive surface plot", we demonstrated that TRAIL was located in the cytoplasm of resting pDC (Colisson, Barblu et al.). In contrast, HTLV-1 stimulated pDC showed a relocalization of TRAIL from cytoplasm to plasma membrane (Figure 6). HTLV-1 exposure induced a relocalization of intracellular stock of TRAIL to the membrane, conferring a killer activity to pDC. Surprinsingly, we did not detect HTLV-1 viruses in pDC. However, chloroquine treated pDC revealed some HTLV-1 particles in cytoplasm. In fact, this latest result provides some indication concerning the pathway by which HTLV-1 particles activate pDC.

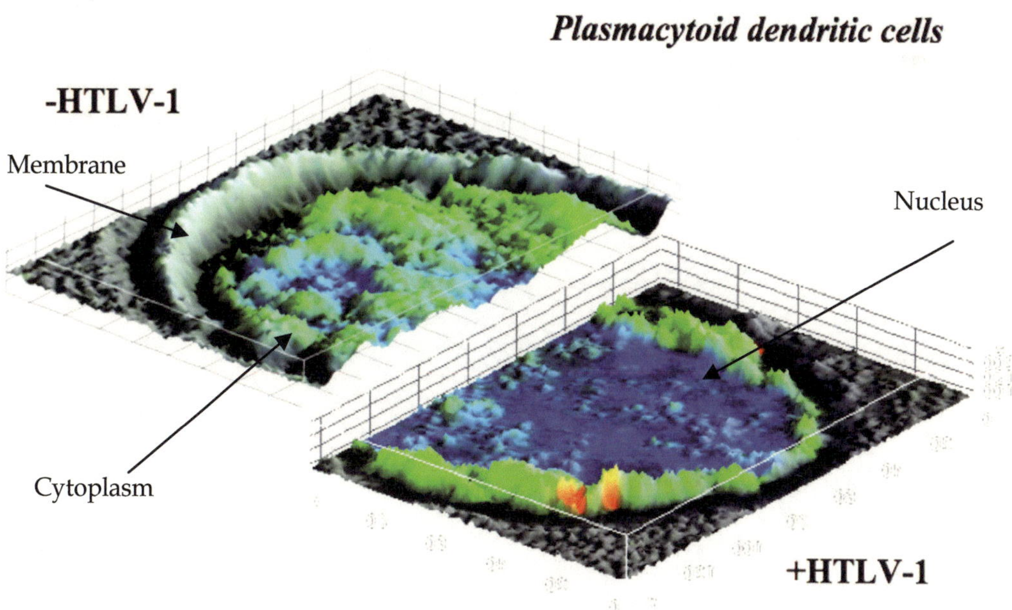

Fig. 6. 3D microscopy of HTLV-1 activated pDC. 3D interactive surface plot was used to precisely delimitated TRAIL in pDC. Upper picture show intracellular TRAIL (green) inside pDC plasma membrane. Bottom picture shows TRAIL relocalization to the membrane that appears green in HTLV-1 exposed pDC. HTLV-1 viruses (red) binds to plasma cell membrane. Adapated from Colisson, Barblu et al 2010.

5.4 HTLV-1 activated endocytosis pathway in pDC

Because pDC express high levels of NRP-1, which is a member of the HTLV-1 complex receptor, they may be productively infected by HTLV-1. However, pDC could aslo activate the endocytosis pathway under viral exposure. Endocytosis pathway is charcaterized by formation of endosomes in which pH get low activating multiple protease. Viral particles are degradated by low pH proteases and genetic material is released into the vesicles. Thus, viral RNA or DNA activate their respective receptors TLR7 or TLR9. Chloroquine inhibits endocytosis by reducing pH acidification in endosomes.

We demonstrated using chloroquine and TLR7 inhibitor that HTLV-1 activated the endocytosis pathway in pDC as demonstrated for other retrovirus like HIV-1 (Beignon, McKenna et al., 2005; Hardy, Graham et al., 2007). Viral particles, after initial binding to HTLV-1 receptor complex, entered into the endosome, which became pH low. This acidification activates endosomal protease that destroyed virus envelop and capsid, leading to single strand RNA (ssRNA) release into the vesicles. This viral ssRNA activates TLR7, which in turn recrutes the adaptor protein MyD88, a central molecule in most of TLR-dependent. The recruitment of MyD88 starts a cascade of activation leading to IFN-α production (due to the recruitment of Inteferon Regulatory factor 7, IRF7). We also showed that TRAIL expression, activation markers (CD40, HLADR) and maturation markers (CD80, CD86) were regulated by TLR7 activation in pDC. These results place TLR7 as the central molecule of HTLV-1-induced pDC response (Figure 7). Thus, endocytosis seems to be the major pathway involved in pDC activation by HTLV-1. However, it should be noticed that our findings do not exclude the possibility that pDC could get productively infected. Our study focused on short time experiments that did not allow us to detect newly synthesized viruses. Jones *et al* showed that coculture of mDC and pDC with HTLV-1 could induce CD4+ T cell infection, while free viruses alone could not infect T cells (Jones, Petrow-Sadowski et al., 2008). Further experiments are needed to determine what is the proportion of infected pDC versus activated IKpDC.

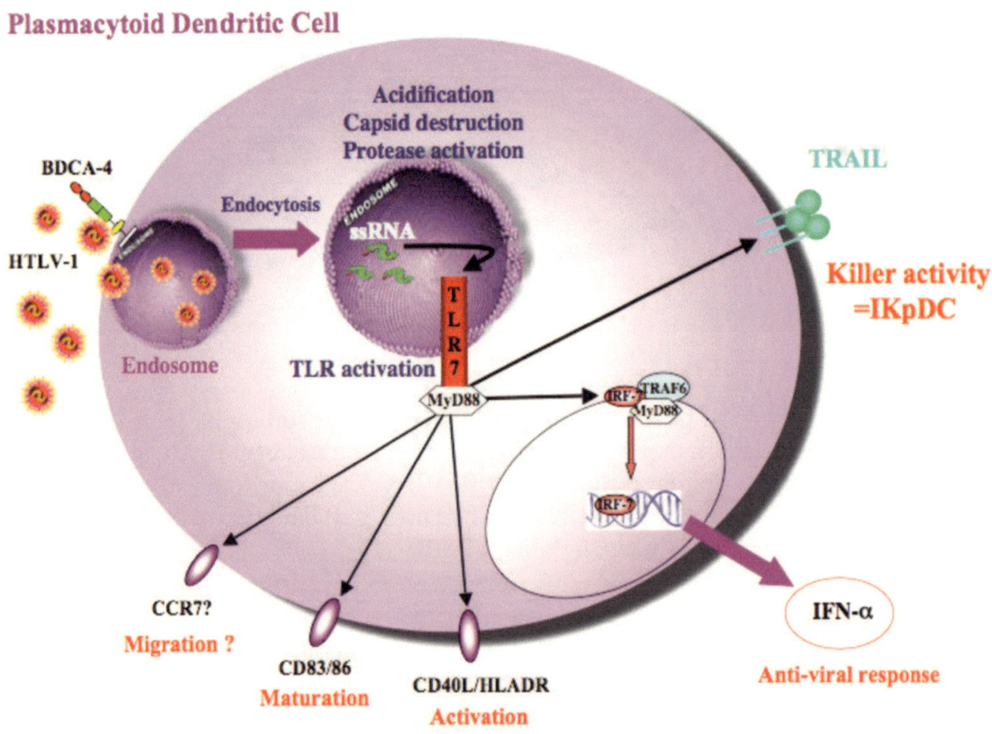

Fig. 7. Transformation of pDC into IKpDC by HTLV-1.

6. Conclusion

Adult T cell leukemia induced by HTLV-1 infection exhibits diverse clinical features. The outcome is directly correlated to ATL subtype, that could range from a very indolent and slowly progressive lymphoma to a very aggressive and nearly uniformaly lethal proliferative lymphoma. Thus, knowledge about HTLV-1 infection and propagation remains essential to better understand pathogenesis consequences.

An important challenge would be to link the pDC phenotype to the different HTLV-1 associated pathologies (ATLL). It would be interesting to determine whether IKpDC persist during chronic infection in order to generate new HTLV-1 progression markers. The characterization of IKpDC *in vivo* opens new area of dendritic cells research in HTLV-1 and other retrovirus-induced immunopathogenesis and in tumor cell biology. Considered together, our data highlight a dual role for pDC in HTLV-1 disease. pDC that become infected may participate in viral spread in the host (Jones, Petrow-Sadowski et al., 2008) and concomitantly express TRAIL, which may select the transformed $CD4^+$ T cell clone, leading to ATLL years later. In this context, it will be of great interest to test TRAIL sensitivity of the persistent clones after HTLV-1 infection that may subsequently be transformed to lymphoma/leukemia. Thus, pDC investigation in HTLV-1 disease will be crucial for understanding complex HTLV-1-associated pathologies. However, detection of primary infection in humans is currently not feasible due to the high latency of HTLV-1 virus before disease symptoms appearance. An alternative way to characterize and understand the early steps of HTLV-1 infection is the development of the pathogenic simian model (STLV-1). However, in addition to selection of TRAIL-resistant clones, one could hypothesize that similar to HIV-1 infection, pDC may participate in and contribute to the immune suppression that occurs in ATLL.

HTLV-1 free particles generate an immune response by professional virus "sentinel" pDC. We then identify and describe the mechanism by which purified HTLV-1 virions stimulate pDC and transform them into functional killer cells. We show that pDC response and activation to HTLV-1 is strictly virus-dose dependent. Finally, purified HTLV-1 particles induced TLR7-mediated relocalization of intracellular TRAIL to the pDC membrane. In conclusion, the physiological function of pDC during the different stages of HTLV-1 infection will represent a new field of investigation and may lead to new therapeutic strategies.

7. Acknowledgment

I would like to thank Pr Olivier Hermine, UMR 8147 Hopital Necker, Paris, for his precious advice and critics and Lucie Barblu for helping me on this manuscript.

8. References

Banchereau, J. and R. M. Steinman (1998). "Dendritic cells and the control of immunity." *Nature* 392 (6673): 245-52

Bangert, C., J. Friedl, et al. (2003). "Immunopathologic features of allergic contact dermatitis in humans: participation of plasmacytoid dendritic cells in the pathogenesis of the disease?" *J Invest Dermatol* 121 (6): 1409-18

Beignon, A. S., K. McKenna, et al. (2005). "Endocytosis of HIV-1 activates plasmacytoid dendritic cells via Toll-like receptor- viral RNA interactions." *J Clin Invest*

Bellail, A. C., M. C. Tse, et al. (2009). "DR5-mediated DISC controls caspase-8 cleavage and initiation of apoptosis in human glioblastomas." *J Cell Mol Med*

Bleumink, M., R. Kohler, et al. "Rocaglamide breaks TRAIL resistance in HTLV-1-associated adult T-cell leukemia/lymphoma by translational suppression of c-FLIP expression." *Cell Death Differ* 18 (2): 362-70

Cao, W., L. Zhang, et al. (2007). "BDCA2/Fc epsilon RI gamma complex signals through a novel BCR-like pathway in human plasmacytoid dendritic cells." *PLoS Biol* 5 (10): e248

Cella, M., D. Jarrossay, et al. (1999). "Plasmacytoid monocytes migrate to inflamed lymph nodes and produce large amounts of type I interferon." *Nat Med* 5 (8): 919-23

Chaperot, L., A. Blum, et al. (2006). "Virus or TLR agonists induce TRAIL-mediated cytotoxic activity of plasmacytoid dendritic cells." *J Immunol* 176 (1): 248-55

Colisson, R., L. Barblu, et al. "Free HTLV-1 induces TLR7-dependent innate immune response and TRAIL relocalization in killer plasmacytoid dendritic cells." *Blood* 115 (11): 2177-85

Collison, A., P. S. Foster, et al. (2009). "Emerging role of tumour necrosis factor-related apoptosis-inducing ligand (TRAIL) as a key regulator of inflammatory responses." *Clin Exp Pharmacol Physiol* 36 (11): 1049-53

Colonna, M. (2006). "Toll-like receptors and IFN-alpha: partners in autoimmunity." *J Clin Invest* 116 (9): 2319-22

Colonna, M., G. Trinchieri, et al. (2004). "Plasmacytoid dendritic cells in immunity." *Nat Immunol* 5 (12): 1219-26

de The, G., L. Gazzolo, et al. (1985). "Viruses as risk factors or causes of human leukaemias and lymphomas?" *Leuk Res* 9 (6): 691-6

Diebold, S. S., T. Kaisho, et al. (2004). "Innate antiviral responses by means of TLR7-mediated recognition of single-stranded RNA." *Science* 303 (5663): 1529-31

Donegan, E., H. Lee, et al. (1994). "Transfusion transmission of retroviruses: human T-lymphotropic virus types I and II compared with human immunodeficiency virus type 1." *Transfusion* 34 (6): 478-83

Duramad, O., K. L. Fearon, et al. (2005). "Inhibitors of TLR-9 act on multiple cell subsets in mouse and man in vitro and prevent death in vivo from systemic inflammation." *Journal of immunology* (Baltimore, Md.: 1950) 174 (9): 5193-5200

Dzionek, A., Y. Inagaki, et al. (2002). "Plasmacytoid dendritic cells: from specific surface markers to specific cellular functions." *Hum Immunol* 63 (12): 1133-48

Dzionek, A., Y. Sohma, et al. (2001). "BDCA-2, a novel plasmacytoid dendritic cell-specific type II C-type lectin, mediates antigen capture and is a potent inhibitor of interferon alpha/beta induction." *J Exp Med* 194 (12): 1823-34

Ehrlich, S., C. Infante-Duarte, et al. (2003). "Regulation of soluble and surface-bound TRAIL in human T cells, B cells, and monocytes." *Cytokine* 24 (6): 244-53

Fonteneau, J. F., M. Larsson, et al. (2004). "Human immunodeficiency virus type 1 activates plasmacytoid dendritic cells and concomitantly induces the bystander maturation of myeloid dendritic cells." *J Virol* 78 (10): 5223-32

Fujino, T. and Y. Nagata (2000). "HTLV-I transmission from mother to child." *J Reprod Immunol* 47 (2): 197-206

Gasper-Smith, N., D. M. Crossman, et al. (2008). "Induction of plasma (TRAIL), TNFR-2, Fas ligand, and plasma microparticles after human immunodeficiency virus type 1 (HIV-1) transmission: implications for HIV-1 vaccine design." *J Virol* 82 (15): 7700-10

Gessain, A., F. Barin, et al. (1985). "Antibodies to human T-lymphotropic virus type-I in patients with tropical spastic paraparesis." *Lancet* 2 (8452): 407-10

Ghez, D., Y. Lepelletier, et al. "Current concepts regarding the HTLV-1 receptor complex." *Retrovirology* 7: 99

Ghez, D., Y. Lepelletier, et al. (2006). "Neuropilin-1 is involved in human T-cell lymphotropic virus type 1 entry." *J Virol 80 (14): 6844-54*

Gibson, S. J., J. M. Lindh, et al. (2002). "Plasmacytoid dendritic cells produce cytokines and mature in response to the TLR7 agonists, imiquimod and resiquimod." *Cell Immunol* 218 (1-2): 74-86

Gomez-Benito, M., M. J. Martinez-Lorenzo, et al. (2007). "Membrane expression of DR4, DR5 and caspase-8 levels, but not Mcl-1, determine sensitivity of human myeloma cells to Apo2L/TRAIL." *Exp Cell Res* 313 (11): 2378-88

Grabbe, S., E. Kampgen, et al. (2000). "Dendritic cells: multi-lineal and multi-functional." *Immunol Today* 21 (9): 431-3

Griffith, T. S., W. A. Chin, et al. (1998). "Intracellular regulation of TRAIL-induced apoptosis in human melanoma cells." *J Immunol* 161 (6): 2833-40

Grouard, G., M. C. Rissoan, et al. (1997). "The enigmatic plasmacytoid T cells develop into dendritic cells with interleukin (IL)-3 and CD40-ligand." *J Exp Med* 185 (6): 1101-11

Grumont, R. J. and S. Gerondakis (2000). "Rel induces interferon regulatory factor 4 (IRF-4) expression in lymphocytes: modulation of interferon-regulated gene expression by rel/nuclear factor kappaB." *J Exp Med* 191 (8): 1281-92

Guiducci, C., C. Ghirelli, et al. (2008). "PI3K is critical for the nuclear translocation of IRF-7 and type I IFN production by human plasmacytoid predendritic cells in response to TLR activation." *J Exp Med*

Guiducci, C., G. Ott, et al. (2006). "Properties regulating the nature of the plasmacytoid dendritic cell response to Toll-like receptor 9 activation." *J Exp Med* 203 (8): 1999-2008

Gura, T. (1997). "How TRAIL kills cancer cells, but not normal cells." *Science* 277 (5327): 768

Hardy, A. W., D. R. Graham, et al. (2007). "HIV turns plasmacytoid dendritic cells (pDC) into TRAIL-expressing killer pDC and down-regulates HIV coreceptors by Toll-like receptor 7-induced IFN-alpha." *Proc Natl Acad Sci U S A* 104 (44): 17453-8

Hasegawa, H., Y. Yamada, et al. (2005). "Sensitivity of adult T-cell leukaemia lymphoma cells to tumour necrosis factor-related apoptosis-inducing ligand." *Br J Haematol* 128 (2): 253-65

Hasegawa, H., Y. Yamada, et al. (2009). "Activation of p53 by Nutlin-3a, an antagonist of MDM2, induces apoptosis and cellular senescence in adult T-cell leukemia cells." *Leukemia* 23 (11): 2090-101

Heil, F., H. Hemmi, et al. (2004). "Species-specific recognition of single-stranded RNA via toll-like receptor 7 and 8." *Science* 303 (5663): 1526-9

Hemmi, H., T. Kaisho, et al. (2002). "Small anti-viral compounds activate immune cells via the TLR7 MyD88-dependent signaling pathway." *Nat Immunol* 3 (2): 196-200

Hemmi, H., O. Takeuchi, et al. (2000). "A Toll-like receptor recognizes bacterial DNA." *Nature* 408 (6813): 740-5

Herbeuval, J. P., A. Boasso, et al. (2005). "TNF-related apoptosis-inducing ligand (TRAIL) in HIV-1-infected patients and its in vitro production by antigen-presenting cells." *Blood* 105 (6): 2458-64

Herbeuval, J. P., J. C. Grivel, et al. (2005). "CD4+ T-cell death induced by infectious and noninfectious HIV-1: role of type 1 interferon-dependent, TRAIL/DR5-mediated apoptosis." *Blood* 106 (10): 3524-31

Herbeuval, J. P., C. Lambert, et al. (2003). "Macrophages From Cancer Patients: Analysis of TRAIL, TRAIL Receptors, and Colon Tumor Cell Apoptosis." *J Natl Cancer Inst* 95 (8): 611-621

Herbeuval, J. P., J. Nilsson, et al. (2009). "HAART reduces death ligand but not death receptors in lymphoid tissue of HIV-infected patients and simian immunodeficiency virus-infected macaques." *Aids* 23 (1): 35-40

Hermine, O., D. Bouscary, et al. (1995). "Brief report: treatment of adult T-cell leukemia-lymphoma with zidovudine and interferon alfa." *N Engl J Med* 332 (26): 1749-51

Hermine, O., H. Dombret, et al. (2004). "Phase II trial of arsenic trioxide and alpha interferon in patients with relapsed/refractory adult T-cell leukemia/lymphoma." *Hematol J* 5 (2): 130-4

Hinuma, Y., Y. Gotoh, et al. (1982). "A retrovirus associated with human adult T-cell leukemia: in vitro activation." *Gann* 73 (2): 341-4

Honda, K., Y. Ohba, et al. (2005). "Spatiotemporal regulation of MyD88-IRF-7 signalling for robust type-I interferon induction." *Nature* 434 (7036): 1035-40

Honda, K., H. Yanai, et al. (2005). "IRF-7 is the master regulator of type-I interferon-dependent immune responses." *Nature* 434 (7034): 772-7

Hoshino, K., T. Sugiyama, et al. (2006). "IkappaB kinase-alpha is critical for interferon-alpha production induced by Toll-like receptors 7 and 9." *Nature* 440 (7086): 949-953

Imaizumi, Y., T. Kohno, et al. (2001). "Possible involvement of interferon regulatory factor 4 (IRF4) in a clinical subtype of adult T-cell leukemia." *Jpn J Cancer Res* 92 (12): 1284-92

Imura, A., T. Hori, et al. (1997). "OX40 expressed on fresh leukemic cells from adult T-cell leukemia patients mediates cell adhesion to vascular endothelial cells: implication for the possible involvement of OX40 in leukemic cell infiltration." *Blood* 89 (8): 2951-8

Jacobson, S. (1996). "Cellular immune responses to HTLV-I: immunopathogenic role in HTLV-I-associated neurologic disease." *J Acquir Immune Defic Syndr Hum Retrovirol* 13 Suppl 1: S100-6

Jarrossay, D., G. Napolitani, et al. (2001). "Specialization and complementarity in microbial molecule recognition by human myeloid and plasmacytoid dendritic cells." *Eur J Immunol* 31 (11): 3388-93

Jin, T. G., A. Kurakin, et al. (2004). "Fas-associated protein with death domain (FADD)-independent recruitment of c-FLIPL to death receptor 5." *J Biol Chem* 279 (53): 55594-601

Jones, K. S., C. Petrow-Sadowski, et al. (2005). "Heparan sulfate proteoglycans mediate attachment and entry of human T-cell leukemia virus type 1 virions into CD4+ T cells." *J Virol* 79 (20): 12692-702

Jones, K. S., C. Petrow-Sadowski, et al. (2008). "Cell-free HTLV-1 infects dendritic cells leading to transmission and transformation of CD4(+) T cells." *Nat Med* 14 (4): 429-36

Kadowaki, N., S. Antonenko, et al. (2000). "Natural interferon alpha/beta-producing cells link innate and adaptive immunity." *J Exp Med* 192 (2): 219-26

Kadowaki, N. and Y. J. Liu (2002). "Natural type I interferon-producing cells as a link between innate and adaptive immunity." *Hum Immunol* 63 (12): 1126-32

Kayagaki, N., N. Yamaguchi, et al. (1999). "Involvement of TNF-related apoptosis-inducing ligand in human CD4+ T cell-mediated cytotoxicity." *J Immunol* 162 (5): 2639-47

Kohno, T., R. Moriuchi, et al. (2000). "Identification of genes associated with the progression of adult T cell leukemia (ATL)." *Jpn J Cancer Res* 91 (11): 1103-10

Koyanagi, Y., Y. Itoyama, et al. (1993). "In vivo infection of human T-cell leukemia virus type I in non-T cells." *Virology* 196 (1): 25-33

Kunitomi, A., T. Hori, et al. (2002). "OX40 signaling renders adult T-cell leukemia cells resistant to Fas-induced apoptosis." *Int J Hematol* 76 (3): 260-6

Lambert, S., M. Bouttier, et al. (2009). "HTLV-1 uses HSPG and neuropilin 1 for entry by molecular mimicry of VEGF165." *Blood*

Lichtner, M., C. Maranon, et al. (2004). "HIV type 1-infected dendritic cells induce apoptotic death in infected and uninfected primary CD4 T lymphocytes." *AIDS Res Hum Retroviruses* 20 (2): 175-82

Liu, Y. J. (2005). "IPC: professional type 1 interferon-producing cells and plasmacytoid dendritic cell precursors." *Annu Rev Immunol* 23: 275-306

Lund, J., A. Sato, et al. (2003). "Toll-like receptor 9-mediated recognition of Herpes simplex virus-2 by plasmacytoid dendritic cells." *J Exp Med* 198 (3): 513-20

Lund, J. M., L. Alexopoulou, et al. (2004). "Recognition of single-stranded RNA viruses by Toll-like receptor 7." *Proc Natl Acad Sci U S A* 101 (15): 5598-603

Macatonia, S. E., J. K. Cruickshank, et al. (1992). "Dendritic cells from patients with tropical spastic paraparesis are infected with HTLV-1 and stimulate autologous lymphocyte proliferation." *AIDS Res Hum Retroviruses* 8 (9): 1699-706

Makino, M., S. Shimokubo, et al. (1999). "The role of human T-lymphotropic virus type 1 (HTLV-1)-infected dendritic cells in the development of HTLV-1-associated myelopathy/tropical spastic paraparesis." *J Virol* 73 (6): 4575-81

Mamane, Y., N. Grandvaux, et al. (2002). "Repression of IRF-4 target genes in human T cell leukemia virus-1 infection." *Oncogene* 21 (44): 6751-65

Mamane, Y., M. Loignon, et al. (2005). "Repression of DNA repair mechanisms in IRF-4-expressing and HTLV-I-infected T lymphocytes." *J Interferon Cytokine Res* 25 (1): 43-51

Manel, N., F. J. Kim, et al. (2003). "The ubiquitous glucose transporter GLUT-1 is a receptor for HTLV." Cell 115 (4): 449-59

Manns, A., W. J. Miley, et al. (1999). "Quantitative proviral DNA and antibody levels in the natural history of HTLV-I infection." *J Infect Dis* 180 (5): 1487-93

Mansky, L. M. (2000). "In vivo analysis of human T-cell leukemia virus type 1 reverse transcription accuracy." *J Virol* 74 (20): 9525-31

Marshak-Rothstein, A. (2006). "Toll-like receptors in systemic autoimmune disease." *Nat Rev Immunol* 6 (11): 823-35

Matsuda, T., A. Almasan, et al. (2005). "Resistance to Apo2 ligand (Apo2L)/tumor necrosis factor-related apoptosis-inducing ligand (TRAIL)-mediated apoptosis and constitutive expression of Apo2L/TRAIL in human T-cell leukemia virus type 1-infected T-cell lines." *J Virol* 79 (3): 1367-78

Matsuoka, M. (2005). "Human T-cell leukemia virus type I (HTLV-I) infection and the onset of adult T-cell leukemia (ATL)." *Retrovirology* 2: 27

Mortreux, F., I. Leclercq, et al. (2001). "Somatic mutation in human T-cell leukemia virus type 1 provirus and flanking cellular sequences during clonal expansion in vivo." *J Natl Cancer Inst* 93 (5): 367-77

Mueller, N., A. Okayama, et al. (1996). "Findings from the Miyazaki Cohort Study." *J Acquir Immune Defic Syndr Hum Retrovirol* 13 Suppl 1: S2-7

Nagai, M., R. Kubota, et al. (2001). "Increased activated human T cell lymphotropic virus type I (HTLV-I) Tax11-19-specific memory and effector CD8+ cells in patients with HTLV-I-associated myelopathy/tropical spastic paraparesis: correlation with HTLV-I provirus load." *J Infect Dis* 183 (2): 197-205

Nestle, F. O., C. Conrad, et al. (2005). "Plasmacytoid predendritic cells initiate psoriasis through interferon-alpha production." *J Exp Med* 202 (1): 135-43

Pais-Correia, A. M., M. Sachse, et al. "Biofilm-like extracellular viral assemblies mediate HTLV-1 cell-to-cell transmission at virological synapses." *Nat Med* 16 (1): 83-9

Poiesz, B. J., F. W. Ruscetti, et al. (1980). "T-cell lines established from human T-lymphocytic neoplasias by direct response to T-cell growth factor." *Proc Natl Acad Sci U S A* 77 (11): 6815-9

Poiesz, B. J., F. W. Ruscetti, et al. (1981). "Isolation of a new type C retrovirus (HTLV) in primary uncultured cells of a patient with Sezary T-cell leukaemia." *Nature* 294 (5838): 268-71

Proietti, F. A., A. B. Carneiro-Proietti, et al. (2005). "Global epidemiology of HTLV-I infection and associated diseases." *Oncogene* 24 (39): 6058-68

Pulendran, B., K. Palucka, et al. (2001). "Sensing pathogens and tuning immune responses." *Science* 293 (5528): 253-6

Richardson, J. H., A. J. Edwards, et al. (1990). "In vivo cellular tropism of human T-cell leukemia virus type 1." *J Virol* 64 (11): 5682-7

Robert-Guroff, M., Y. Nakao, et al. (1982). "Natural antibodies to human retrovirus HTLV in a cluster of Japanese patients with adult T cell leukemia." *Science* 215 (4535): 975-8

Salio, M., M. Cella, et al. (2003). "Plasmacytoid dendritic cells prime IFN-gamma-secreting melanoma-specific CD8 lymphocytes and are found in primary melanoma lesions." *Eur J Immunol* 33 (4): 1052-62

Sato, K., S. Hida, et al. (2001). "Antiviral response by natural killer cells through TRAIL gene induction by IFN-alpha/beta." *Eur J Immunol* 31 (11): 3138-46

Sharma, S., N. Grandvaux, et al. (2002). "Regulation of IFN regulatory factor 4 expression in human T cell leukemia virus-I-transformed T cells." *J Immunol* 169 (6): 3120-30

Sharma, S., Y. Mamane, et al. (2000). "Activation and regulation of interferon regulatory factor 4 in HTLV type 1-infected T lymphocytes." *AIDS Res Hum Retroviruses* 16 (16): 1613-22

Sheikh, M. S., T. F. Burns, et al. (1998). "p53-dependent and -independent regulation of the death receptor KILLER/DR5 gene expression in response to genotoxic stress and tumor necrosis factor alpha." *Cancer Res* 58 (8): 1593-8

Sheridan, J. P., S. A. Marsters, et al. (1997). "Control of TRAIL-induced apoptosis by a family of signaling and decoy receptors." *Science* 277 (5327): 818-21.

Siegal, F. P., N. Kadowaki, et al. (1999). "The nature of the principal type 1 interferon-producing cells in human blood." *Science* 284 (5421): 1835-7

Smyth, M. J., E. Cretney, et al. (2001). "Tumor necrosis factor-related apoptosis-inducing ligand (TRAIL) contributes to interferon gamma-dependent natural killer cell protection from tumor metastasis." *J Exp Med* 193 (6): 661-70

Stary, G., I. Klein, et al. (2009). "Plasmacytoid dendritic cells express TRAIL and induce CD4+ T-cell apoptosis in HIV-1 viremic patients." *Blood* 114 (18): 3854-63

Takenouchi, N., K. S. Jones, et al. (2007). "GLUT1 is not the primary binding receptor but is associated with cell-to-cell transmission of human T-cell leukemia virus type 1." *J Virol* 81 (3): 1506-10

Tecchio, C., V. Huber, et al. (2004). "IFNalpha-stimulated neutrophils and monocytes release a soluble form of TNF-related apoptosis-inducing ligand (TRAIL/Apo-2 ligand) displaying apoptotic activity on leukemic cells." *Blood* 103 (10): 3837-44

Tendler, C. L., S. J. Greenberg, et al. (1991). "Cytokine induction in HTLV-I associated myelopathy and adult T-cell leukemia: alternate molecular mechanisms underlying retroviral pathogenesis." *J Cell Biochem* 46 (4): 302-11

Tordjman, R., Y. Lepelletier, et al. (2002). "A neuronal receptor, neuropilin-1, is essential for the initiation of the primary immune response." *Nat Immunol* 3 (5): 477-82

Uematsu, S., S. Sato, et al. (2005). "Interleukin-1 receptor-associated kinase-1 plays an essential role for Toll-like receptor (TLR)7- and TLR9-mediated interferon-{alpha} induction." *J ex Med* 201 (6): 915-923

Uozumi, K. "Treatment of adult T-cell leukemia." *J Clin Exp Hematop* 50 (1): 9-25

Valledor, A. F., F. E. Borras, et al. (1998). "Transcription factors that regulate monocyte/macrophage differentiation." *J Leukoc Biol* 63 (4): 405-17

Verdonck, K., E. Gonzalez, et al. (2007). "Human T-lymphotropic virus 1: recent knowledge about an ancient infection." *Lancet Infect Dis* 7 (4): 266-81

Vidalain, P. O., O. Azocar, et al. (2000). "Measles virus induces functional TRAIL production by human dendritic cells." *J Virol* 74 (1): 556-9

Vidalain, P. O., O. Azocar, et al. (2001). "Measle virus-infected dendritic cells develop immunosuppressive and cytotoxic activities." *Immunobiology* 204 (5): 629-38

Walczak, H. and T. L. Haas (2008). "Biochemical analysis of the native TRAIL death-inducing signaling complex." *Methods Mol Biol* 414: 221-39

Walczak, H., R. E. Miller, et al. (1999). "Tumoricidal activity of tumor necrosis factor-related apoptosis-inducing ligand in vivo." *Nat Med* 5 (2): 157-63

Wiley, S. R., K. Schooley, et al. (1995). "Identification and characterization of a new member of the TNF family that induces apoptosis." *Immunity* 3 (6): 673-82

Wu, G. S., T. F. Burns, et al. (1997). "KILLER/DR5 is a DNA damage-inducible p53-regulated death receptor gene." *Nat Genet* 17 (2): 141-3

Yamaguchi, K. (1994). "Human T-lymphotropic virus type I in Japan." *Lancet* 343 (8891): 213-6

Yang, G. X., Z. X. Lian, et al. (2005). "Plasmacytoid dendritic cells of different origins have distinct characteristics and function: studies of lymphoid progenitors versus myeloid progenitors." *J Immunol* 175 (11): 7281-7

Yoshie, O. (2005). "Expression of CCR4 in adult T-cell leukemia." *Leuk Lymphoma* 46 (2): 185-90

2

Human T-Cell Lymphotropic Virus (HTLV-1) and Adult T-Cell Leukemia

Mohammad R. Abbaszadegan and Mehran Gholamin
Division of Human Genetics, Immunology Research Center
Avicenna Research Institute, Mashhad University of Medical Sciences, Mashhad
Iran

1. Introduction

Human T-cell Lymphotropic Viruses (HTLVs) and Simian T-cell Lymphotropic Viruses (STLVs) are anciently related primate T-cell leukemia viruses (PTLVs) that share molecular and virological features. Human T-cell Lymphotropic Virus (HTLV-1) is believed to be repeatedly transmitted in separate independent events from simians to humans beginning 50,000 ± 10,000 years ago; this course has resulted in the formation of several viral subtypes around the world. There are four known strains of HTLV, of which HTLV-1 and HTLV-2 are the most prevalent worldwide. Newer HTLVs, HTLV-3 and 4 have been identified recently from bush meat hunters in central Africa(Matsuoka and Jeang 2007).

HTLV-1, the first human retrovirus was discovered by two independent investigating groups in 1980 and 1981. A geographical clustering of leukaemias in southwestern Japan led to the description of a unique clinical entity termed adult T-cell leukemia (ATL), where Japanese investigators identified HTLV-1 as an etiologic agent of newly described ATL, and the U.S. investigators detected HTLV-1 retrovirus in human cell lines (Yoshida 2010).

HTLV-1 belongs to the Deltaretrovirus genera of the Orthoretrovirinae subfamily, the first discovered human retrovirus, isolated in the early 1980s from peripheral blood samples of a patient with cutaneous T-cell lymphoma (Poiesz et al, 1980). It is the etiologic agent of two predominant distinct human diseases, ATL or adult T-cell leukemia lymphoma (ATLL) and a chronic, progressive demyelinating disorder known as HTLV-1-associated myelopathy/tropical spastic paraparesis (HAM/TSP)(Zanjani et al. 2010).

The major findings that support the etiologic association of HTLV-1 are: 1) All patients with ATL have antibodies against HTLV-1, 2) The areas of high incidence of ATL patients correspond closely with those of high incidence of HTLV-1 carriers, 3) HTLV-1 immortalizes human T cells *in vitro,* 4) Monoclonal integration of HTLV-1 proviral DNA was demonstrated in ATL cells. Thus, HTLV-1 is the first retrovirus directly associated with human malignancy (Takatsuki 2005). HTLV-1 is a complex leukemogenic retrovirus with a single stranded positive sense RNA genome that expresses unique proteins with oncogenic potential. HTLV-1 can infect T cells, B cells, monocytes, dendritic cells and endothelial cells with equal efficiency; yet, it can transform only primary T cells (Hanon et al. 2000).

HTLV-2 was identified in a CD8+ T cell line derived from a patient with a variant form of hairy T cell leukemia. Since then, HTLV-2 has not been associated with leukemia/lymphoma; nevertheless, it has been associated with a few sporadic cases of neurological disorders and chronic encephalomyelopathy (Hjelle et al. 1992). The clinical symptoms presented are similar to those of HAM/TSP. The prevalence of HTLV-2-associated myelopathy was reported to be 1% compared to 3.7% for HTLV-1 associated HAM/TSP in the United State. Although other neurological disorders have been reported, their clear association with HTLV-2 is hampered by confounding factors such as intravenous drug use or concomitant HIV infection. To date, HTLV-3 and HTLV-4 have not been associated with any known clinical conditions (Kannian 2010).

In 1985, Gessain et al., demonstrated that 68% of patients with tropical spastic paraparesis (TSP) in Martinique had positive serology for HTLV-1. In 1986, a similar neurological condition was described in Japan and named HTLV-1 associated myelopathy (HAM). Later, Román and Osame (1988) concluded that they were dealing with the same disease, and the term HTLV associated myelopathy/tropical spastic paraparesis (HAM/TSP) came to be used. Since then, countless other diseases have been correlated with this infection: uveitis, Sjögren's syndrome, infectious dermatitis, polymyositis, arthropathies, thyroiditis, polyneuropathies, lymphocytic alveolitis, cutaneous T-cell lymphoma, strongyloidiasis, scabies, Hansen's disease and tuberculosis. The importance of the possible clinical manifestations of the HTLV virus has now become clear in several different medical specialties such as oncology, neurology, internal medicine, dermatology, and ophthalmology (Romanelli, Caramelli and Proietti 2010).

Only HTLV-1-infected individuals develop ATL, and all ATL cells contain integrated HTLV-1 provirus, supporting the causal etiology of the virus for leukaemogenesis. Nevertheless, only a small minority of HTLV-1-infected individuals progress to ATL. Indeed, the cumulative risks of developing ATL among virus carriers are estimated to be approximately 6.6% for males and 2.1% for females (Matsuoka and Jeang 2007).

A long period of latency from HTLV-1 infection to ATL development suggests a multistep process of T-lymphocyte transformation. In ATL patients, the malignant cells typically consist of oligoclonal or monoclonal outgrowths of CD4+ and CD25+ T lymphocytes carrying a complete or defective provirus of HTLV-1. Four clinical subtypes of ATL include acute, lymphoma, chronic and smoldering (Noula Shembade 2010).

2. Worldwide distribution

Approximately 15-25 million people worldwide are infected with HTLV-1. The virus is endemic in southwestern Japan, Africa, the Caribbean Islands and South America and is frequently found in Melanesia, Papua New Guinea, Solomon Islands and Australian aborigines. HTLV-1 is also prevalent in certain populations in the Middle East (Iran) and India. HTLV-2 is more prevalent among intravenous drug users (IDUs), and is endemic among IDUs in the USA, Europe, South America and Southeast Asia. HTLV-3 and HTLV-4 have been identified only in African primate hunters (Kannian 2010). HTLV-1 infection is endemic in northeastern Iran (Khorasan province) and the prevalence of HTLV-1 infection is estimated to be 2-3% in the whole population and 0.78% in blood donors (Abbaszadegan et al. 2003; Safai et al. 1996).

High prevalence rates in the general population are observed in the South of Japan (10%), in Jamaica and Trinidad and Tobago (6%). In South America (Argentina, Brazil, Colombia and Peru) a 2% prevalence of seropositivity was observed among blood donors. It is known that the prevalence of HITLV-1 in population of blood donors represents an underestimation of prevalence in the general population. In absolute terms, Brazil may have the largest number of seropositive people in the world. In non-endemic areas, certain groups should be considered as at risk, such as immigrants from endemic areas, the sexual partners and descendents of people known to be infected, sex professionals and drug users(Romanelli, Caramelli and Proietti 2010).

HTLV-1 carriers are mostly asymptomatic in their life spans. The lifetime risks of developing ATL and HAM/TSP are about 2.5 to 5% and 0.3 to 2%, respectively (Silva et al. 2007). Among HTLV-1 infected individuals in Japan, a small proportion of carriers (6% for males and 2% for females) develop ATL. The majority of HTLV-1 carriers do not develop HTLV-1-associated diseases. The latency period from the initial infection until onset of ATL is about 60 years in Japan and 40 years in Jamaica. These determinations indicate a multistep leukemogenic mechanism in the generation of ATL.

3. Genomic structure of HTLV-1

HTLV-1 virions are complex type C particles, spherical, enveloped and 100–110 nm in diameter. The inner membrane of the virion envelope is lined by the viral matrix protein (MA). This structure encloses the viral capsid (CA), which carries two identical strands of the genomic RNA as well as functional protease (Pro), integrase (IN), and reverse transcriptase (RT) enzymes. A newly synthesized viral particle attaches to the target cell receptor through the viral envelope (Env) and enters via fusion, which is followed by the uncoating of the capsid and the release of its contents into the cell cytoplasm. The viral genome consists of a linear, positive sense, ssRNA held together by hydrogen bonds. Each monomer has about 9032 nucleotides. The 3′ terminal viral genome is polyadenylated and its 5′- terminal is capped. Each unit is associated with a specific molecule of tRNA that is base paired to a region, primer binding site, near the 5′ end of the RNA. Proviral forms are flanked at both termini by long terminal repeats (LTRs) of 754 nucleotides. The genomic structure encodes structural and enzymatic proteins: gag, pol, env, reverse transcriptase, protease, and integrase. In addition, HTLV-1 has a region at the 3′ end of the virus, called pX, which encodes four partially overlapping reading frames (ORFs). These ORFs code for regulatory proteins which impact the expression and replication of the virus (Figure 1) (Boxus and Willems 2009).

The viral RNA is reverse transcribed into double stranded DNA by the RT. This double stranded DNA is then transported to the nucleus and becomes integrated into the host chromosome forming the provirus. The provirus contains the promoter and enhancer elements for transcription initiation in the long terminal repeats (LTR); the polyadenylation signal for plus strand transcription are located in the 3'LTR (Kannian 2010).

The initial round of HTLV-1 transcription is dependent on cellular factors. The complex retroviral genome codes for the structural proteins Gag (capsid, nucleocapsid, and matrix), Pro, polymerase (Pol) and Env from unspliced/singly spliced mRNAs. Alternatively spliced mRNA transcripts encode regulatory and accessory proteins. The two regulatory genes rex and tax are encoded by open reading frames (ORF) III and IV, respectively, and share a common doubly spliced transcript. Tax is the transactivator gene, which increases the rate of viral LTR-mediated transcription and modulates the transcription of numerous cellular genes involved in cell proliferation and differentiation, cell cycle control and DNA repair. Tax has displayed oncogenic potential in several experimental systems and is essential for HTLV-1 and HTLV-2-mediated transformation of primary human T cells. Rex acts post-transcriptionally by preferentially binding, stabilizing exporting intron-containing viral

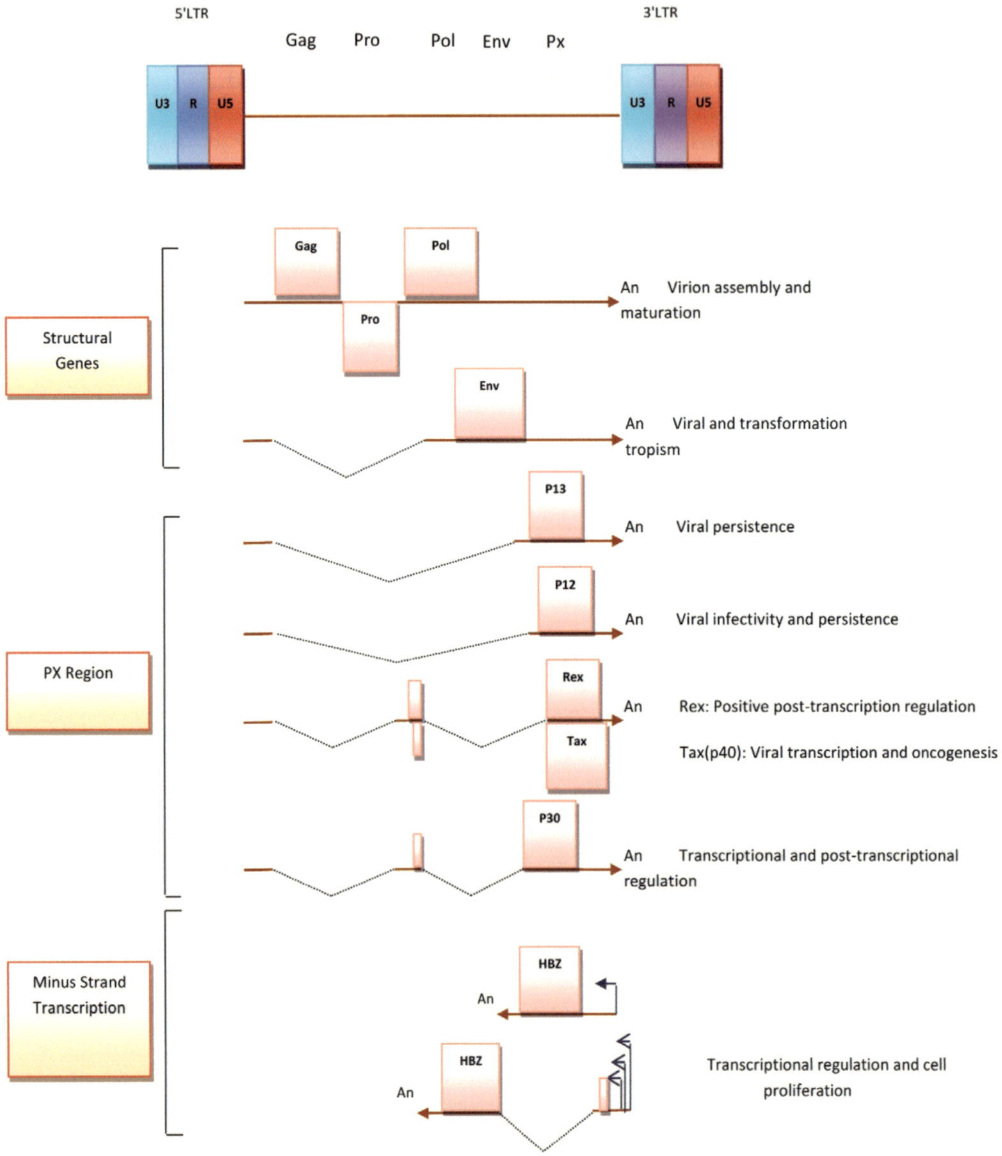

Fig. 1. HTLV-1 genome structure and gene product

mRNAs from the nucleus to the cytoplasm. The accessory genes, p12/p8 encoded by ORF I and p30/p13 encoded by ORF II is not necessary in standard immortalization assays in culture. However, these genes are essential for initiation of viral infection and the establishment of persistence in animal models. P8 is a proteolytic cleavage product of the p12 parent molecule, whereas the p13 polypeptide, comprised of the carboxy terminus of p30, is expressed from a distinct mRNA. These accessory proteins may also play a role in gene regulation and contribute to the productive infection of quiescent T lymphocytes *in vitro*. The minus strand of the proviral genome encodes several isoforms (generated from unspliced and spliced mRNAs) of the HTLV-1 basic leucine zipper factor (HBZ). HBZ interacts with cellular factors JunB, c-Jun, JunD, cAMP response element binding (CREB) and CREB binding protein (CBP)/p300to modulate both viral and cellular gene transcription. HBZ also plays a crucial role in T cell proliferation. Although research data indicate that Tax, among all the viral proteins, is the viral oncoprotein, but emerging data suggests a supporting role for HBZ in the oncogenic process (Kannian 2010).

4. Transmission

HTLV-1 can infect various cell types, including T-lymphocytes, B-lymphocytes, monocytes, dendritic cells (DC) and fibroblasts. Glucose transporter 1 (GLUT-1) is ubiquitously expressed cell surface receptor targeted by HTLV-1 (Manel et al. 2003). Other cell surface receptors such as neuropilin 1 (NRP1) and surface heparan sulfate proteoglycans (HSPGs) have been reported to be target of HTLV-1 and are required for efficient entry (Boxus and Willems 2009). There is also evidence for cell-type specific receptors since a recent study has reported that HTLV-1 enters DCs by binding to the receptor DC-SIGN (Noula Shembade 2010.). However, the HTLV-1 provirus is mainly detected in CD4-positive lymphocytes, with about 10% in CD8-positive T-lymphocytes. This situation possibly arises because of Tax transformation of CD4-positive T-lymphocytes in vivo causing enhanced proliferation and suppressed apoptosis. In HTLV-1-infected individuals, no virions are detected in the serum. In addition, the infectivity of free virions is very poor compared with that of infected cells suggesting that HTLV-1 spreads through cell-to-cell transmission, rather than by free virions. *In vitro* analyses of HTLV-1 infected cells revealed that HTLV-1-infected cells form "virological synapses" with uninfected cells. The viral proteins Gag and Env, viral RNA and microtubules are accumulated as an infected cell is in contact with a target cell, and the viral complex subsequently transfers into the target cell. HTLV-1 also spreads in a cell- to-cell manner via such virological synapses *in vivo* (Igakura et al. 2003).

In either route, HTLV-1-infected cells are essential for transmission. This was supported by the findings that fresh frozen plasma from carriers did not cause transmission and freeze-thawing of breast milk reduced vertical transmission (Matsuoka 2005).

Transplacental transmission is also suspected. Cellular blood products are the main source of transfusion- associated HTLV transmission, whereas fresh frozen plasma, cryoprecipitate, or coagulation factor concentrates appear not to cause infection (Abbaszadegan et al. 2003).

The efficiency of virus transmission is from males to females during sexually active years causing a higher seroprevalence of about more than twice in females. The HTLV-1 infection tends to be more within family members and three to four times greater than its rate in general population. It is proposed that repeated close contact and shared environment could be significant in HTLV-1 transmission (Rafatpanah et al. 2006). Viral antigens expressed by infected cell are quickly targeted by cytotoxic T cells; hence the viral load is maintained predominantly by cells harboring silent provirus spread by mitotic transmission. HTLV-1 transmission by free virions is very inefficient, at least in T cells, however, recent studies indicate that cell-free HTLV-1 virions are highly infectious for DCs (Noula Shembade 2010).

4.1 Transmission of HTLV-1 occurs through three main routes

HTLV-1 is mainly transmitted via three routes: 1) mother- to-infant transmission, mainly through breast feeding; 2) sexual transmission, mainly from male-to- female; and 3) parenteral transmission (blood transfusion or intravenous drug use).

Mother to child: One of the main modes of HTLV-1 transmition from mother to child is by breast feeding. Studies in Japan showed that the prevalence of HTLV-1 infection in children of carrier mothers was significantly higher (21%) than in children in the general population (1%). More than 85% of infected mothers had infected their children. The length of breast-feeding affects the risk of HTLV-1 transmission. The duration of breast-feeding affects the risk of HTLV-1 transmission. HTLV-1 antigen in cord blood lymphocytes of babies born to healthy carriers raised a possibility to consider intrauterine transmission as an alternative pathway. However, the HTLV-1 provirus in the cord blood circulation is derived from migrated maternal cells that are not a part of blood circulation of the baby. Thus, intrauterine transmission could not be a major pathway of transmission.

Only ~3%–4% of children become infected if they are not breast-fed or are breast- fed for <6 months, and the transmission risk increases with the duration of breast-feeding. The cumulative risk of infection in children who are regularly breast-fed is ~20%. Furthermore, the transmission risk increases with the amount of provirus in breast milk. Breast milk proviral levels also correlate with proviral levels in maternal peripheral blood mononuclear cells (PBMCs) and with antibody titers. It is therefore not surprising that the transmission risk correlates with proviral and antibody levels in maternal peripheral blood. However, this is contradictory to the fact that the majority of children who are breastfed for long periods do not become infected. HIV can also be transmitted by breast-feeding, however, it is more commonly transmitted in utero or perinatally, As with HTLV-1, transmission occurs in proportion to the duration of breast-feeding, and the risk increases when mothers have high HIV provirus levels in breast milk, which are also directly correlated with peripheral blood provirus levels. Mother- to-child in utero and perinatal HIV transmission was more likely when children were more concordant with their mothers in HLA class I type. Children with HLA class I type A*02 (later reported to be the A2 supertype) have a decreased risk of early infection. HLA class I type variability is not associated with HIV transmission via breast-feeding, whereas, with HTLV-1, vertical transmission almost always occurs via breast-feeding. However, unlike HIV, HTLV-1 is transmitted primarily by cell- to-cell contact rather than by free virus. We reasoned that factors affecting cellular immunity might be more important for the vertical transmission of HTLV-1 than for HIV (Biggar et al. 2006).

Transmission rates are 16% for children born to infected mothers, 27% for children nursed by infected mothers for more than three months and 5% for children nursed by infected mothers for less than three months (Ureta-Vidal et al. 1999). It is Interesting that HTLV is transmitted to about 13% of bottle-fed children from their infected mother suggesting a different route than breast-feeding. The infants seroconvert within 1-3 years of age (Ureta-Vidal et al. 1999). The infants seroconvert within 1-3 years of age (Ureta-Vidal et al. 1999).

Sexual: HTLV-1 can also be transmitted through sexual contact. Heterosexual transmission is able to introduce HTLV-1 infection into previously uninfected groups. Transmission from man to woman is more frequent (60%) than woman to man (0.4%). Like HIV, HTLV-1 can be transmitted through homosexual activity. Predisposing factors associated with sexual transmission include the presence of genital ulcers, high viral loads and high antibody titers in the donor (Kaplan et al. 1996). Sexual transmission is a more common mode in non-drug user sexual partners of IDUs than parenteral transmission. Among IDUs, blood and blood products are the most significant source of infection (Roucoux and Murphy 2004).

Blood transfusion: is the third mode of HTLV-1 transmission. The proviral DNA in donor's blood lymphocytes acts as an infectious agent. The probability of seroconversion in a recipient of contaminated blood is about 44%. Thus, it is essential to have an efficient blood screening system for HTLV-1 in endemic areas to limit the HTLV-1 transmission. Whole blood components, platelets and packed red blood cells, but not fresh frozen plasma, are the sources of virus transmission. White blood cells are reservoirs of HTLV-1. The probability of transmission of HTLV-1 decreases, if infected units of blood are stored for more than one week HTLV-1. Approximately 12% of HTLV infections occur by blood transfusion. Unlike HIV-1, whole cell transfusion is required for transmission of the virus, with a seroconversion rate of approximately 50%. The development of HAM/TSP has been noted as early as six months after transfusion of an individual with infected blood. In 1988, concerns about transmission of HTLV through blood components led to mandatory blood donor screening for HTLV resulting in a significant decrease in transmission via this mode. Cell-free infection with HTLV-1 is very inefficient; and efficient transmission depends on cell-to-cell transfer through direct cell contact, polarization of the microtubule-organizing center (MTOC), which is triggered by Tax, and the formation of a virological synapse, which allows the entry of viral particles, viral proteins and genomic RNA into fresh target cells. Similar to HIV-1 infection, dendritic cells (DCs) have been demonstrated to play a biphasic role in cell-to-cell transmission of HTLV-1. DCs can capture and transfer the virions to fresh T cells in a trans fashion or transmit de novo synthesized virions upon infection to fresh T cells in a cis fashion (Kannian 2010). Transmission via organ transplantation has been described and is associated with rapidly progressing HAM/TSP, possibly because of the immunosuppression that transplant patients undergo (Romanelli, Caramelli and Proietti 2010).

Contaminated needles from Drug addicts: HTLV-1 can also be transmitted by sharing of needles among drug addicts (Rafatpanah et al. 2006). In the United States, HTLV infection of intravenous drug users (IVDUs) was first reported from Queens, New York, and was mainly attributed to HTLV-II (Robert-Guroff et al. 1986). Subsequently, others have reported prevalence rates of HTLV antibody among IVDUs ranging from 0.4% to 24.0% (Lee et al. 1990).

5. Diagnosis

HTLV-1 is usually detected by carrying out laboratory tests because of clinical suspicion, screening at the blood bank or due to concerns by family members of HTLV-1 positive patients. The antibodies can be detected by enzyme-linked immunosorbent assay (ELISA). ELISA kits have high sensitivity and low specificity; thus, it may not be a reliable screening tool. Therefore, positive ELISA results should be confirmed by western blot analysis and or polymerase chain reaction (PCR) (Andrade et al. 2010).

For the diagnosis of HTLV-1/2 infection, the first immunoassays used HTLV-1 whole-viral lysate as the only antigen. Then, assays were based on recombinant and/or synthetic peptide antigens only or in combination with viral lysates. Furthermore, HTLV-2 specific antigens were included, which improved the sensitivity for detection of HTLV- 2 antibodies. At present, the initial diagnosis of HTLV-1/2 infection is based mainly on screening for antibodies by ELISA. Even the lack of Food and Drug Administration (FDA) licensure for HTLV-1/2 Western blot (WB) assay, it is generally applied to all repeatedly reactive samples for further confirmation of HTLV-1/2 infection (CDC, 1988). The WB assay reduces the number of false positive transmembrane results thereby increasing the specificity for serological confirmation of HTLV-1/2. This assay contains viral lysates and recombinant proteins. MTA-1 is a unique HTLV-1 envelope recombinant protein (rgp46-I), K-55 is a unique HTLV-2 envelope recombinant protein (rgp46-II), and GD21 is a common yet specific HTLV-1 and HTLV-2 epitope recombinant envelope protein. An HTLV-1 positive sample was considered when there were bands for the gag proteins p19 and p24, and the env proteins GD21 and rgp46-I; HTLV-2 positive if p24, GD21, and rgp46-II bands were present; an indeterminate sample when there were specific bands for the virus that did not meet the HTLV-1/2 positivity criteria, and a negative result for those samples that did not exhibit any specific band. In some cases, however, it is necessary to perform a complementary assay such as a nested-polymerase chain reaction (nested-PCR) in order to confirm true HTLV-1/2 infection and to obtain a conclusive diagnosis. When WB is used for confirmation, a significant proportion of the samples reports indeterminate results, ranging from0.02% in non-endemic areas to 50% in endemic ones , although it has been observed that indeterminate samples could result in true HTLV-1/2 infection, even in non-endemic areas. Several studies have shown that most low-risk HTLV-seroindeterminate and asymptomatic individuals are negative for HTLV-1/2 infection after testing with a highly sensitive nested-PCR. It is known that the use of highly efficient screening assays may reduce significantly false reactive results, diminishing the amount of samples further submitted to WB and/or nested-PCR analysis for confirmation. One of the strategies proposed to reduce the number of samples requiring confirmatory testing is the use of a dual ELISA algorithm (Yoshida 2010).

A pitfall in ELISA-based immunoassay may exist in HTLV-1 detection due to truncated MTA-1 envelope glycoprotein. This report describes experiments designed to determine whether some discrepancies between ELISA and PCR results could be due to truncation of immunodominant epitopes using immunoassay method. Recombinant envelope glycoprotein is used in production of diagnostic enzyme-linked immunosorbent assay (ELISA) kit. There are some reports that a significant percentage of Iranian HTLV-1 infected patients showed no seroreactivity with MTA-1 peptide, while HTLV-1 had been confirmed by PCR detection methods or ELISA kits containing a cocktail of HTLV-1 specific peptides. Some discrepancies between ELISA and PCR results could be due to truncation of immunodominant epitopes using immunoassay method. This is because of an insertion of a cytosine in position 271 causing a stop codon in the MTA-1 protein translation. SDS-PAGE analysis also failed to reveal the presence of the desired protein. Subjects with a mutant HTLV-1 env gene were shown to be seronegative using ELISA, but positive with PCR (Abbaszadegan et al. 2008).

Three diagnostic criteria for ATL have been defined. The first is the presence of morphologically proven lymphoid malignancy with T-cell surface antigens (typically CD4+, CD25+). These abnormal T lymphocytes have hyperlobulated nuclei in acute ATL and are known as "flower cells." On the other hand, in the indolent types of ATL, smoldering and chronic types, the abnormality of the nuclear shape is generally milder than that in the acute form of the disease. The second criteria is the presence of antibodies to HTLV-1 in the sera, and the third is the demonstration of monoclonal integration of HTLV-1 provirus in tumor cells by Southern blotting (Yasunaga and Matsuoka 2007).

6. HTLV-1 and the host immune system

HTLV-1 is a complex retrovirus that may have been transmitted to humans from monkeys more than ten thousands years ago. The human host has several immune mechanisms that eliminate foreign pathogens, and like other successful pathogens, HTLV-1 must have strategies for escaping the host immune response.

Like HIV, HTLV-1 mainly infects CD4 T cells, which are the central regulators of the acquired immune response. To establish persistent infection, HTLV-1 perturbs the regulation of CD4 T cells, sometimes leading to diseases such as ATL or chronic inflammatory diseases such as HAM/TSP, uveitis, arthritis, and alveolitis. Since the discovery of HTLV-1, extensive studies have been performed using various experimental approaches to elucidate the exact pathogenesis of this virus. However, the nature of HTLV-1 pathogenesis still remains elusive. This problem is a serious obstacle to establishing effective therapies for HTLV-1 associated diseases. Precise insight into HTLV-1 mediated pathogenesis requires careful consideration of the host cells and the effect HTLV-1 has on them. A better understanding of the interactions between HTLV-1 and the host immune system should provide additional clues to effective therapies for HTLV-1- associated diseases (Satou and Matsuoka 2010).

The host immune system, especially the cellular response, against HTLV-1 exerts critical control over virus replication and the proliferation of infected cells. CTLs against the virus have been extensively studied, and Tax protein was found to be the dominant antigen recognized by CTLs in vivo. HTLV-1-specific CD8-positive CTLs are abundant and chronically activated. The paradox is that the frequency of Tax-specific CTLs is much higher in HAM/TSP patients than in carriers. Since the provirus load is higher in HAM/TSP patients, this finding suggests that the CTLs in HAM/TSP cannot control the number of infected cells. One explanation for this is that the CTLs in HAM/TSP patients show less efficient cytolytic activity toward infected cells, whereas CTLs in carriers can suppress the proliferation of infected cells. Hence, the gene expression profiles of circulating CD4+ and CD8+ lymphocytes were compared between carriers with high and low provirus loads. The results revealed that CD8+ lymphocytes from individuals with a low HTLV-1 provirus load show higher expressions of genes associated with cytolytic activities or antigen recognition than those from carriers with a high provirus load. Thus, CD8+ T-lymphocytes in individuals with a low provirus load successfully control the number of HTLV-1-infected cells due to their higher CTL activities. Thus, the major determinant of the provirus load is thought to be the CTL response to HTLV-1. As mentioned above, the provirus load is considered to be controlled by host factors. Considering that the cellular immune responses are critically implicated in the control of HTLV-1 infection, human leukocyte antigen (HLA) should be a candidate for such a host genetic factor. From analyses of HAM/TSP patients and asymptomatic carriers, HLA-A02, and Cw08 are independently associated with a lower provirus load and a lower risk of HAM/TSP. In addition, polymorphisms of other genes including TNF-α, SDF-1, HLA- B54, HLA-DRB-10101 and IL-15 are also associated with the provirus load, however with a lower significance than with HLA-A02, and Cw08. Regarding the onset of ATL, only a polymorphism of TNF- α gene was reported to show an association. However, familial clustering of ATL cases is a well-known phenomenon, strongly suggesting that genetic factors are implicated in the onset of ATL. Spontaneous remission is more frequently observed in patients with ATL than those with other hematological malignancies. Usually, this phenomenon is associated with infectious diseases, suggesting that immune activation of the host enhances the immune response against ATL cells. If the immune response against HTLV-1 is implicated in spontaneous remission, this suggests the possibility of immunotherapy for ATL patients by the induction of an immune response to HTLV-1, for example via antigen-stimulated dendritic cells. Immunodeficiency in ATL patients is pronounced, and results in frequent opportunistic infections by various pathogens, including Pneumocystis carinii, cytomegalovirus, fungus, Strongyloides and bacteria, due to the inevitable impairment of the T-cell functions. To a lesser extent, impaired cell-mediated immunity has also been demonstrated in HTLV-1 carriers. Such immunodeficiency in the carrier state may be associated with the leukemogenesis of ATL by allowing the proliferation of HTLV-1-infected cells. A prospective study of HTLV-1-infected individuals found that carriers who later develop ATL have a higher anti-HTLV-1 antibody and a low anti-Tax antibody level for up to 10 years preceding their diagnosis. This finding indicates that HTLV-1 carriers with a higher anti-HTLV-1 titer, which is roughly correlated with the HTLV-1 provirus load and a lower anti-Tax reactivity, may be at the greatest risk of developing ATL. The anti-HTLV-1 antibody and soluble IL-2 receptor (sIL-2R) levels are correlated with the HTLV-1 provirus load, and a high antibody titer and high sIL-2R level are risk factors for developing ATL among carriers. Taken together, these findings suggest that a higher proliferation of HTLV-1-infected cells and a low immune response against Tax may be associated with the onset of ATL. Given these findings, potentiation of CTLs against Tax via a vaccine strategy may be useful for preventing the onset of ATL. EBV-associated lymphomas frequently develop in individuals with an immunodeficient state associated with transplantation or AIDS. This has also been reported in an ATL patient. Does such an immunodeficient state influence the onset of ATL? Among 24 patients with post- transplantation lymphoproliferative disorders (PT-LPDs) after renal transplantation in Japan, 5 cases of ATL have been reported. Considering that most PT-LPDs are of B- cell origin in Western countries, this frequency of ATL in Japan is quite high. Although the high HTLV-1 seroprevalence is due to blood transfusion during hemodialysis, the immunodeficient state during renal transplantation apparently promotes the onset of ATL. In addition, when experimental allogeneic transplantation was performed to 12 rhesus monkeys and immunosuppressive agents (cyclosporine, prednisolone or lymphocyte-specific monoclonal antibodies) were administered to prevent rejection, 4 of the 7 monkeys that died during the experiment showed PT-LPDs. Importantly, the STLV pro- virus was detected in all PT-LPD samples. These observations emphasize that transplantation into HTLV-1- infected individuals or from HTLV-1 positive donors require special attention. Although the mechanism of immunodeficiency remains unknown, some previous reports have provided important clues. One mechanism for immunodeficiency is that HTLV-1 infects CD8-positive T-lymphocytes, which may impair their functions. Indeed, the immune response against Tax via HTLV-1-infected CD8-positive T-cells renders these cells susceptible to fratricide mediated by autologous HTLV-1-specific CD8-positive T-lymphocytes. Fratricide among virus-specific CTLs could impair the immune control of HTLV-1. Another mechanism for immunodeficiency is based on the observation that the number of naive T-cells decreases in individuals infected with HTLV-1 via decreased thymopoiesis [48]. In addition, CD4+ and CD25+ T-lymphocytes are classified as immunoregulatory T-cells that control the host immune system. Regulatory T-cells suppress the immune reaction via the expression of immunoregulatory molecules on their surfaces. The FOXP3 gene has been identified as a master gene that controls gene expressions specific to regulatory T-cells. FOXP3 gene transcription can be detected in some ATL cases (10/17;

59%). Such ATL cells are thought to suppress the immune response via expression of immunoregulatory molecules on their surfaces, and production of immunosuppressive cytokines (Matsuoka 2005).

7. Mechanism of oncogenesis by HTLV 1

In 1977, Takatsuki et al. reported ATL as a distinct clinical entity. This disease is characterized by its aggressive clinical course, infiltrations into skin, liver, gastrointestinal tract and lung, hypercalcemia and the presence of leukemic cells with multilobulated nuclei, flower cell (Figure 2). The linkage between ATL and HTLV-1 was proven by Hinuma et al., who demonstrated the presence of an antibody against HTLV-1 in patient sera. Thereafter, Seiki et al. determined the whole sequence of HTLV-1 and revealed the presence of a unique region, designated pX. The pX region encodes several accessory genes, which control viral replication and the proliferation of infected cells (Matsuoka 2005).

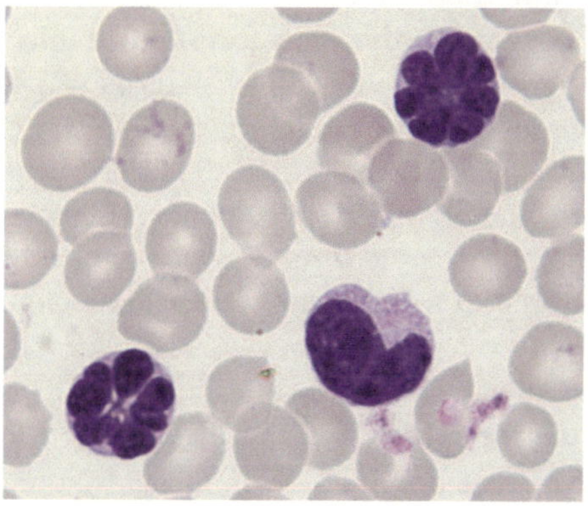

Fig. 2. Typical "**flower cell**", Morphological findings of typical ATL cells, leukemic cells with multilobulated nuclei was Shawn.

Several molecular biologic studies have reported that various cellular dysfunctions induced by viral genes (eg, tax and HBZ), genetic and epigenetic alterations, and the host immune system may be involved in the leukemogenesis of ATL. Clinical and epidemiologic studies have also reported a variety of possible risk factors for ATL, including vertical transmission of HTLV-1 infection, male gender, a long latent period, increased leukocyte counts or abnormal lymphocyte counts, and higher levels of anti-HTLV-1 antibody titers and soluble interleukin-2 receptor. However, there are no clear determinants that separate those who develop ATL from those who remain healthy carriers. Recently, HTLV-1 proviral load levels have been evaluated as important predictors of development of ATL and HAM/TSP. Some cross-sectional studies showed that HTLV-1 proviral load levels were higher in ATL and HAM/TSP compared with asymptomatic HTLV-1 carriers. In conclusion, the cohort study of 1218 asymptomatic HTLV-1 carriers provided detailed distributions for HTLV-1 proviral loads regarding the host-specific characteristics and the associations with the development of ATL. A higher proviral load levels (especially > 4 copies/100 PBMCs), advanced age, family history of ATL, and having the first opportunity to learn of HTLV-1 infection during treatment of other diseases are independent risk factors for progression from carrier status to ATL.

Further large-scale epidemiologic studies are needed to clearly identify the determinants of ATL for early detection and rapid cure for HTLV-1–associated diseases(Silva et al. 2007). Genetic and immunological factors in the host are the principal determinants of the emergence of associated diseases(Romanelli, Caramelli and Proietti 2010).

7.1 Etiology of ATL

The most important aspect of the new retroviral isolation was not just novelty but an etiology for a human leukemia. However, etiological proof for a human disease is generally not easy unless an animal model is available. The most critical question thereafter was whether 'close association of HTLV-1 with ATL' reflects its causative role or whether the virus was just a passenger. The nature of provirus integration of the retroviruses provided a critical tool for the discrimination. The retroviral genomes are generally reverse-transcribed into provirus DNA, and the proviral genomes are integrated into host cell DNA at random sites. Since a tumor originates from unlimited expansion of a single malignant cell, the site for the proviral integration into tumor cells would be uniform in individuals if the retroviral infection plays a causative role; but if the virus fortuitously infects leukemic cells, then the integration sites would be random. Southern blot analysis of patients' leukemic cell DNA clearly indicated clonal integration in each patient revealing two distinct bands with cellular flanking sequences. This finding clearly supported the virus playing a causative role in ATL. Virtually all ATL cases were clonally infected leukemic cells; therefore, the conclusion for a 'causative role' became generally accepted. As controls, the sites for the integration in viral carriers are random except only in a few cases which show clonal integration with higher viral burden (Yoshida 2005).

7.2 Pathogenesis of HTLV-1 infection

ATL cells are derived from activated helper T-lymphocytes, which play central roles in the immune system by elaborating cytokines and expressing immunoregulatory molecules. ATL cells are known to retain such features and this cytokine production or surface molecule expression may modify the pathogenesis. ATL is well known to infiltrate various organs and tissues, such as the skin, lungs, liver, gastrointestinal tract, central nervous system and bone (Takatsuki 1995). This infiltrative tendency of leukemic cells is possibly attributable to the expressions of various surface molecules, such as chemokine receptors and adhesion molecules. Skin-homing memory T-cells uniformly expresses CCR4, and its ligands are thymus and activation-regulated chemokine (TARC) and macrophage- derived chemokine (MDC). CCR4 is expressed on most ATL cells. In addition, TARC and MDC are expressed in skin lesions in ATL patients. Thus, CCR4 expression should be implicated in the skin infiltration (Yoshie et al. 2002). On the other hand, CCR7 expression is associated with lymph node involvement (Hasegawa et al. 2000). OX40 is a member of the tumor necrosis factor family, and was reported to be expressed on ATL cells (Higashimura et al. 1996). It was also identified as a gene associated with the adhesion of ATL cells to endothelial cells by a functional cloning system using a monoclonal antibody that inhibited the attachment of ATL cells (Imura et al. 1996). Thus, OX40 is also implicated in the cell adhesion and infiltration of ATL cells. Thus, ATL cells express various molecules that can modify their phenotypic properties, thereby modifying the clinical disease manifestation, and facilitating the survival of ATL cells (Matsuoka 2003). Hypercalcemia is frequently complicated in patients with acute ATL (more than 70% during the whole clinical course)

(Kiyokawa et al. 1987). In hypercalcemic patients, the number of osteoclasts increases in the bone. RANK ligand, which is expressed on osteoblasts, and M-CSF act synergistically on hematopoietic precursor cells, and induce the differentiation into osteoclasts (Arai et al. 1999). ATL cells from hypercalcemic ATL patients express RANK ligand, and induced the differentiation of hematopoietic stem cells into osteoclasts when ATL cells were co-cultured with hematopoietic stem cells (Nosaka et al. 2002). In addition, the serum level of parathyroid hormone-related peptide (PTH-rP) is also elevated in most of hypercalcemic ATL patients. PTH- rP indirectly increases the number of osteoclasts, as well as activating them (Watanabe et al. 1990), which is also implicated in mechanisms of hypercalcemia.

7.3 Role of Tax in HTLV-1 induced oncogenesis

Tax, a transactivator protein, triggers a plethora of events like cell signaling, cell cycle regulation and interference with checkpoint control and inhibition of DNA repair. Tax is expressed from a doubly spliced mRNA transcript. Although Tax shares the same mRNA transcript with Rex, translation of Tax is favored over Rex due to a stronger Kozak sequence. Tax made in the cytoplasm is translocated into the nucleus, where it binds to its response element and activates viral LTR-mediated transcription. (Boxus and Willems 2009).

The tax gene plays central roles in viral gene transcription, viral replication and the proliferation of HTLV-1-infected cells. Tax enhances viral gene transcription from the 5'-LTR via interaction with cyclic AMP responsive element binding protein (CREB). Tax also interacts with cellular factors and activates transcriptional pathways, such as NF-κB, AP-1 and SRF (Yoshida 2001). For example, activation of NF-κB induces the transcription of various cytokines and their receptor genes, as well as anti-apoptotic genes such as bcl- xL and survivin (Tsukahara et al. 1999). The activation of NF-κB has been demonstrated to be critical for tumorigenesis both in vitro and in vivo (Mori et al. 1999). On the other hand, Tax variant without activation of NF-κB has also been reported to immortalize primary T-lymphocytes in vitro, suggesting that mechanisms of immortalization are complex. In addition to NF-κB, activation of other transcriptional pathways such as CREB by Tax should be implicated in the immortalization and leukemogenesis. Tax also interferes with the functions of p53, p16 and MAD1 (Ariumi et al. 2000). These interactions enable HTLV-1-infected cells to escape from apoptosis, and also induce genetic instability. Although inactivation of p53 function by Tax is reported to be mediated by p300/CBP or NF- κB activation (Pise-Masison et al. 2000), Tax can still repress p53's activity in spite of loss of p300/CBP binding or in cells lacking NF- κB activation (Miyazato et al. 2005), indicating the mechanism of p53 inactivation by Tax needs further investigation. Although Tax promotes the proliferation of infected cells, it is also the major target of cytotoxic T-lymphocytes (CTLs) *in vivo*. Moreover, excess expression of Tax protein is considered to be harmful to infected cells. Therefore, HTLV-1 has redundant mechanisms to suppress Tax expression. Rex binds to Rex-responsive element (RxRE) in the U3 and R regions of the 3'-LTR, and enhances the transport of the unspliced gag/pol and the singly spliced env transcripts. By this mechanism, double-spliced tax/rex mRNA decreases, resulting in suppressed expression of Tax (Inoue, Yoshida and Seiki 1987). Additionally, p30 binds to tax/rex transcripts, and retains them in the nucleus. The HBZ gene is encoded by the complementary strand of HTLV-1, and contains a leucine zipper domain. HBZ directly interacts with c-Jun or JunB (Basbous et al. 2003), or enhances their degradation, resulting in the suppression of Tax-mediated viral transcription from the LTR. Transforming growth factor-β (TGF-β) is an inhibitory cytokine that plays important roles in development, the immune system and oncogenesis. Since TGF-β generally suppresses the growth of tumor cells, most tumor cells acquire escape mechanisms that inhibit TGF-β signaling, including mutations in its receptor and in the Smad molecules that transduce the signal from the receptor. Tax has also been reported to inhibit TGF-β signaling by binding to Smad2, 3 and 4 or CBP/p300 (Mori et al. 2001). Inhibition of TGF-β signaling enables HTLV-1-infected cells to escape TGF-β-mediated growth inhibition. ATL cells have been reported to show remarkable chromosomal abnormalities (Sanada et al. 1986), implicated in the disease progression. Tax has been reported to interact with the checkpoint protein MAD1, which forms a complex with MAD2 and controls the mitotic checkpoint. This functional hindrance of MAD1 by Tax protein causes chromosomal instability, suggesting the involvement of this mechanism in oncogenesis. Recently, Tax has been reported to interact with Cdc20 and activate Cdc20- associated anaphase-promoting complex, an E3 ubiquitin ligase that controls the metaphase-to-anaphase transition, thereby resulting in mitotic abnormalities (Liu et al. 2005). In contrast to HTLV-1, HTLV-2 promotes the proliferation of CD8-positive T-lymphocytes in vivo. Although it was first discovered in a patient with variant hairy cell leukemia, HTLV-2 is less likely to have oncogenic properties since there is no obvious association between HTLV-2 infections and cancers. Regardless of the homology of their tax sequences, the oncogenic potential of Tax1 (HTLV-1 Tax) is more prominent than that of Tax2 (HTLV- 2 Tax). The most striking difference is that Tax2 lacks the binding motif at C-terminal end to PDZ domain proteins, while Tax 1 retains it. When the PDZ domain of Tax1 is added to Tax2, the latter acquires oncogenic properties in the rat fibroblast cell line Rat-1, indicating that this domain is responsible for the transforming activity of HTLV-1. To understand the pleiotropic actions of Tax protein more clearly, transcriptome analyses are essential. The transcriptional changes induced by Tax expression have been studied using DNA microarrays, which revealed that Tax upregulated the expression of the mixed-lineage kinase MLK3. MLK3 is involved in NF-κB activation by Tax as well as NIK and MEKK1. In addition to transcriptional changes, Tax is also well known to interact with cellular proteins and impair or alter their functions. For example, proteomic analyses of Tax-associated complexes showed that Tax could interact with cellular proteins, including the active forms of small GTPases, such as Cdc42, RhoA and Rac1, which should be implicated in the migration, invasion and adhesion of T-cells, as well as in the activation of the Jun-kinase (JNK) pathway (figure 3) (Matsuoka 2005).

Tax1 upregulates the expression of genes encoding cytokines, chemokines, cell surface ligands, and their receptors, in an NF-κB, AP-1, CREB/ATF and/or NFAT dependent manner. They include IL-2 receptor (IL-2R) α-chain, IL-9, IL-13, IL-15/IL-15R, IL-21/IL-21R, IL-8, CCL2, CCL5, CCL22, CCR9, CXCR7, CD40, OX40/OX40L, and 4-1BB/4-1BBL. Among these, the IL-2R α-chain is crucially important for T-cell immortalization by Tax, since the immortalized cells are dependent on IL-2 for their growth.

ATL cells are well known to infiltrate into various organs or tissues, frequently invading skin or lymphoid tissues. Analysis of chemokine receptor expression revealed that CCR4 was frequently expressed on HTLV-1-transformed cell lines and fresh ATL cells. CCR4-positive T lymphocytes contain skin-seeking memory T cells, accounting for frequent infiltration of ATL cells into skin. On the other hand, expression of CCR7 was reported to be associated with the involvement of lymphoid tissues, and lymph node enlargement. A subtraction strategy between ATL cell lines and activated T cells identified I-309 as a secreted chemokine from ATL cells, and I-309 expression was remarkably enhanced in ATL cell lines. I-309 showed anti apoptotic effect via its receptor CCR8, invoking that an autocrine mechanism via I-309/CCR8 allowed ATL cells to survive in vivo (Matsuoka 2003).

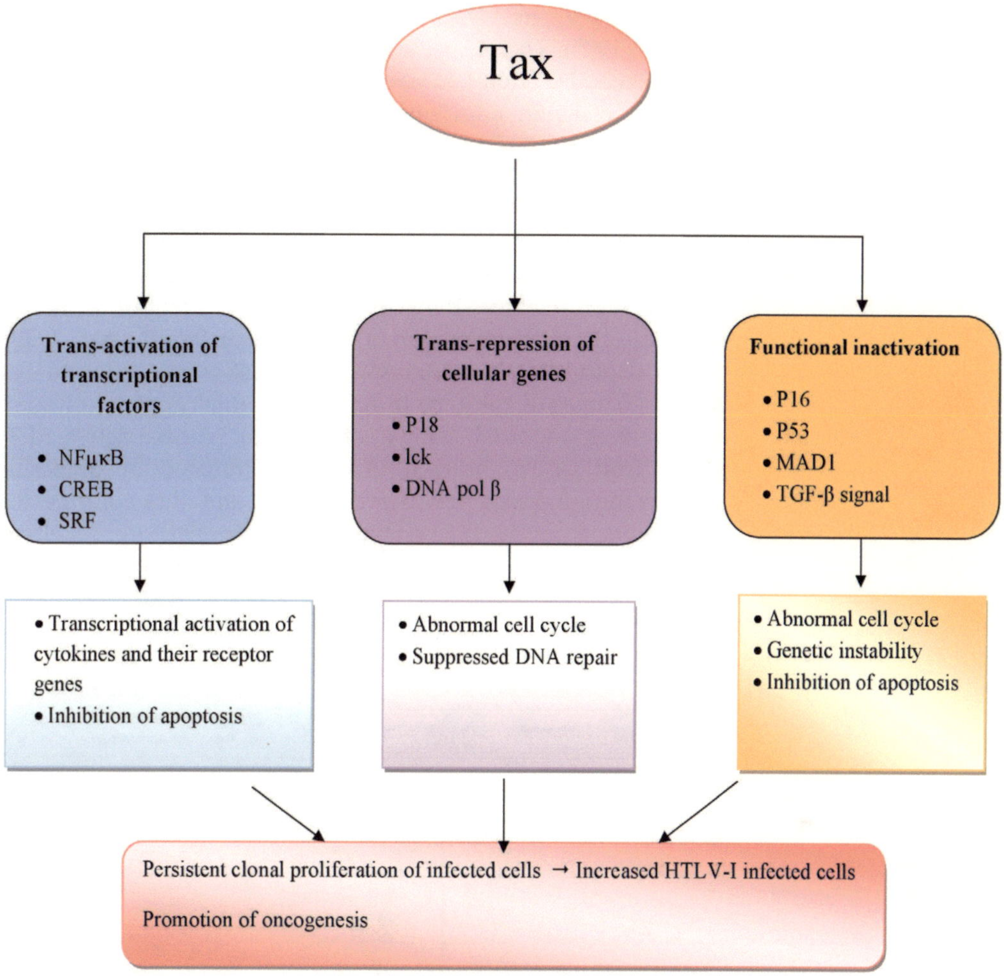

Fig. 3. Pleiotropic actions of Tax. Pleiotropic actions of Tax proteins are summarized

7.4 Inactivation of Tax expression in ATL cells

As mentioned above, Tax expression confers advantages and disadvantages on HTLV-1-infected cells. Although the proliferation of infected cells is promoted by Tax expression, CTLs attack the Tax-expressing cells since Tax is their major target. In HTLV-1-infected cells, Rex, p30 and HBZ suppress Tax expression. On the other hand, loss of Tax expression is frequently observed in leukemic cells. Three mechanisms have been identified for inactivation of Tax expression: 1) genetic changes of the tax gene (non- sense mutations, deletions or insertions); 2) DNA methylation of the 5'-LTR; and 3) deletion of the 5'-LTR. Among fresh leukemic cells isolated from ATL patients, about 60% of cases do not express the tax gene transcript. Interestingly, ATL cells with genetic changes of the tax gene expressed its transcripts, suggesting that ATL cells do not silence the transcription when the tax gene is abortive. Loss of Tax expression gives ATL cells advantage for their survival since they can escape from CTLs (Figure 4) (Matsuoka 2005).

Some ATL cells can proliferate without functional Tax protein, suggesting that somatic (genetic and epigenetic) alterations cause transcriptional or functional changes to the host genes. The mutation rate of the p53 gene in ATL cells has been reported to be 36% (4/11) and 30% (3/10) (Nishimura et al. 1995). The p16 gene is an inhibitor of cyclin-dependent kinase 4/6, and blocks the cell cycle. Deletion and aberrant methylation of the p16 gene has also been reported in ATL cells. In addition, genetic changes in the p27KIP1, RB1/p105 and RB2/p130 genes have been reported in ATL, although they are relatively rare: 2/42 (4.8%) for the p27KIP1 gene; 2/40 (5%) for the RB1/p105 gene; and 1/41 (2.4%) for the RB2/p130 gene) (Morosetti et al. 1995). The fact that higher frequencies of genetic changes in these tumor suppressor genes are observed among aggressive forms of ATL suggests that such genetic changes are implicated in disease progression. Fas antigen was the first identified death receptor. It transduces the death signal by binding of its ligand, Fas ligand (FasL). ATL cells highly express Fas antigen on their cell surface (Nagata 1999), and are highly susceptible to death signals mediated by agonistic antibodies to Fas antigen, such as CH-11. Genetic changes of Fas gene in ATL cells, which confer resistance to the Fas-mediated signal, have been reported (Tamiya et al. 1998). Normal activated T-lymphocytes express FasL as well as Fas antigen. Apoptosis induced by autocrine mechanisms is designated activation-induced cell death (AICD) and this controls the

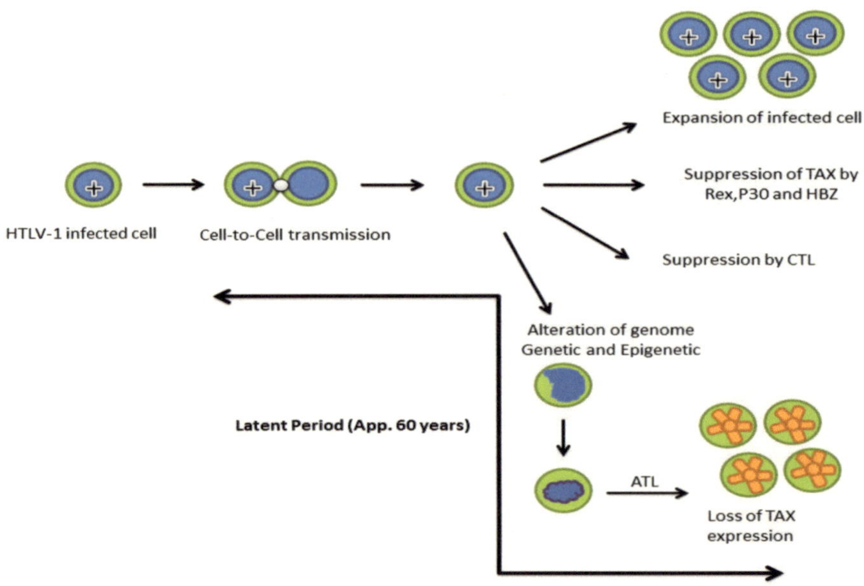

Fig. 4. Natural course from the infection of HTLV-I to onset of ATL

immune response (Krueger et al. 2003). Although ATL cells express Fas antigen, they do not produce FasL, thereby enabling ATL cells to escape from AICD. Attempts to isolate hypermethylated genes from ATL cells identified the EGR3 gene as a hypermethylated gene compared to PBMCs from carriers (Yasunaga et al. 2004). EGR3 is a transcriptional factor with a zinc finger domain, which is essential for transcription of the FasL gene. The finding that EGR3 gene transcription is silenced in ATL cells could account for the loss of FasL expression, and the escape of ATL cells from AICD. Thus, alterations of the Fas (genetic) and EGR3 (epigenetic) genes are examples of ATL cell evolution *in vivo*. Disordered DNA methylation has been identified in the genome of ATL cells compared with that of PBMCs from carriers: hypomethylation is associated with aberrant expression of the MEL1S gene (Yoshida et al. 2004), while hypermethylation silences transcription of the p16 (Nosaka et al. 2000), EGR3 and KLF4 genes as well as many others. It is reasonable to consider that other currently unidentified genes are involved in such alterations of the genome in ATL cells, and play roles in leukemogenesis. Transcriptome analyses using DNA microarrays have revealed transcriptional changes that are specific to ATL cells. Among 192 up-regulated genes, the expressions of the tumor suppressor in lung cancer 1 (TSLC1), caveolin 1 and prostaglandin D2 synthase genes were increased more than 30-fold in fresh ATL cells compared with normal CD4+ and CD4+, CD45RO+ T-cells (Sasaki et al. 2005). TSLC1 is a cell adhesion molecule that acts as a tumor suppressor in lung cancer. Although TSLC1 is not expressed on normal T- lymphocytes, all acute ATL cells show ectopic TSLC1 expression. Enforced expression of TSLC1 enhances both the self-aggregation and adhesion abilities to vascular endothelial cells in ATL cells. Thus, TSLC1 expression is implicated in the adhesion or infiltration of ATL cells. A retrovirus cDNA library screening from ATL cells, a gene with oncogenic potency was identified in NIH3T3 cells, and designated the Tgat gene. Ectopic expression of the Tgat gene is observed in aggressive forms of ATL, and in vitro experiments showed that its expression is associated with an invasive phenotype (Matsuoka 2005).

7.5 Role of HBZ in HTLV-1-induced oncogenesis

The pathogenesis of ATL involves four stages: infection, polyclonal proliferation, clinical latency and tumorigenesis. HTLV-1 induced ATL after a long latent period. Previous studies suggested the significance of the tax gene. However, Tax is not expressed in approximately 60% of ATL cases by three mechanisms: 1) deletion of 5' long terminal repeat (LTR), 2) DNA methylation of 5 LTR, and 3) genetic changes of the tax gene. Recent studies, demonstrated that the HTLV-1 basic leucine zipper factor (HBZ) encoded by the virus in an antisense orientation may play a critical role in the malignant proliferation of ATL cells. The expression of HBZ gene is detected in all ATL cases, and this is due to the usage of the promoter in the 3' LTR of HTLV-1 gene which is not inactivated in the ATL cells. HBZ interacts with various host factors, including c-Jun, JunB, JunD, and p65. Thus, HBZ modulates cellular signal pathways in addition to promoted proliferation. These findings indicate that HBZ is an essential viral gene for oncogenesis by HTLV-1(Boxus and Willems 2009).

Short hairpin RNA mediated knockdowns of HBZ expression in both ATL and HTLV-1 transformed cell lines reduce their proliferation. Moreover, transgenic mice expressing HBZ under the control of the CD4 promoter/enhancer display increased numbers of CD4-positive T-cells in the spleen, and augmented proliferation of thymocytes after anti-CD3 stimulation. Thus, these findings indicate that HBZ has a growth promoting activity, and could be involved in the malignant proliferation of ATL cells *in vivo*, although the precise molecular mechanism for these findings is still unclear. HTLV-2 also encodes a HBZ like protein, designated as the antisense protein of HTLV-2 (APH-2). Interestingly, unlike HBZ, APH-2 does not have a leucine zipper motif which is essential for various HBZ functions. Thus, it is important to study whether the HTLV-2 APH-2 protein has a growth promoting activity in T-cells like HBZ in order to understand better how these two viruses show distinct pathogenicities (Higuchi and Fujii 2009).

Both the HBZ and Tax genes are found in the genome of the simian T-cell leukemia virus type 1 (STLV-1), which shares a common ancestor with HTLV-1, indicating that HBZ has not been recently acquired; that is once the virus adapted to humans (STLV-1 and HTLV-1 are considered to have diverged around 50 000 years ago. it did not tolerate genetic drift resulting in its silencing. In the HTLV-2 genome, a human retrovirus related to HTLV-1, Tax also exists but, surprisingly, HTLV-2 lacks the HBZ-ORF. Moreover, in contrast to HTLV-1 and STLV-1, which both cause lymphoid malignancy in the host, no association between HTLV-2 infection and cancer has been yet evidenced. There has been only one reported case of a patient carrying HTLV-2 who developed a variant of hairy cell leukemia (Mesnard, Barbeau and Devaux 2006).

8. ATL treatment: Current state and new strategies

In spite of intensive chemotherapies, the prognosis of ATL patients has not improved. The median survival time of acute or lymphoma-type ATL was reported to be *13 months* with the most intensive chemotherapy. Such a poor prognosis might be due to: 1) the resistance of ATL cells to anti-cancer drugs; and 2) the immunodeficient state and complicated opportunistic infections. One mechanism of resistance to anti-cancer drugs is the activated NF-κB pathway in ATL cells (Mori et al. 1999), which increases the transcription of anti-apoptotic genes such as bcl-xL and survivin.

A proteasome inhibitor, Bortezomib, is currently used for the treatment of multiple myeloma. One of its mechanisms is suppression of the NF-κB pathway by inhibiting the proteasomal degradation of IκB protein. Several groups have shown that Bortezomib is effective against ATL cells both *in vitro* and *in vivo* (Mitra-Kaushik et al. 2004). The sensitivity to Bortezomib is well correlated with the extent of NF-κB activation. Depsipeptide is a histone deacetylase inhibitor, and a clinical trial on its use in cutaneous T-cell lymphoma has commenced. This drug also inhibits the activation of NF-κB and AP-1 in ATL cells, and it induces apoptosis (Mori et al. 2004).

An alternative approach to the therapy of ATL is to target cell-surface markers on the malignant cells with monoclonal antibodies. Anti- CD25 (anti-Tac) monoclonal antibody, which was first administered to patients with ATL in the late 1980s, was reported to be effective in some patients, with a complete response in 2 of 19 patients and a partial response in 4 of 19 patients (Waldmann et al. 1993). Another antibody, anti- CD52 monoclonal antibody (Campath-1H), is being evaluated in a phase II clinical trial by the National Institutes of Health (Protocol 03-C-0194). Humanized anti-CD2 antibody (MEDI-507) has also been shown to be effective *in vivo* (Zhang et al. 2003). Bortezomib effect could be enhanced by combined use of anti-CD25 antibody (Tan and Waldmann 2002). During chemotherapy for ATL, chemotherapeutic agents worsens the immunodeficient state of ATL patients. Antibody therapy against ATL cells has advantages due to its decreased adverse effects.

As described above, most ATL cells express CCR4 antigen on their surfaces, and a humanized antibody against CCR4 is being developed as an anti-ATL agent (Ishida et al. 2004). Advances in the treatment of ATL were brought about by allogeneic bone marrow or stem cell transplantation (Borg et al. 1996; Yamada et al. 2001). Absence of graft-versus-host disease (GVHD) was linked with relapse of ATL, suggesting that GVHD or graft-versus-ATL may be implicated in the clinical effects of allogeneic stem cell transplantation (Borg et al. 1996). Furthermore, 16 patients with ATL, who were over 50 years of age, were treated with allogeneic stem cell transplantation with reduced conditioning intensity (RIST) from HLA-matched sibling donors (Okamura et al. 2005). Among 9 patients in whom ATL relapsed after transplantation, 3 achieved a second complete remission after rapid discontinuation of cyclosporine A. This finding strongly suggests the presence of a graft-versus-ATL effect in these patients. In addition, Tax peptide-recognizing cells were detected by a tetramer assay (HLA-A2/Tax 11–19 or HLA-A24/Tax 301–309) in patients after allogeneic stem cell transplantation (Harashima et al. 2004). In 8 patients, the provirus became undetectable by real- time PCR. Among these, 2 patients who received grafts from HTLV-1-positive donors also became provirus-negative after RIST. Since the provirus load is relatively constant in HTLV-1-infected individuals (Etoh et al. 1999), this finding indicates an enhanced immune response against HTLV-1 after RIST, which suppresses the provirus load. This may account for the effectiveness of allogeneic stem cell transplantation to ATL. However, Tax expression is frequently lost in ATL cells as described above. Many questions arise, such as whether the tax gene status is correlated with the effect of allogeneic stem cell transplantation, and whether the effectiveness of the anti-HTLV-1 immune response is against leukemic cells or non-leukemic HTLV-1-infected cells. Nevertheless, these data suggest that potentiation of the immune response against viral proteins such as Tax may be an attractive way to treat ATL patients. Such strategies may enable preventive treatment of high-risk HTLV-1 carriers, such as those with familial ATL history, predisposing genetic factors to ATL, a higher provirus load, etc (Matsuoka 2005).

The leukemic phase of ATL tends to spare the bone marrow; accentuated anemia and thrombocytopenia are not observed. White blood cell counts are always elevated and can be as high as 100,000/mm^3. Heightened leukocyte counts and elevated lactate dehydrogenase (DHL) and calcium levels are markers of worse prognosis. Atypical lymphocytes that are pleomorphic and lobulated and have significant nuclear abnormalities (flower cells) are found in peripheral blood. If left untreated it is rapidly fatal, with death caused by pulmonary complications, opportunistic infections, sepsis and uncontrolled hypercalcemia. The chronic and indolent forms of ATL are less common, but after a number of years they will evolve into the acute form. Treatment of the indolent and chronic forms can be postponed until they evolve into the acute form; despite a less aggressive clinical course, prognosis for survival over the long term is poor. Some studies, with small patient samples and short follow-up periods, have demonstrated a satisfactory response and moderate toxicity using zidovudine in combination with interferon alpha, and both of these in combination with arsenic. In the more aggressive acute and lymphomatous forms, treatment should be started as early as possible using, CHOP chemotherapy regimens (cyclophosphamide, doxorubicin, vincristine and prednisolone). More powerful regimens such as VCAP (vincristine, cyclophosphamide, doxorubicin and prednisolone) or AMP (doxorubicin, ranimustine and prednisolone), offer a better response and prognosis, but mortality is higher. Other treatment options described in the literature include allogeneic stem cell transplant, inhibition of the NF-kappa Beta protein and monoclonal antibodies (Romanelli, Caramelli and Proietti 2010).

Regardless of the extensive progress in virology, immunology and molecular biology of ATL and HTLV-1, the prognosis of patients with ATL remains poor. ATL is generally treated with aggressive combination chemotherapy, but long-term success has been less than 10%. The acute form, with hypercalcemia, high LDH levels and an elevated white blood cell count shows a particularly poor prognosis. Although G-CSF supported combination chemotherapy with eight drugs improved the survival (mean survival time 13 months), the prognosis of aggressive ATL remains poor with deaths usually being the result of severe infection or hypercalcemia, often associated with drug resistance. After successful allogeneic bone marrow transplantation (alloBMT) for a patient with ATL was reported, more patients with ATL were treated with alloBMT. The low risk of relapse in cases with graftversus-host disease, suggested that graft-versus-leukemia was effective against ATL cells. CTLs attack ATL cells via Fas ligand, perforin or granzyme. These results are consistent with the finding that ATL cells are highly susceptible to the signal via Fas antigen. Thus, the signal through Fas antigen might be a good target in therapy against ATL (Matsuoka 2003).

In a phase II study, combination of zidovudine and interferon-alpha presented promising results. Chronic ATL has a relatively better out-come, but poor long-term survival is noted when patients are managed with a watchful-waiting policy or with chemotherapy. In ATL cell lines, arsenic trioxide shuts off constitutive NF-κB activation and potentiates interferon-alpha apoptotic effects through proteasomal degradation of Tax. In conclusion, treatment of chronic ATL with arsenic, interferon- alpha, and zidovudine is feasible and exhibits an impressive response rate with moderate toxicity. Viral replication (AZT) and Tax degradation (As/IFN) may eradicate the disease through this treatment. These clinical results strengthen the concept of oncogene-targeted cancer therapy (Kchour et al. 2009).

Key Words: HTLV-1, ATL, Leukemia, Molecular pathogenesis, Diagnosis, Novel treatements, Oncogenesis, Mutation, Arsenic, Interferon-alpha, Zidovudine

9. References

Abbaszadegan, M. R., M. Gholamin, A. Tabatabaee, R. Farid, M. Houshmand, and M. Abbaszadegan. 2003. "Prevalence of human T-lymphotropic virus type 1 among blood donors from Mashhad, Iran." *J Clin Microbiol* 41(6):2593-5.

Abbaszadegan, M. R., N. Jafarzadeh, M. Sankian, A. Varasteh, M. Mahmoudi, M. Sadeghizadeh, F. Khatami, and N. Mehramiz. 2008. "Truncated MTA-1: a pitfall in ELISA-based immunoassay of HTLV-1 infection." *J Biomed Biotechnol* 2008: 846371.

Andrade, R. G., M. A. Ribeiro, M. S. Namen-Lopes, S. M. Silva, F. V. Basques, J. G. Ribas, A. B. Carneiro-Proietti, and M. L. Martins. 2010. "Evaluation of the use of real-time PCR for human T cell lymphotropic virus 1 and 2 as a confirmatory test in screening for blood donors." *Rev Soc Bras Med Trop* 43(2):111-5.

Arai, F., T. Miyamoto, O. Ohneda, T. Inada, T. Sudo, K. Brasel, T. Miyata, D. M. Anderson, and T. Suda. 1999. "Commitment and differentiation of osteoclast precursor cells by the sequential expression of c-Fms and receptor activator of nuclear factor kappaB (RANK) receptors." *J Exp Med* 190(12):1741-54.

Ariumi, Y., A. Kaida, J. Y. Lin, M. Hirota, O. Masui, S. Yamaoka, Y. Taya, and K. Shimotohno. 2000. "HTLV-1 tax oncoprotein represses the p53-mediated trans-activation function through coactivator CBP sequestration." *Oncogene* 19(12): 1491-9.

Basbous, J., C. Arpin, G. Gaudray, M. Piechaczyk, C. Devaux, and J. M. Mesnard. 2003. "The HBZ factor of human T-cell leukemia virus type I dimerizes with transcription factors JunB and c-Jun and modulates their transcriptional activity." *J Biol Chem* 278(44):43620-7.

Biggar, R. J., J. Ng, N. Kim, M. Hisada, H. C. Li, B. Cranston, B. Hanchard, and E. M. Maloney. 2006. "Human leukocyte antigen concordance and the transmission risk via breast-feeding of human T cell lymphotropic virus type I." *J Infect Dis* 193(2):277-82.

Borg, A., J. A. Yin, P. R. Johnson, J. Tosswill, M. Saunders, and D. Morris. 1996. "Successful treatment of HTLV-1-associated acute adult T-cell leukaemia lymphoma by allogeneic bone marrow transplantation." *Br J Haematol* 94(4):713-5.

Boxus, M., and L. Willems. 2009. "Mechanisms of HTLV-1 persistence and transformation." *Br J Cancer* 101(9):1497-501.

Etoh, K., K. Yamaguchi, S. Tokudome, T. Watanabe, A. Okayama, S. Stuver, N. Mueller, K. Takatsuki, and M. Matsuoka. 1999. "Rapid quantification of HTLV-I provirus load: detection of monoclonal proliferation of HTLV-I-infected cells among blood donors." *Int J Cancer* 81(6):859-64.

Hanon, E., J. C. Stinchcombe, M. Saito, B. E. Asquith, G. P. Taylor, Y. Tanaka, J. N. Weber, G. M. Griffiths, and C. R. Bangham. 2000. "Fratricide among CD8(+) T lymphocytes naturally infected with human T cell lymphotropic virus type I." *Immunity* 13(5):657-64.

Harashima, N., K. Kurihara, A. Utsunomiya, R. Tanosaki, S. Hanabuchi, M. Masuda, T. Ohashi, F. Fukui, A. Hasegawa, T. Masuda, Y. Takaue, J. Okamura, and M. Kannagi. 2004. "Graft-versus-Tax response in adult T-cell leukemia patients after hematopoietic stem cell transplantation." *Cancer Res* 64(1):391-9.

Hasegawa, H., T. Nomura, M. Kohno, N. Tateishi, Y. Suzuki, N. Maeda, R. Fujisawa, O. Yoshie, and S. Fujita. 2000. "Increased chemokine receptor CCR7/EBI1 expression enhances the infiltration of lymphoid organs by adult T-cell leukemia cells." *Blood* 95(1):30-8.

Higashimura, N., N. Takasawa, Y. Tanaka, M. Nakamura, and K. Sugamura. 1996. "Induction of OX40, a receptor of gp34, on T cells by trans-acting transcriptional activator, Tax, of human T-cell leukemia virus type I." *Jpn J Cancer Res* 87(3): 227-31.

Higuchi, M., and M. Fujii. 2009. "Distinct functions of HTLV-1 Tax1 from HTLV-2 Tax2 contribute key roles to viral pathogenesis." *Retrovirology* 6:117.

Hjelle, B., O. Appenzeller, R. Mills, S. Alexander, N. Torrez-Martinez, R. Jahnke, and G. Ross. 1992. "Chronic neurodegenerative disease associated with HTLV-II infection." *Lancet* 339(8794):645-6.

Igakura, T., J. C. Stinchcombe, P. K. Goon, G. P. Taylor, J. N. Weber, G. M. Griffiths, Y. Tanaka, M. Osame, and C. R. Bangham. 2003. "Spread of HTLV-I between lymphocytes by virus-induced polarization of the cytoskeleton." *Science* 299(5613):1713-6.

Imura, A., T. Hori, K. Imada, T. Ishikawa, Y. Tanaka, M. Maeda, S. Imamura, and T. Uchiyama. 1996. "The human OX40/gp34 system directly mediates adhesion of activated T cells to vascular endothelial cells." *J Exp Med* 183(5):2185-95.

Inoue, J., M. Yoshida, and M. Seiki. 1987. "Transcriptional (p40x) and post-transcriptional (p27x-III) regulators are required for the expression and replication of human T-cell leukemia virus type I genes." *Proc Natl Acad Sci U S A* 84(11):3653-7.

Ishida, T., S. Iida, Y. Akatsuka, T. Ishii, M. Miyazaki, H. Komatsu, H. Inagaki, N. Okada, T. Fujita, K. Shitara, S. Akinaga, T. Takahashi, A. Utsunomiya, and R. Ueda. 2004. "The CC chemokine receptor 4 as a novel specific molecular target for immunotherapy in adult T-Cell leukemia/lymphoma." *Clin Cancer Res* 10(22): 7529-39.

Kannian, Priya. 2010. "Human T Lymphotropic Virus Type 1 (HTLV-1): Molecular Biology and Oncogenesis " *Viruses* 2.

Kaplan, J. E., R. F. Khabbaz, E. L. Murphy, S. Hermansen, C. Roberts, R. Lal, W. Heneine, D. Wright, L. Matijas, R. Thomson, D. Rudolph, W. M. Switzer, S. Kleinman, M. Busch, and G. B. Schreiber. 1996. "Male-to-female transmission of human T-cell lymphotropic virus types I and II: association with viral load. The Retrovirus Epidemiology Donor Study Group." *J Acquir Immune Defic Syndr Hum Retrovirol* 12(2):193-201.

Karin, M. 2006. "Nuclear factor-kappaB in cancer development and progression." *Nature* 441(7092):431-6.

Kchour, G., M. Tarhini, M. M. Kooshyar, H. El Hajj, E. Wattel, M. Mahmoudi, H. Hatoum, H. Rahimi, M. Maleki, H. Rafatpanah, S. A. Rezaee, M. T. Yazdi, A. Shirdel, H. de The, O. Hermine, R. Farid, and A. Bazarbachi. 2009. "Phase 2 study of the efficacy and safety of the combination of arsenic trioxide, interferon alpha, and zidovudine in newly diagnosed chronic adult T-cell leukemia/lymphoma (ATL)." *Blood* 113(26):6528-32.

Kiyokawa, T., K. Yamaguchi, M. Takeya, K. Takahashi, T. Watanabe, T. Matsumoto, S. Y. Lee, and K. Takatsuki. 1987. "Hypercalcemia and osteoclast proliferation in adult T-cell leukemia." *Cancer* 59(6):1187-91.

Krueger, A., S. C. Fas, S. Baumann, and P. H. Krammer. 2003. "The role of CD95 in the regulation of peripheral T-cell apoptosis." *Immunol Rev* 193:58-69.

Lee, H. H., S. H. Weiss, L. S. Brown, D. Mildvan, V. Shorty, L. Saravolatz, A. Chu, H. M. Ginzburg, N. Markowitz, D. C. Des Jarlais, and et al. 1990. "Patterns of HIV-1 and HTLV-I/II in intravenous drug abusers from the middle atlantic and central regions of the USA." *J Infect Dis* 162(2):347-52.

Liu, B., S. Hong, Z. Tang, H. Yu, and C. Z. Giam. 2005. "HTLV-I Tax directly binds the Cdc20-associated anaphase-promoting complex and activates it ahead of schedule." *Proc Natl Acad Sci U S A* 102(1):63-8.

Manel, N., F. J. Kim, S. Kinet, N. Taylor, M. Sitbon, and J. L. Battini. 2003. "The ubiquitous glucose transporter GLUT-1 is a receptor for HTLV." *Cell* 115(4):449-59.

Matsuoka, M. 2003. "Human T-cell leukemia virus type I and adult T-cell leukemia." *Oncogene* 22(33):5131-40.

Matsuoka, M. 2005. "Human T-cell leukemia virus type I (HTLV-I) infection and the onset of adult T-cell leukemia (ATL)." *Retrovirology* 2:27.

Matsuoka, M., and K. T. Jeang. 2007. "Human T-cell leukaemia virus type 1 (HTLV-1) infectivity and cellular transformation 5." *Nat Rev Cancer* 7(4):270-80.

Mesnard, J. M., B. Barbeau, and C. Devaux. 2006. "HBZ, a new important player in the mystery of adult T-cell leukemia." *Blood* 108(13):3979-82.

Mitra-Kaushik, S., J. C. Harding, J. L. Hess, and L. Ratner. 2004. "Effects of the proteasome inhibitor PS-341 on tumor growth in HTLV-1 Tax transgenic mice and Tax tumor transplants." *Blood* 104(3):802-9.

Miyazato, A., S. Sheleg, H. Iha, Y. Li, and K. T. Jeang. 2005. "Evidence for NF-kappaB- and CBP-independent repression of p53's transcriptional activity by human T-cell leukemia virus type 1 Tax in mouse embryo and primary human fibroblasts." *J Virol* 79(14):9346-50.

Mori, N., M. Fujii, S. Ikeda, Y. Yamada, M. Tomonaga, D. W. Ballard, and N. Yamamoto. 1999. "Constitutive activation of NF-kappaB in primary adult T-cell leukemia cells." *Blood* 93(7):2360-8.

Mori, N., T. Matsuda, M. Tadano, T. Kinjo, Y. Yamada, K. Tsukasaki, S. Ikeda, Y. Yamasaki, Y. Tanaka, T. Ohta, T. Iwamasa, M. Tomonaga, and N. Yamamoto. 2004. "Apoptosis induced by the histone deacetylase inhibitor FR901228 in human T-cell leukemia virus type 1-infected T-cell lines and primary adult T-cell leukemia cells." *J Virol* 78(9):4582-90.

Mori, N., M. Morishita, T. Tsukazaki, C. Z. Giam, A. Kumatori, Y. Tanaka, and N. Yamamoto. 2001. "Human T-cell leukemia virus type I oncoprotein Tax represses Smad-dependent transforming growth factor beta signaling through interaction with CREB-binding protein/p300." *Blood* 97(7):2137-44.

Morosetti, R., N. Kawamata, A. F. Gombart, C. W. Miller, Y. Hatta, T. Hirama, J. W. Said, M. Tomonaga, and H. P. Koeffler. 1995. "Alterations of the p27KIP1 gene in non-Hodgkin's lymphomas and adult T-cell leukemia/lymphoma." *Blood* 86(5): 1924-30.

Nagata, S. 1999. "Fas ligand-induced apoptosis." *Annu Rev Genet* 33:29-55.

Nishimura, S., N. Asou, H. Suzushima, T. Okubo, T. Fujimoto, M. Osato, H. Yamasaki, L. Lisha, and K. Takatsuki. 1995. "p53 gene mutation and loss of heterozygosity are associated with increased risk of disease progression in adult T cell leukemia." *Leukemia* 9(4):598-604.

Nosaka, K., M. Maeda, S. Tamiya, T. Sakai, H. Mitsuya, and M. Matsuoka. 2000. "Increasing methylation of the CDKN2A gene is associated with the progression of adult T-cell leukemia." *Cancer Res* 60(4):1043-8.

Nosaka, K., T. Miyamoto, T. Sakai, H. Mitsuya, T. Suda, and M. Matsuoka. 2002. "Mechanism of hypercalcemia in adult T-cell leukemia: overexpression of receptor activator of nuclear factor kappaB ligand on adult T-cell leukemia cells." *Blood* 99(2):634-40.

Noula Shembade, Edward W Harhaj. 2010. "Role of post-translational modifications of HTLV-1 Tax in NF-κB activation." *World Journal of Biological Chemistry* 26(1): 13-20.

Okamura, J., A. Utsunomiya, R. Tanosaki, N. Uike, S. Sonoda, M. Kannagi, M. Tomonaga, M. Harada, N. Kimura, M. Masuda, F. Kawano, Y. Yufu, H. Hattori, H. Kikuchi, and Y. Saburi. 2005. "Allogeneic stem-cell transplantation with reduced conditioning intensity as a novel immunotherapy and antiviral therapy for adult T-cell leukemia/lymphoma." *Blood* 105(10):4143-5.

Pise-Masison, C. A., R. Mahieux, H. Jiang, M. Ashcroft, M. Radonovich, J. Duvall, C. Guillerm, and J. N. Brady. 2000. "Inactivation of p53 by human T-cell lymphotropic virus type 1 Tax requires activation of the NF-kappaB pathway and is dependent on p53 phosphorylation." *Mol Cell Biol* 20(10):3377-86.

Rafatpanah, H., R. Farid, G. Golanbar, and F. Jabbari Azad. 2006. "HTLV-I Infection: virus structure, immune response to the virus and genetic association studies in HTLV-I-infected individuals." *Iran J Allergy Asthma Immunol* 5(4):153-66.

Robert-Guroff, M., S. H. Weiss, J. A. Giron, A. M. Jennings, H. M. Ginzburg, I. B. Margolis, W. A. Blattner, and R. C. Gallo. 1986. "Prevalence of antibodies to HTLV-I, -II, and -III in intravenous drug abusers from an AIDS endemic region." *JAMA* 255(22): 3133-7.

Romanelli, L. C., P. Caramelli, and A. B. Proietti. 2010. "[Human T cell lymphotropic virus (HTLV)1: When should infection be suspected?]." *Rev Assoc Med Bras* 56(3): 340-7.

Roucoux, D. F., and E. L. Murphy. 2004. "The epidemiology and disease outcomes of human T-lymphotropic virus type II." *AIDS Rev* 6(3):144-54.

Sabouri, A. H., M. Saito, K. Usuku, S. N. Bajestan, M. Mahmoudi, M. Forughipour, Z. Sabouri, Z. Abbaspour, M. E. Goharjoo, E. Khayami, A. Hasani, S. Izumo, K. Arimura, R. Farid, and M. Osame. 2005. "Differences in viral and host genetic risk factors for development of human T-cell lymphotropic virus type 1 (HTLV-1)-associated myelopathy/tropical spastic paraparesis between Iranian and Japanese HTLV-1-infected individuals." *J Gen Virol* 86(Pt 3):773-81.

Safai, B., J. L. Huang, E. Boeri, R. Farid, J. Raafat, P. Schutzer, R. Ahkami, and G. Franchini. 1996. "Prevalence of HTLV type I infection in Iran: a serological and genetic study." *AIDS Res Hum Retroviruses* 12(12):1185-90.

Sanada, I., K. Nakada, S. Furugen, E. Kumagai, K. Yamaguchi, M. Yoshida, and K. Takatsuki. 1986. "Chromosomal abnormalities in a patient with smoldering adult T-cell leukemia: evidence for a multistep pathogenesis." *Leuk Res* 10(12):1377-82.

Sasaki, H., I. Nishikata, T. Shiraga, E. Akamatsu, T. Fukami, T. Hidaka, Y. Kubuki, A. Okayama, K. Hamada, H. Okabe, Y. Murakami, H. Tsubouchi, and K. Morishita. 2005. "Overexpression of a cell adhesion molecule, TSLC1, as a possible molecular marker for acute-type adult T-cell leukemia." *Blood* 105(3):1204-13.

Satou, Y., and M. Matsuoka. 2010. "HTLV-1 and the host immune system: how the virus disrupts immune regulation, leading to HTLV-1 associated diseases." *J Clin Exp Hematop* 50(1):1-8.

Silva, M. T., R. C. Harab, A. C. Leite, D. Schor, A. Araujo, and M. J. Andrada-Serpa. 2007. "Human T lymphotropic virus type 1 (HTLV-1) proviral load in asymptomatic carriers, HTLV-1-associated myelopathy/tropical spastic paraparesis, and other neurological abnormalities associated with HTLV-1 infection." *Clin Infect Dis* 44(5):689-92.

Takatsuki, K. 1995. "Adult T-cell leukemia." *Intern Med* 34(10):947-52.

Takatsuki, K. 2005. "Discovery of adult T-cell leukemia." *Retrovirology* 2:16.

Tamiya, S., K. Etoh, H. Suzushima, K. Takatsuki, and M. Matsuoka. 1998. "Mutation of CD95 (Fas/Apo-1) gene in adult T-cell leukemia cells." *Blood* 91(10):3935-42.

Tan, C., and T. A. Waldmann. 2002. "Proteasome inhibitor PS-341, a potential therapeutic agent for adult T-cell leukemia." *Cancer Res* 62(4):1083-6.

Tsukahara, T., M. Kannagi, T. Ohashi, H. Kato, M. Arai, G. Nunez, Y. Iwanaga, N. Yamamoto, K. Ohtani, M. Nakamura, and M. Fujii. 1999. "Induction of Bcl-x(L) expression by human T-cell leukemia virus type 1 Tax through NF-kappaB in apoptosis-resistant T-cell transfectants with Tax." *J Virol* 73(10):7981-7.

Ureta-Vidal, A., C. Angelin-Duclos, P. Tortevoye, E. Murphy, J. F. Lepere, R. P. Buigues, N. Jolly, M. Joubert, G. Carles, J. F. Pouliquen, G. de The, J. P. Moreau, and A. Gessain. 1999. "Mother-to-child transmission of human T-cell-leukemia/lymphoma virus type I: implication of high antiviral antibody titer and high proviral load in carrier mothers." *Int J Cancer* 82(6):832-6.

Waldmann, T. A., J. D. White, C. K. Goldman, L. Top, A. Grant, R. Bamford, E. Roessler, I. D. Horak, S. Zaknoen, C. Kasten-Sportes, and et al. 1993. "The interleukin-2 receptor: a target for monoclonal antibody treatment of human T-cell lymphotrophic virus I-induced adult T-cell leukemia." *Blood* 82(6):1701-12.

Watanabe, T., K. Yamaguchi, K. Takatsuki, M. Osame, and M. Yoshida. 1990. "Constitutive expression of parathyroid hormone-related protein gene in human T cell leukemia virus type 1 (HTLV-1) carriers and adult T cell leukemia patients that can be trans-activated by HTLV-1 tax gene." *J Exp Med* 172(3):759-65.

Yamada, Y., M. Tomonaga, H. Fukuda, S. Hanada, A. Utsunomiya, M. Tara, M. Sano, S. Ikeda, K. Takatsuki, M. Kozuru, K. Araki, F. Kawano, M. Niimi, K. Tobinai, T. Hotta, and M. Shimoyama. 2001. "A new G-CSF-supported combination chemotherapy, LSG15, for adult T-cell leukaemia-lymphoma: Japan Clinical Oncology Group Study 9303." *Br J Haematol* 113(2):375-82.

Yasunaga, J., and M. Matsuoka. 2007. "Human T-cell leukemia virus type I induces adult T-cell leukemia: from clinical aspects to molecular mechanisms." *Cancer Control* 14(2):133-40.

Yasunaga, J., Y. Taniguchi, K. Nosaka, M. Yoshida, Y. Satou, T. Sakai, H. Mitsuya, and M. Matsuoka. 2004. "Identification of aberrantly methylated genes in association with adult T-cell leukemia." *Cancer Res* 64(17):6002-9.

Yoshida, M. 2001. "Multiple viral strategies of HTLV-1 for dysregulation of cell growth control." *Annu Rev Immunol* 19:475-96.

Yoshida, M. 2005. "Discovery of HTLV-1, the first human retrovirus, its unique regulatory mechanisms, and insights into pathogenesis." *Oncogene* 24(39):5931-7.

Yoshida, M. 2010. "Molecular approach to human leukemia: isolation and characterization of the first human retrovirus HTLV-1 and its impact on tumorigenesis in adult T-cell leukemia." *Proc Jpn Acad Ser B Phys Biol Sci* 86(2):117-30.

Yoshida, M., K. Nosaka, J. Yasunaga, I. Nishikata, K. Morishita, and M. Matsuoka. 2004. "Aberrant expression of the MEL1S gene identified in association with hypomethylation in adult T-cell leukemia cells." *Blood* 103(7):2753-60.

Yoshie, O., R. Fujisawa, T. Nakayama, H. Harasawa, H. Tago, D. Izawa, K. Hieshima, Y. Tatsumi, K. Matsushima, H. Hasegawa, A. Kanamaru, S. Kamihira, and Y. Yamada.

2002. "Frequent expression of CCR4 in adult T-cell leukemia and human T-cell leukemia virus type 1-transformed T cells." *Blood* 99(5):1505-11.

Zanjani, D. S., M. Shahabi, N. Talaei, M. Afzalaghaee, F. Tehranian, and R. Bazargani. 2010. "Molecular Analysis of Human T Cell Lymphotropic Virus Type 1 and 2 (HTLV-1/2) Seroindeterminate Blood Donors from Northeast Iran: Evidence of Proviral tax, env, and gag Sequences." *AIDS Res Hum Retroviruses.*

Zhang, Z., M. Zhang, J. V. Ravetch, C. Goldman, and T. A. Waldmann. 2003. "Effective therapy for a murine model of adult T-cell leukemia with the humanized anti-CD2 monoclonal antibody, MEDI-507." *Blood* 102(1):284-8.

3

Roles of HTLV-1 Tax in Leukemogenesis of Human T-Cells

Mariko Mizuguchi, Toshifumi Hara and Masataka Nakamura
Human Gene Sciences Center, Tokyo Medical and Dental University, Yushima, Bunkyo-ku, Tokyo
Japan

1. Introduction

Human T-cell leukemia/lymphoma virus type 1 (HTLV-1), a member of the delta-retrovirus family, is an oncogenic retrovirus that is etiologically associated with adult T-cell leukemia (ATL) (Hinuma et al., 1981, Poiesz et al., 1980, Yoshida et al., 1982) and HTLV-1-associated myelopathy/tropical spastic paraparesis (HAM/TSP) (Gessain et al., 1985, Osame et al., 1986). ATL is characterized by an aggressive $CD4^{+}$ T-cell malignancy with resistance to anti-cancer therapeutics. It is currently estimated that HTLV-1 infects 10-20 million people in the world, endemically southwestern Japan, Africa, South America and the Caribbean basin (Proietti et al., 2005). HTLV-1 transmission mainly occurs from mother to child through breast milk followed by infection to child cells in a cell-cell contact manner (Kinoshita et al., 1987). Approximately 2-5% of HTLV-1-infected individuals develop ATL after a long latent period. The average Japanese ATL patients are 60 years old. Accumulation of genetic and epigenetic changes in provirus and host genes during the latent period is thought to be essential for immortalization and transformation of T-cells. However the pathogenesis of ATL by HTLV-1 remains incompletely understood.

Like other retroviruses, HTLV-1 provirus genome structure genes, gag, pro, pol, and env are flanked by 5′ and 3′ long terminal repeat (LTR). Besides the prototype genes, the HTLV-1 genome has the 1.6 kb pX region in the 3′ terminal region. The pX region codes for several non-structural molecules Tax1, Rex, p12, p13, p30, p21 and HBZ by combination of the reading frames and alternative splicing (Figure 1) (Nicot et al., 2005). Tax1 was initially identified as a trans-acting transcriptional activator of the HTLV-1 promoter in LTR, leading to virus replication (Fujisawa et al., 1985, Sodroski et al., 1984). Tax1 has the ability to modulate transcription of cellular genes through activation of at least three cellular transcriptional factors NF-κB, CREB/ATF and AP-1 (Yoshida, 2001). Tax1-mediated dysregulation of gene expression is believed to be implicated in cellular immortalization and transformation through multistep processes. Cell immortaliztion and transformation generally require at least three steps: cell growth promotion, prevention of apoptosis and escape from senescence. Involvement of Tax1 in three steps has been studies intensively and extensively; Introduction of the Tax1 gene induces phenotypic transformation in fibroblast cell lines (Tanaka et al., 1990), neoplastic transformation of primary rat fibroblast in co-operation with the ras oncogene, persistent interleukin (IL) 2-dependent growth of primary T-cells in vitro (Akagi et al., 1995, Grassmann et al., 1989), and development of tumors and leukemia in mice (Grassmann et al., 1989, Nerenberg et al., 1987). Tax1 exertion may be important for the early stage of the development of ATL, because some ATL cells do not express Tax1. The disturbance of normal cellular environment by Tax1 may be an initial step of ATL development. This chapter focuses on recent advances in molecular basis of Tax1 implication in leukemogenesis.

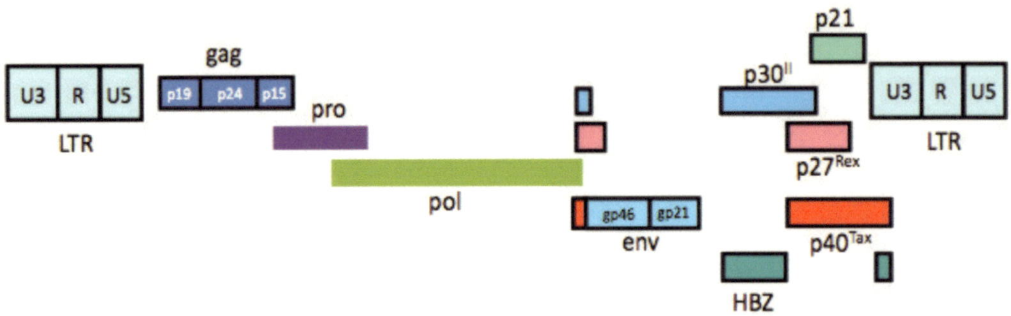

Fig. 1. Structure of HTLV-1 proviral genome

2. Effect of Tax1 on cell growth promotion

2.1 Cell cycle progression

Dysregulated cell cycle progression is potential for cellular transformation (Trimarchi and Lees, 2002). Cell growth is primarily controlled by the cell cycle, which in divided into five phases for convenience: the first gap (G1) phase, the DNA synthetic (S) phase, the second gap (G2) phase, the mitotic (M) phase and the resting (G0) phase. Mitogenic stimulation induces cell cycle progression by going through the restriction point between G1 and S phases (Trimarchi and Lees, 2002). Once they pass the restriction point, cells are destined to undergo one round of the cell cycle without further mitogenic stimulation. Most somatic cells usually stay at G0 or G1 phase. G1 cyclins and cyclin-dependent kinase (CDK) complexes (cyclin D1-CDK4, 6 and cyclin E-CDK2) control G1 to S transition (Dyson, 1998, Nevins, 1998, Trimarchi and Lees, 2002). Mitogenic stimulation activates cyclin-CDK complexes, which phosphorylates the retinoblastoma tumor suppressor protein (pRb), releasing active E2F that functions as a transcription factor to produce gene products required for G0/G1 to S transition (Figure 2).

Previous studies including our findings indicate that Tax1 is directly implicated in cell cycle control (Liang et al., 2002, Neuveut et al., 1998, Ohtani et al., 2000, Schmitt et al., 1998). Tax1 induces cell cycle progression from G0/G1 to S phases in normal peripheral blood lymphocytes (PBLs) and IL-2-dependent human T-cell line Kit 225 cells (Iwanaga et al., 2001, Ohtani et al., 2000). The advantage of Kit 225 cells is that their growth is arrested at the G1 phase by depletion of IL-2 without significant apoptosis, and growth promotion can be re-induced by the addition of IL-2 (Hori et al., 1987). Tax1 is known not to have the ability to bind directly to DNA elements and to perturb expression of a lot of cellular genes through interaction with cellular transcription factors NF-κB, CREB and AP-1 (Yoshida, 2001). Ectopic introduction of Tax1 into resting Kit 225 cells by recombinant adenoviruses revealed that a Tax1 mutant lacking the ability to activate NF-κB fails to cell cycle progression, suggesting that NF-κB is important for Tax1-mediated cell cycle progression (Iwanaga et al., 2001). To address the molecular mechanism underlying Tax1-induced cell cycle progression, effects of Tax1 on expression of cell cycle regulators have been examined. Tax1 up-regulates expression of genes for cyclin D2, cyclin E, E2F1, CDK2, CDK4 and CDK6, while Tax1 reduced expression of genes for CDK inhibitors $p19^{INK4d}$ and $p27^{Kip1}$ in resting Kit 225 cells (Iwanaga et al., 2001, Ohtani et al., 2000). These results indicate that Tax1-dependent deregulation of cell cycle regulators is directly associated with abnormal cell cycle progression.

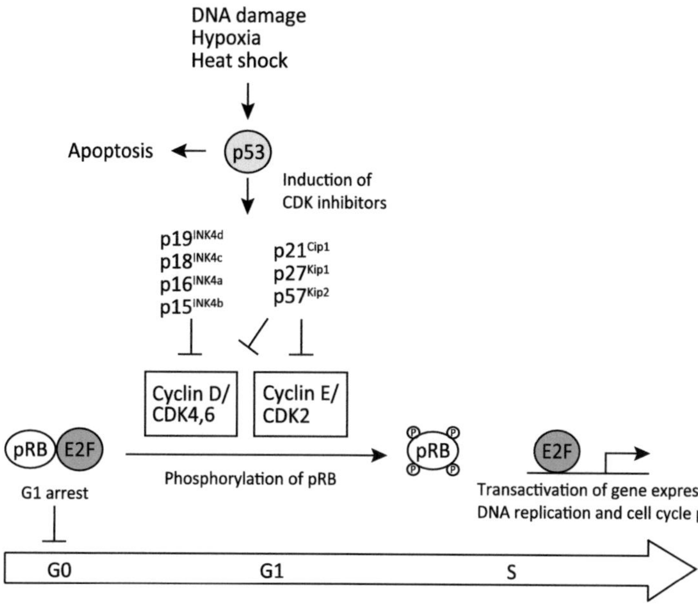

Fig. 2. Regulation of G1/S transition

2.2 Activation of E2F

E2F plays crucial roles in induction of the S phase by regulating expression of genes that encode a set of molecules involved in DNA replication and cell cycle progression (Figure 2) (Nevins et al., 1997). Thus it is important to understand how Tax1 affects E2F activity. Tax1-dependnt phosphorylation of pRb results in activation of E2F1 (Iwanaga et al., 2001). Active E2F1 enhances own transcription by direct interaction to the E2F promoter in Kit 225 cells, whereas the E2F gene promoter is not activated by Tax1 in rat embryonic fibroblast REF52 cells (Ohtani et al., 2000). This finding suggests that Tax1 induces a positive feedback loop of E2F in a cell lineage-dependent manner. Indeed Tax1 increases transcript levels of genes carrying the E2F binding sites in their promoters. The HsOrc1, DHFR, DNA polymerase α and Cdc6 gene are examples, all of which are necessary for DNA replication in S phase (Ohtani et al., 2000). The activity of Tax1 to activate NF-κB and/or NFAT is indispensable for E2F activation (Ohtani et al., 2000). Tax1 also trans-activated promoters with E2F sites of cell cycle regulatory genes such as c-myc, cyclin D2, cyclin E and cyclin A (Huang et al., 2001, Ohtani et al., 2000, Santiago et al., 1999). These results demonstrate that Tax1 induces cell cycle progression, partly by releasing active E2F molecules.

2.3 Interfere with mitosis

Surprisingly and interestingly, primary T-cells or Kit 225 cells transduced with Tax1 show the cellular G1/S entry, but proliferation of such cells is not observed (Iwanaga et al., 2001,

Ohtani et al., 2000), perhaps suggesting blockage of mitosis by Tax1. Similarly induction of Tax1 in PA18G-BHK-21 cells, which are Tax1-inducible syrian hamster kidney cell line, revealed cell cycle transition from G1 to S phase, but further progression to mitosis was not seen (Liang et al., 2002). In addition, Tax1-transduced cells show nuclear abnormalities and cytokinesis defects, which are similar to symptoms observed in ATL patients (Jin et al., 1998, Majone et al., 1993, Semmes and Jeang, 1996). However the exact roles of Tax1 in entire cell cycle progression will be elucidated by future studies.

3. Deregulation of cellular signaling by Tax1

3.1 Induction of cytokines and their receptors

Growth stimuli for T-cells are usually delivered by cytokines, in particular IL-2 acts as an effective growth factor for T-cells (Asao et al., 1994, Tanaka et al., 1994). Cytokines, which are expressed inducibly and transiently, bind to their specific receptors, transducing intracellular signalings important not only for cellular proliferation, but for differentiation and survival of lymphocytes (Rochman et al., 2009). Expression of cytokines is crucial for proliferation of lymphocytes. The α-chain of IL-2 receptor (IL-2Rα) is also induced by immune stimulation and its gene is the first identified cellular gene that is activated by Tax1 (Ballard et al., 1988, Ruben et al., 1988). Together with IL-2Rα, IL-2Rβ and the common γ-chain form the high affinity IL-2 receptor complex that is an actual growth signal transducer of T-cells (Takeshita et al., 1992). Furthermore, transient transfection studies showed that the IL-2 promoter is activated by Tax1 in an NF-AT and NF-κB pathway-dependent manner (Good et al., 1996, Hoyos et al., 1989, McGuire et al., 1993). These led to the hypothesis that Tax1 makes T-cells proliferative through autocrine and/or paracrine action of induced IL-2 and IL-2R. However recent studies revealed that Tax1-expressing T-cells do not produce either the IL-2 mRNA or protein (Akagi and Shimotohno, 1993, Chung et al., 2003). Hence, the IL-2/IL-2R autocrine loop mediated by Tax1 in transformation of T-cells has been reconsidered.

Tax1 trans-activates transcription of genes for other cytokines related to T-cell growth such as IL-9, IL-13, IL-15 and IL-21 (Azimi et al., 1998, Chen et al., 2008, Mizuguchi et al., 2009, Silbermann et al., 2008, Waldele et al., 2004). Notably, IL-21 is produced by activated $CD4^+$ T-cells and effectively promotes proliferation of T-cells in co-operation with IL-15 (Onoda et al., 2007, Parrish-Novak et al., 2000). IL-21 is similar to IL-2 and IL-15 in terms of biological activity and receptor constitution, which is composed of itself specific receptor(s) and the common γ-chain (Asao et al., 2001, Onoda et al., 2007, Parrish-Novak et al., 2000). The common γ-chain is a target of Tax1 at transcription (Ohbo et al., 1995). These observations suggest that incomplete progression of the cell cycle by Tax1 may be complemented by action of cytokines and their receptors induced by Tax1. Coordination between IL-21 and IL-15 induced by Tax1 may deliver more effective growth signals in T-cells. This notion does not exclude the possibility of implication of IL-2 in Tax1-mediated cell growth. IL-21 may function as a powerful inducer for T-cell growth in the presence of IL-2, which is released in immune responses to HTLV-1 infection.

3.2 Intracellular signaling

Cytokines deliver more effective growth signals in T-cells. Interaction of cytokines with their receptors activates Janus kinase (JAK)/signal transducer and activator of transcription (STAT) and PI3 kinase growth signaling pathways (Kelly-Welch et al., 2003,

Marzec et al., 2008, Zeng et al., 2007). The JAK/STAT pathway is one of the major cytokine signaling pathways. JAK-mediated phosphorylation of receptor subunits increases phosphorylation and dimerization of STATs, resulting in activation of downstream genes essential for cell growth and immunity (Levy and Darnell, 2002). JAK and STAT proteins are unphosphorylated and inactive in normal quiescent lymphocytes. STAT3 and STAT5 in HTLV-1 infected T-cells are reported to be constitutively activated (Hall and Fujii, 2005, Migone et al., 1995). Persistent activation of STAT3 is shown to increase proliferation, survival, angiogenesis and metastasis in various human cancers (Yu et al., 2009). IL-21 preferentially activates STAT1 and STAT3, while IL-2 and IL-15 primarily activate STAT5 (Asao et al., 2001, Zeng et al., 2007). Co-operation of intrinsic cell cycle promotion with cytokine-dependent signal transduction may be essential for cell proliferation induced by Tax1.

The pathway involving phosphoinositide 3-kinase (PI3K) and its downstream kinase Akt provides cell survival and growth signals in T-cells (Cantley, 2002). PI3K primarily phosphorylates phosphatidylinositol-4,5-bisphosphate (PIP_2) to generate the second messenger, phosphatidylinositol-3,4,5-trisphosphate (PIP_3), which form a complex with Akt and phosphoinositide-dependent protein kinese 1 (PDK1) on the plasma membrane, where Akt is activated by phosphorylation by PDK1 and mTOR complex 2 (mTORC2) (Sarbassov et al., 2005). Active Akt phosphorylates several cellular proteins for cell survival and cell cycle entry. Tensin homolog deleted on chromosome 10 (PTEN) and Src homology 2 domain containing inositol polyphosphate phosphatase-1 (SHIP-1) inhibit the pathway by phosphorylation of PIP_3 (Cantley and Neel, 1999, Rohrschneider et al., 2000). The PI3K/Akt pathway is constitutively active in HTLV-1 transformed cells and ATL cells (Fukuda et al., 2005, Peloponese and Jeang, 2006). Tax1 induces the phosphorylation of Akt that is linked to NF-κB activation and p53 inhibition (Jeong et al., 2005). Inhibition of PI3K or Akt induces cell cycle arrest and apoptosis with accumulation of $p27^{Kip1}$ and caspase-9 activation in HTLV-1 transformed T-cells (Jeong et al., 2008). In addition, Tax1 down-regulates transcription for PTEN and SHIP-1 through NF-κB-mediated inhibition of the transcriptional coactivator p300 (Fukuda et al., 2009). These findings indicate that the PI3K/Akt pathway activated by Tax1 is involved in cell cycle progression and survive.

4. Modification of apoptosis by Tax1

Tax1 inactivates p53 (Tabakin-Fix et al., 2006). The transcription factor p53 is critical for prevention of abnormal cell proliferation. When DNA is damaged by γ radiation, ultraviolet and carcinostatic, cells express high amount of active p53, resulting in expression of genes essential for cell cycle arrest, DNA repair or apoptosis (Figure 2). The p53 gene is mutated in roughly 50% of various human cancers (Grassmann et al., 2005). Mutation of p53 is poorly defined in ATL cells. Tax1 neither binds p53 nor represses p53 gene expression. Two major findings have been reported regarding inactivation of p53 by Tax1. First, Tax1 and p53 competes with each other for binding to the coactivator CREB binding protein (CBP)/p300 and p53 loses the ability to activate transcription (Ariumi et al., 2000, Van Orden et al., 1999). Second, Tax1-mediated p53 inactivation is dependent on NF-κB activation. Tax1 facilitates the formation of functionally inactive complexes containing p65 (RelA) and p53, and this interaction requires p53 phosphorylation at serine-15, a site is preferentially phosphorylated in Tax1-expressing cells (Pise-Masison et al., 2000). Tax1-mediated interference with tumor suppressor p53 has been thought to facilitate resistance to apoptosis. Apoptosis is an

important mechanism with intrinsic active processes of programmed cell death, by which cells keep themselves from uncontrolled cell death. As p53 is one of pivotal molecules to trigger apoptosis, Tax1-mediated inactivation of p53 may predispose HTLV-1 infected cells to survive. In addition to Tax1-mediated inactivation of p53, Tax1 induces anti-apoptotic molecules such as Bcl-χL, XIAP and survivin (Tsukahara et al., 1999, Yoshida, 2001). In tumor cells, prevention of apoptosis is essential for their continuous growth. Anti-apoptotic effects of Tax1 may lead to cellular immortalization and contribute to accumulation of genetic mutations.
Conversely, perevious studies reported that Tax1 expression is closely linked to the induction of apoptosis (Chlichlia et al., 1995, Chlichlia et al., 1997, Kao et al., 2000). Tax1-mediated apoptosis occurs in Tax1-inducible cell line JPX-9 by activation of the Fas/FasL pathway (Chen et al., 1997). Tax1 has been reported to sensitize cells to apoptosis induced by DNA damaging agents. The results from human cDNA expression array analysis with HTLV-1 infected Tax1-expressing T-cells (C81) treated with γ irradiation show up-regulation of various genes for cell cycle inducers and inhibitors, anti- and pro-apoptotic molecules (de la Fuente et al., 2003). Upon γ irradiation, S and G2/M phase-enriched population increases in cell numbers with apoptosis, while little, if any, or no induction of apoptosis is associated with G0/G1 population (de la Fuente et al., 2003). The apparent paradox of the opposite effects of Tax1 on cell death remains to be elucidated. The choice between proliferation and cell death by Tax1 may be influenced by cell cycle state or intracellular status.

5. Immortalization by Tax1

Telomeres are DNA-protein complex structures located at the end of chromosomes (Blackburn, 1991). The structures are thought to contribute to the stabilization of linear chromosomes (Blackburn, 1991, Counter et al., 1992). Each cell division leads to the shortening of telomere length by the end-replication problem (Olovnikov, 1973, Watson, 1972). The shortening of telomeres results in chromosome instability, which is closely related to cellular senescence (Allsopp et al., 1992). Thus most human somatic cells have a limited replicative life span due to shortening of the telomere length. To avoid telomere shortening, transformed cells and germline cells appear to have certain compensatory mechanisms (Counter et al., 1994, Kim et al., 1994). One mechanism synthesizing terminal telomere sequences is mediated by the reibonucleoprotein enzyme telomerase, whose activity is restricted by expression of its catalytic subunit human telomerase reverse transcriptase (hTERT) (Meyerson et al., 1997, Nakamura et al., 1997). Development and maintenance of ATL probably require telomerase activity and indeed ATL cells carry telomerase activity (Uchida et al., 1999). Therefore activation of telomerase seems to be one of key events in development of ATL.
Effects of Tax1 on expression of telomerase in human T-cells remains controversial. An early report concerning this issue suggested that Tax1 reduced telomerase activity in human T-cell line Jurkat cells and Tax1 negatively regulated hTERT promoter activity (Gabet et al., 2003). In contrast, other group showed that Tax1 stimulated the endogenous hTERT promoter through NF-κB activation (Sinha-Datta et al., 2004). Recent studies may provide systemic solution to the discrepancy. Tax1 activates hTERT gene expression only in resting T-cells, while hTERT expression is not significantly changed by Tax1 in growing cells (Hara et al., 2008). Thus, the cell cycle state may differentially influence action of Tax1 on hTERT expression in human T-cells. The activity of Tax1 to promote cell cycle progression may be critically linked to regulation of expression of the hTERT gene, because kinetics of Tax1-mediated activation of

the hTERT promoter parallels Tax1-mediated cell cycle progression (Matsumura-Arioka et al., 2005). In leukemia cells, Tax1 may be negatively associated with or independent of regulation of hTERT expression, rather epigenetic changes in the promoter in leukemia cells may significantly contribute to constitutive activation of the hTERT promoter. It may be important that strict repression of telomerase expression in normal T-cells to avoid undesirable immune responses and malignant transformation. An element involved in repression in the promoter is suggested (Gabet et al., 2003, Hara et al., 2008).

6. HTLV-1 Tax and HTLV-2 Tax

HTLV-2 is close to HTLV-1 in genetic and biological terms, showing ~70% sequence homology with each other (Feuer and Green, 2005). HTLV-2 encodes Tax2, which shows ~75% sequence homology to Tax1 (Feuer and Green, 2005). Tax1 and Tax2 have been shown to important roles in immortalization of T-cells in an IL-2 dependent manner, though HTLV-2 has not been linked with development of hematological malignant diseases (Feuer and Green, 2005). Differences in functional domains between Tax1 and Tax2 has been demonstrated. Tax1 possesses a leucine zipper like region (LZR) within amino acids 225-232 and the PDZ binding motif (PBM) at C-terminus, which are responsible for Tax1-mediated p100 processing and p52 nuclear translocation (Higuchi et al., 2007, Shoji et al., 2009).

The NF-κB pathway is tightly controlled in normal T-cells, and transiently activated upon immune stimulation. On the other hand, aberrant NF-κB activation is implicated in many types of cancer, especially hematological malignancies such as leukemia, lymphoma and myeloma (Karin, 2006). In HTLV-1 infected T-cells, NF-κB is constitutively activated, which is also thought to be linked to immortalization of T-cell by HTLV-1 and HTLV-2 (Mori et al., 1999, Robek and Ratner, 1999, Ross et al., 2000). Tax1 activates both the canonical (mainly consisting of the p50 and p65 subunits) and non-canonical (mainly consisting of the p52 and RelB subunits) NF-κB pathways. These are consequences of interaction of Tax1 with IKK complex. In contrast, although Tax2 can activate the canonical pathway to a level comparable to Tax1, Tax2 rarely induces the p100 processing because of lacking the LZR and PBM regions (Higuchi et al., 2007, Shoji et al., 2009).

Recent studies demonstrate that Tax2 induces expression of IL-2, but Tax1 fails to induce IL-2 production (Figure 3) (Niinuma et al., 2005). This finding prompted us to search for

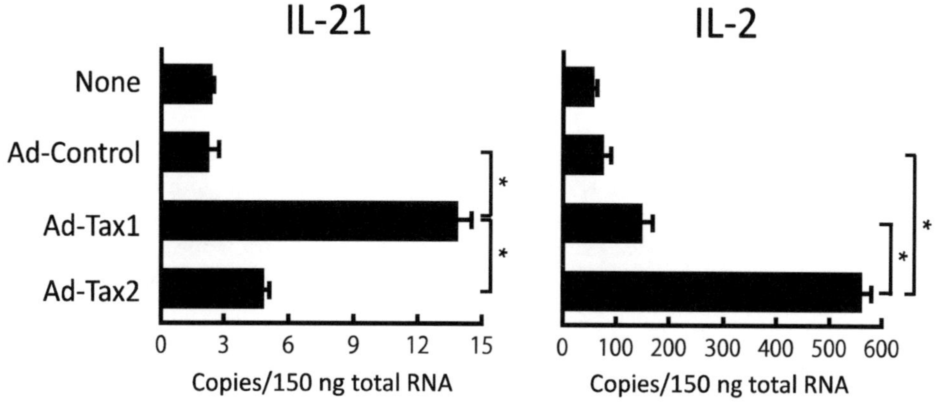

Fig. 3. Differential cytokine expression by Tax

another factor(s), which is differently induced between Tax1 and Tax2. In contrast to IL-2 induction, Tax1 induced IL-21 expression in $CD4^+$ T-cells, but Tax2 did not (Figure 3) (Miuguchi et al., 2009). The IL-21 promoter NF-κB binding site is activated by the p52/RelB complex by direct binding in a Tax1-dependent manner, probably reflecting the difference in NF-κB activation between Tax1 and Tax2. The functional differences between Tax1 and Tax2 causes different profiles of cytokine production, and may be related to phathogenesis between HTLV-1 and HTLV-2.

7. Conclusion

HTLV-1 is the first human retrovirus, which causes leukemia/lymphoma. Before the discovery of HTLV-1, many oncogenic retroviruses have been found, which induce malignant tumors in animals such as avian and rodent (Maeda et al., 2008). Most animal oncogenic retroviruses carry oncogenes, but they are totally different from the HTLV-1 oncogene for Tax1. Oncogenes, called v-onc, in animal retroviruses are usually derived from host cells, while Tax1 has no identity in host cells in terms of the origin of oncogene. Action of oncogenes are also different, unlikely to animal oncogenes, whose products are directly integrated cellular signaling pathways with dysregulated activities, Tax1 acts as transcriptional modulator that indirectly affects transcription of cellular genes related to immortalization and transformation. Therefore literature studies concerning animal retrovirus oncogenes was not much helpful in analyzes of mode of action of Tax1 in leukemogenesis.

Tax1 is a molecule of HTLV-1 products that shows strong immunogenicity (Kannagi et al., 1991). Human $CD8^+$ T-cells target Tax1-expressing cells. It is probably expected that most Tax1-expressing cells are killed by this mechanism. Thus Tax1 functions as a molecule both advantageous and disadvantageous to virus survive in vivo. Only cells escaped from immune attack further require genetic and epigenetic changes to become full transformants. These are may be reasons why ATL occurs after the long latent period at low frequency. In summary, Tax1 provides cells abilities of cell growth promotion, apoptosis prevention and senescence avoidance, but Tax1 alone may be insufficient for ATL development.

8. Acknowledgements

We are indebted to H. Asao, M. Higuchi and M. Fujii for support and discussion. This study was supported in part by Grants-in-Aid for scientific research from the Ministry of Education, Culture, Sports, Science and Technology of Japan.

9. References

Akagi, T., Ono, H. & Shimotohno, K. 1995. Characterization of T cells immortalized by Tax1 of human T-cell leukemia virus type 1. *Blood,* 86, 4243-9.

Akagi, T. & Shimotohno, K. 1993. Proliferative response of Tax1-transduced primary human T cells to anti-CD3 antibody stimulation by an interleukin-2-independent pathway. *J Virol,* 67, 1211-7.

Allsopp, R. C., Vaziri, H., Patterson, C., Goldstein, S., Younglai, E. V., Futcher, A. B., Greider, C. W. & Harley, C. B. 1992. Telomere length predicts replicative capacity of human fibroblasts. *Proc Natl Acad Sci USA,* 89, 10114-8.

Ariumi, Y., Kaida, A., Lin, J. Y., Hirota, M., Masui, O., Yamaoka, S., Taya, Y. & Shimotohno, K. 2000. HTLV-1 tax oncoprotein represses the p53-mediated trans-activation function through coactivator CBP sequestration. *Oncogene,* 19, 1491-9.

Asao, H., Okuyama, C., Kumaki, S., Ishii, N., Tsuchiya, S., Foster, D. & Sugamura, K. 2001. The common γ-chain is an indispensable subunit of the IL-21 receptor complex. *J Immunol,* 167, 1-5.

Asao, H., Tanaka, N., Ishii, N., Higuchi, M., Takeshita, T., Nakamura, M., Shirasawa, T. & Sugamura, K. 1994. Interleukin 2-induced activation of JAK3: possible involvement in signal transduction for c-myc induction and cell proliferation. *FEBS Lett,* 351, 201-6.

Azimi, N., Brown, K., Bamford, R. N., Tagaya, Y., Siebenlist, U. & Waldmann, T. A. 1998. Human T cell lymphotropic virus type I Tax protein trans-activates interleukin 15 gene transcription through an NF-κB site. *Proc Natl Acad Sci USA,* 95, 2452-7.

Ballard, D. W., Bohnlein, E., Lowenthal, J. W., Wano, Y., Franza, B. R. & Greene, W. C. 1988. HTLV-I tax induces cellular proteins that activate the κB element in the IL-2 receptor α gene. *Science,* 241, 1652-5.

Blackburn, E. H. 1991. Structure and function of telomeres. *Nature,* 350, 569-73.

Cantley, L. C. 2002. The phosphoinositide 3-kinase pathway. *Science,* 296, 1655-7.

Cantley, L. C. & Neel, B. G. 1999. New insights into tumor suppression: PTEN suppresses tumor formation by restraining the phosphoinositide 3-kinase/AKT pathway. *Proc Natl Acad Sci USA,* 96, 4240-5.

Chen, J., Petrus, M., Bryant, B. R., Phuc Nguyen, V., Stamer, M., Goldman, C. K., Bamford, R., Morris, J. C., Janik, J. E. & Waldmann, T. A. 2008. Induction of the IL-9 gene by HTLV-I Tax stimulates the spontaneous proliferation of primary adult T-cell leukemia cells by a paracrine mechanism. *Blood,* 111,5163-72.

Chen, X., Zachar, V., Zdravkovic, M., Guo, M., Ebbesen, P. & Liu, X. 1997. Role of the Fas/Fas ligand pathway in apoptotic cell death induced by the human T cell lymphotropic virus type I Tax transactivator. *J Gen Virol,* 78, 3277-85.

Chlichlia, K., Busslinger, M., Peter, M. E., Walczak, H., Krammer, P. H., Schirrmacher, V. & Khazaie, K. 1997. ICE-proteases mediate HTLV-I Tax-induced apoptotic T-cell death. *Oncogene,* 14, 2265-72.

Chlichlia, K., Moldenhauer, G., Daniel, P. T., Busslinger, M., Gazzolo, L., Schirrmacher, V. & Khazaie, K. 1995. Immediate effects of reversible HTLV-1 tax function: T-cell activation and apoptosis. *Oncogene,* 10, 269-77.

Chung, H. K., Young, H. A., Goon, P. K., Heidecker, G., Princler, G. L., Shimozato, O., Taylor, G. P., Bangham, C. R. & Derse, D. 2003. Activation of interleukin-13 expression in T cells from HTLV-1-infected individuals and in chronically infected cell lines. *Blood,* 102, 4130-6.

Counter, C. M., Avilion, A. A., Lefeuvre, C. E., Stewart, N. G., Greider, C. W., Harley, C. B. & Bacchetti, S. 1992. Telomere shortening associated with chromosome instability is arrested in immortal cells which express telomerase activity. *EMBO J,* 11, 1921-9.

Counter, C. M., Hirte, H. W., Bacchetti, S. & Harley, C. B. 1994. Telomerase activity in human ovarian carcinoma. *Proc Natl Acad Sci USA,* 91, 2900-4.

De La Fuente, C., Wang, L., Wang, D., Deng, L., Wu, K., Li, H., Stein, L. D., Denny, T., Coffman, F., Kehn, K., Baylor, S., Maddukuri, A., Pumfery, A. & Kashanchi, F. 2003. Paradoxical effects of a stress signal on pro- and anti-apoptotic machinery in HTLV-1 Tax expressing cells. *Mol Cell Biochem,* 245, 99-113.

Dyson, N. 1998. The regulation of E2F by pRB-family proteins. *Genes Dev,* 12, 2245-62.

Feuer, G. & Green, P. L. 2005. Comparative biology of human T-cell lymphotropic virus type 1 (HTLV-1) and HTLV-2. *Oncogene,* 24, 5996-6004.

Fujisawa, J., Seiki, M., Kiyokawa, T. & Yoshida, M. 1985. Functional activation of the long terminal repeat of human T-cell leukemia-virus type-I by a trans-acting factor. *Proc Natl Acad Sci USA,* 82, 2277-2281.

Fukuda, R., Hayashi, A., Utsunomiya, A., Nukada, Y., Fukui, R., Itoh, K., Tezuka, K., Ohashi, K., Mizuno, K., Sakamoto, M., Hamanoue, M. & Tsuji, T. 2005. Alteration of phosphatidylinositol 3-kinase cascade in the multilobulated nuclear formation of adult T cell leukemia/lymphoma (ATLL). *Proc Natl Acad Sci USA,* 102, 15213-8.

Fukuda, R. I., Tsuchiya, K., Suzuki, K., Itoh, K., Fujita, J., Utsunomiya, A. & Tsuji, T. 2009. Human T-cell leukemia virus type I tax down-regulates the expression of phosphatidylinositol 3,4,5-trisphosphate inositol phosphatases via the NF-κB pathway. *J Biol Chem,* 284, 2680-9.

Gabet, A. S., Mortreux, F., Charneau, P., Riou, P., Duc-Dodon, M., Wu, Y., Jeang, K. T. & Wattel, E. 2003. Inactivation of hTERT transcription by Tax. *Oncogene,* 22, 3734-41.

Gessain, A., Barin, F., Vernant, J. C., Gout, O., Maurs, L., Calender, A. & De The, G. 1985. Antibodies to human T-lymphotropic virus type-I in patients with tropical spastic paraparesis. *Lancet,* 2, 407-10.

Good, L., Maggirwar, S. B. & Sun, S. C. 1996. Activation of the IL-2 gene promoter by HTLV-I tax involves induction of NF-AT complexes bound to the CD28-responsive element. *EMBO J,* 15, 3744-50.

Grassmann, R., Aboud, M. & Jeang, K. T. 2005. Molecular mechanisms of cellular transformation by HTLV-1 Tax. *Oncogene,* 24, 5976-85.

Grassmann, R., Dengler, C., Muller-Fleckenstein, I., Fleckenstein, B., Mcguire, K., Dokhelar, M. C., Sodroski, J. G. & Haseltine, W. A. 1989. Transformation to continuous growth of primary human T lymphocytes by human T-cell leukemia virus type I X-region genes transduced by a Herpesvirus saimiri vector. *Proc Natl Acad Sci USA,* 86, 3351-5.

Hall, W. W. & Fujii, M. 2005. Deregulation of cell-signaling pathways in HTLV-1 infection. *Oncogene,* 24, 5965-75.

Hara, T., Matsumura-Arioka, Y., Ohtani, K. & Nakamura, M. 2008. Role of human T-cell leukemia virus type I Tax in expression of the human telomerase reverse transcriptase (hTERT) gene in human T-cells. *Cancer Sci,* 99, 1155-63.

Higuchi, M., Tsubata, C., Kondo, R., Yoshida, S., Takahashi, M., Oie, M., Tanaka, Y., Mahieux, R., Matsuoka, M. & Fujii, M. 2007. Cooperation of NF-κB2/p100 activation and the PDZ domain binding motif signal in human T-cell leukemia virus type 1 (HTLV-1) Tax1 but not HTLV-2 Tax2 is crucial for interleukin-2-independent growth transformation of a T-cell line. *J Virol,* 81,11900-7.

HINUMA, Y., NAGATA, K., HANAOKA, M., NAKAI, M., MATSUMOTO, T., KINOSHITA, K. I., SHIRAKAWA, S. & MIYOSHI, I. 1981. Adult T-cell leukemia: antigen in an ATL cell line and detection of antibodies to the antigen in human sera. *Proc Natl Acad Sci USA,* 78, 6476–80.

Hori, T., Uchiyama, T., Tsudo, M., Umadome, H., Ohno, H., Fukuhara, S., Kita, K. & Uchino, H. 1987. Establishment of an interleukin 2-dependent human T cell line from a patient with T cell chronic lymphocytic leukemia who is not infected with human T cell leukemia/lymphoma virus. *Blood,* 70, 1069-72.

Hoyos, B., Ballard, D. W., Bohnlein, E., Siekevitz, M. & Greene, W. C. 1989. κB-specific DNA binding proteins: role in the regulation of human interleukin-2 gene expression. *Science,* 244, 457-60.

Huang, Y., Ohtani, K., Iwanaga, R., Matsumura, Y. & Nakamura, M. 2001. Direct transactivation of the human cyclin D2 gene by the oncogene product Tax of human T-cell leukemia virus type I. *Oncogene,* 20, 1094-102.

Iwanaga, R., Ohtani, K., Hayashi, T. & Nakamura, M. 2001. Molecular mechanism of cell cycle progression induced by the oncogene product Tax of human T-cell leukemia virus type I. *Oncogene,* 20, 2055-67.

Jeong, S. J., Dasgupta, A., Jung, K. J., Um, J. H., Burke, A., Park, H. U. & Brady, J. N. 2008. PI3K/AKT inhibition induces caspase-dependent apoptosis in HTLV-1-transformed cells. *Virology,* 370, 264-72.

Jeong, S. J., Pise-Masison, C. A., Radonovich, M. F., Park, H. U. & Brady, J. N. 2005. Activated AKT regulates NF-κB activation, p53 inhibition and cell survival in HTLV-1-transformed cells. *Oncogene,* 24, 6719-28.

Jin, D. Y., Spencer, F. & Jeang, K. T. 1998. Human T cell leukemia virus type 1 oncoprotein Tax targets the human mitotic checkpoint protein MAD1. *Cell,* 93,81-91.

Kannagi, M., Harada, S., Maruyama, I., Inoko, H., Igarashi, H., Kuwashima, G., Sato, S., Morita, M., Kidokoro, M., Sugimoto, M. & ET AL. 1991. Predominant recognition of human T cell leukemia virus type I (HTLV-I) pX gene products by human $CD8^+$ cytotoxic T cells directed against HTLV-I-infected cells. *Int Immunol,* 3, 761-7.

Kao, S. Y., Lemoine, F. J. & Mariott, S. J. 2000. HTLV-1 Tax protein sensitizes cells to apoptotic cell death induced by DNA damaging agents. *Oncogene,* 19, 2240-8.

Karin, M. 2006. Nuclear factor-κB in cancer development and progression. *Nature,* 441, 431-6.

Kelly-Welch, A. E., Hanson, E. M., Boothby, M. R. & Keegan, A. D. 2003. Interleukin-4 and interleukin-13 signaling connections maps. *Science,* 300, 1527-8.

Kim, N. W., Piatyszek, M. A., Prowse, K. R., Harley, C. B., West, M. D., Ho, P. L., Coviello, G. M., Wright, W. E., Weinrich, S. L. & Shay, J. W. 1994. Specific association of human telomerase activity with immortal cells and cancer. *Science,* 266, 2011-5.

Kinoshita, K., Amagasaki, T., Hino, S., Doi, H., Yamanouchi, K., Ban, N., Momita, S., Ikeda, S., Kamihira, S., Ichimaru, M., Katamine, S., Miyamoto, T., Tsuji, Y., Ishimaru, T., Yamabe, T., Ito, M., Kamura, S. & Tsuda, T. 1987. Milk-Borne Transmission of Htlv-I from Carrier Mothers to Their Children. *Jap J Cancer Res,* 78, 674-680.

Levy, D. E. & Darnell, J. E., Jr. 2002. Stats: transcriptional control and biological impact. *Nat Rev Mol Cell Biol,* 3, 651-62.

Liang, M. H., Geisbert, T., Yao, Y., Hinrichs, S. H. & Giam, C. Z. 2002. Human T-lymphotropic virus type 1 oncoprotein tax promotes S-phase entry but blocks mitosis. *J Virol,* 76, 4022-33.

Maeda, N., Fan, H. & Yoshikai, Y. 2008. Oncogenesis by retroviruses: old and new paradigms. *Rev Med Virol,* 18, 387-405.

Majone, F., Semmes, O. J. & Jeang, K. T. 1993. Induction of micronuclei by HTLV-I Tax: a cellular assay for function. *Virology,* 193, 456-9.

Marzec, M., Liu, X., Kasprzycka, M., Witkiewicz, A., Raghunath, P. N., El-Salem, M., Robertson, E., Odum, N. & Wasik, M. A. 2008. IL-2- and IL-15-induced activation of the rapamycin-sensitive mTORC1 pathway in malignant $CD4^+$ T lymphocytes. *Blood,* 111, 2181-9.

Matsumura-Arioka, Y., Ohtani, K., Hara, T., Iwanaga, R. & Nakamura, M. 2005. Identification of two distinct elements mediating activation of telomerase (hTERT) gene expression in association with cell growth in human T cells. *Int Immunol,* 17, 207-15.

Mcguire, K. L., Curtiss, V. E., Larson, E. L. & Haseltine, W. A. 1993. Influence of human T-cell leukemia virus type I tax and rex on interleukin-2 gene expression. *J Virol,* 67, 1590-9.

Meyerson, M., Counter, C. M., Eaton, E. N., Ellisen, L. W., Steiner, P., Caddle, S. D., Ziaugra, L., Beijersbergen, R. L., Davidoff, M. J., Liu, Q., Bacchetti, S., Haber, D. A. & Weinberg, R. A. 1997. hEST2, the putative human telomerase catalytic subunit gene, is up-regulated in tumor cells and during immortalization. *Cell*, 90, 785-95.

Migone, T. S., Lin, J. X., Cereseto, A., Mulloy, J. C., O'shea, J. J., Franchini, G. & Leonard, W. J. 1995. Constitutively activated Jak-STAT pathway in T cells transformed with HTLV-I. *Science*, 269, 79-81.

Mizuguchi, M., Asao, H., Hara, T., Higuchi, M., Fujii, M. & Nakamura, M. 2009. Transcriptional activation of the interleukin-21 gene and its receptor gene by human T-cell leukemia virus type 1 Tax in human T-cells. *J Biol Chem*, 284, 25501-11.

Mori, N., Fujii, M., Ikeda, S., Yamada, Y., Tomonaga, M., Ballard, D. W. & Yamamoto, N. 1999. Constitutive activation of NF-κB in primary adult T-cell leukemia cells. *Blood*, 93, 2360-8.

Nakamura, T. M., Morin, G. B., Chapman, K. B., Weinrich, S. L., Andrews, W. H., Lingner, J., Harley, C. B. & Cech, T. R. 1997. Telomerase catalytic subunit homologs from fission yeast and human. *Science*, 277, 955-9.

Nerenberg, M., Hinrichs, S. H., Reynolds, R. K., Khoury, G. & Jay, G. 1987. The tat gene of human T-lymphotropic virus type 1 induces mesenchymal tumors in transgenic mice. *Science*, 237, 1324-9.

Neuveut, C., Low, K. G., Maldarelli, F., Schmitt, I., Majone, F., Grassmann, R. & Jeang, K. T. 1998. Human T-cell leukemia virus type 1 Tax and cell cycle progression: role of cyclin D-cdk and p110Rb. *Mol Cell Biol*, 18, 3620-32.

Nevins, J. R. 1998. Toward an understanding of the functional complexity of the E2F and retinoblastoma families. *Cell Growth Differ*, 9, 585-93.

Nevins, J. R., Leone, G., Degregori, J. & Jakoi, L. 1997. Role of the Rb/E2F pathway in cell growth control. *J Cell Physiol*, 173, 233-6.

Nicot, C., Harrod, R. L., Ciminale, V. & Franchini, G. 2005. Human T-cell leukemia/lymphoma virus type 1 nonstructural genes and their functions. *Oncogene*, 24, 6026-6034.

Niinuma, A., Higuchi, M., Takahashi, M., Oie, M., Tanaka, Y., Gejyo, F., Tanaka, N., Sugamura, K., Xie, L., Green, P. L. & Fujii, M. 2005. Aberrant activation of the interleukin-2 autocrine loop through the nuclear factor of activated T cells by nonleukemogenic human T-cell leukemia virus type 2 but not by leukemogenic type 1 virus. *J Virol*, 79, 11925-34.

Ohbo, K., Takasawa, N., Ishii, N., Tanaka, N., Nakamura, M. & Sugamura, K. 1995. Functional analysis of the human interleukin 2 receptor γ chain gene promoter. *J Biol Chem*, 270, 7479-86.

Ohtani, K., Iwanaga, R., Arai, M., Huang, Y., Matsumura, Y. & Nakamura, M. 2000. Cell type-specific E2F activation and cell cycle progression induced by the oncogene product Tax of human T-cell leukemia virus type I. *J Biol Chem*, 275, 11154-63.

Olovnikov, A. M. 1973. A theory of marginotomy. The incomplete copying of template margin in enzymic synthesis of polynucleotides and biological significance of the phenomenon. *J Theor Biol*, 41, 181-90.

Onoda, T., Rahman, M., Nara, H., Araki, A., Makabe, K., Tsumoto, K., Kumagai, I., Kudo, T., Ishii, N., Tanaka, N., Sugamura, K., Hayasaka, K. & Asao, H. 2007. Human $CD4^+$ central and effector memory T cells produce IL-21: effect on cytokine-driven proliferation of CD4+ T cell subsets. *Int Immunol*, 19, 1191-9.

Osame, M., Usuku, K., Izumo, S., Ijichi, N., Amitani, H., Igata, A., Matsumoto, M. & Tara, M. 1986. HTLV-I associated myelopathy, a new clinical entity. *Lancet*, 1, 1031-2.

Parrish-Novak, J., Dillon, S. R., Nelson, A., Hammond, A., Sprecher, C., Gross, J. A., Johnston, J., Madden, K., Xu, W., West, J., Schrader, S., Burkhead, S., Heipel, M., Brandt, C., Kuijper, J. L., Kramer, J., Conklin, D., Presnell, S. R., Berry, J., Shiota, F., Bort, S., Hambly, K., Mudri, S., Clegg, C., Moore, M., Grant, F. J., Lofton-Day, C., Gilbert, T., Rayond, F., Ching, A., Yao, L., Smith, D., Webster, P., Whitmore, T., Maurer, M., Kaushansky, K., Holly, R. D. & Foster, D. 2000. Interleukin 21 and its receptor are involved in NK cell expansion and regulation of lymphocyte function. *Nature,* 408, 57-63.

Peloponese, J. M., Jr. & Jeang, K. T. 2006. Role for Akt/protein kinase B and activator protein-1 in cellular proliferation induced by the human T-cell leukemia virus type 1 tax oncoprotein. *J Biol Chem,* 281, 8927-38.

Pise-Masison, C. A., Mahieux, R., Jiang, H., Ashcroft, M., Radonovich, M., Duvall, J., Guillerm, C. & Brady, J. N. 2000. Inactivation of p53 by human T-cell lymphotropic virus type 1 Tax requires activation of the NF-κB pathway and is dependent on p53 phosphorylation. *Mol Cell Biol,* 20, 3377-86.

Poiesz, B. J., Ruscetti, F. W., Gazdar, A. F., Bunn, P. A., Minna, J. D. & Gallo, R. C. 1980. Detection and isolation of type C retrovirus particles from fresh and cultured lymphocytes of a patient with cutaneous T-cell lymphoma. *Proc Natl Acad Sci USA,* 77, 7415-9.

Proietti, F. A., Carneiro-Proietti, A. B., Catalan-Soares, B. C. & Murphy, E. L. 2005. Global epidemiology of HTLV-I infection and associated diseases. *Oncogene,* 24, 6058-68.

Robek, M. D. & Ratner, L. 1999. Immortalization of $CD4^+$ and $CD8^+$ T lymphocytes by human T-cell leukemia virus type 1 Tax mutants expressed in a functional molecular clone. *J Virol,* 73, 4856-65.

Rochman, Y., Spolski, R. & Leonard, W. J. 2009. New insights into the regulation of T cells by γc family cytokines. *Nat Rev Immunol,* 9, 480-90.

Rohrschneider, L. R., Fuller, J. F., Wolf, I., Liu, Y. & Lucas, D. M. 2000. Structure, function, and biology of SHIP proteins. *Genes Dev,* 14, 505-20.

Ross, T. M., Narayan, M., Fang, Z. Y., Minella, A. C. & Green, P. L. 2000. Human T-cell leukemia virus type 2 tax mutants that selectively abrogate NFκB or CREB/ATF activation fail to transform primary human T cells. *J Virol,* 74, 2655-62.

Ruben, S., Poteat, H., Tan, T. H., Kawakami, K., Roeder, R., Haseltine, W. & Rosen, C. A. 1988. Cellular transcription factors and regulation of IL-2 receptor gene expression by HTLV-I tax gene product. *Science,* 241, 89-92.

Santiago, F., Clark, E., Chong, S., Molina, C., Mozafari, F., Mahieux, R., Fujii, M., Azimi, N. & Kashanchi, F. 1999. Transcriptional up-regulation of the cyclin D2 gene and acquisition of new cyclin-dependent kinase partners in human T-cell leukemia virus type 1-infected cells. *J Virol,* 73, 9917-27.

Sarbassov, D. D., Guertin, D. A., Ali, S. M. & Sabatini, D. M. 2005. Phosphorylation and regulation of Akt/PKB by the rictor-mTOR complex. *Science,* 307, 1098-101.

Schmitt, I., Rosin, O., Rohwer, P., Gossen, M. & Grassmann, R. 1998. Stimulation of cyclin-dependent kinase activity and G1- to S-phase transition in human lymphocytes by the human T-cell leukemia/lymphotropic virus type 1 Tax protein. *J Virol,* 72, 633-40.

Semmes, O. J. & Jeang, K. T. 1996. Localization of human T-cell leukemia virus type 1 tax to subnuclear compartments that overlap with interchromatin speckles. *J Virol,* 70, 6347-57.

Shoji, T., Higuchi, M., Kondo, R., Takahashi, M., Oie, M., Tanaka, Y., Aoyagi, Y. & Fujii, M. 2009. Identification of a novel motif responsible for the distinctive transforming activity of human T-cell leukemia virus (HTLV) type 1 Tax1 protein from HTLV-2 Tax2. *Retrovirology,* 6, 83.

Silbermann, K., Schneider, G. & Grassmann, R. 2008. Stimulation of interleukin-13 expression by human T-cell leukemia virus type 1 oncoprotein Tax via a dually active promoter element responsive to NF-κB and NFAT. *J Gen Virol,* 89, 2788-98.

Sinha-Datta, U., Horikawa, I., Michishita, E., Datta, A., Sigler-Nicot, J. C., Brown, M., Kazanji, M., Barrett, J. C. & Nicot, C. 2004. Transcriptional activation of hTERT through the NF-κB pathway in HTLV-I-transformed cells. *Blood,* 104, 2523-31.

Sodroski, J. G., Rosen, C. A. & Haseltine, W. A. 1984. Trans-acting transcriptional activation of the long terminal repeat of human T-lymphotropic viruses in infected-cells. *Science,* 225, 381-385.

Tabakin-Fix, Y., Azran, I., Schavinky-Khrapunsky, Y., Levy, O. & Aboud, M. 2006. Functional inactivation of p53 by human T-cell leukemia virus type 1 Tax protein: mechanisms and clinical implications. *Carcinogenesis,* 27, 673-81.

Takeshita, T., Asao, H., Ohtani, K., Ishii, N., Kumaki, S., Tanaka, N., Munakata, H., Nakamura, M. & Sugamura, K. 1992. Cloning of the γ chain of the human IL-2 receptor. *Science,* 257, 379-82.

Tanaka, A., Takahashi, C., Yamaoka, S., Nosaka, T., Maki, M. & Hatanaka, M. 1990. Oncogenic transformation by the tax gene of human T-cell leukemia virus type I in vitro. *Proc Natl Acad Sci USA,* 87, 1071-5.

Tanaka, N., Asao, H., Ohbo, K., Ishii, N., Takeshita, T., Nakamura, M., Sasaki, H. & Sugamura, K. 1994. Physical association of JAK1 and JAK2 tyrosine kinases with the interleukin 2 receptor β and γ chains. *Proc Natl Acad Sci USA,* 91, 7271-5.

Trimarchi, J. M. & Lees, J. A. 2002. Sibling rivalry in the E2F family. *Nat Rev Mol Cell Biol,* 3, 11-20.

Tsukahara, T., Kannagi, M., Ohashi, T., Kato, H., Arai, M., Nunez, G., Iwanaga, Y., Yamamoto, N., Ohtani, K., Nakamura, M. & Fujii, M. 1999. Induction of Bcl-xL expression by human T-cell leukemia virus type 1 Tax through NF-κB in apoptosis-resistant T-cell transfectants with Tax. *J Virol,* 73,7981-7.

Uchida, N., Otsuka, T., Arima, F., Shigematsu, H., Fukuyama, T., Maeda, M., Sugio, Y., Itoh, Y. & Niho, Y. 1999. Correlation of telomerase activity with development and progression of adult T-cell leukemia. *Leuk Res,* 23, 311-6.

Van Orden, K., Yan, J. P., Ulloa, A. & Nyborg, J. K. 1999. Binding of the human T-cell leukemia virus Tax protein to the coactivator CBP interferes with CBP-mediated transcriptional control. *Oncogene,* 18, 3766-72.

Waldele, K., Schneider, G., Ruckes, T. & Grassmann, R. 2004. Interleukin-13 overexpression by tax transactivation: a potential autocrine stimulus in human T-cell leukemia virus-infected lymphocytes. *J Virol,* 78, 6081-90.

Watson, J. D. 1972. Origin of concatemeric T7 DNA. *Nat New Biol,* 239, 197-201.

Yoshida, M. 2001. Multiple viral strategies of HTLV-1 for dysregulation of cell growth control. *Annu Rev Immunol,* 19, 475-496.

Yoshida, M., Miyoshi, I. & Hinuma, Y. 1982. Isolation and characterization of retrovirus from cell lines of human adult T-cell leukemia and its implication in the disease. *Proc Natl Acad Sci USA,* 79, 2031-5.

Yu, H., Pardoll, D. & Jove, R. 2009. STATs in cancer inflammation and immunity: a leading role for STAT3. *Nat Rev Cancer,* 9, 798-809.

Zeng, R., Spolski, R., Casas, E., Zhu, W., Levy, D. E. & Leonard, W. J. 2007. The molecular basis of IL-21-mediated proliferation. *Blood,* 109, 4135-42.

4

Host Immune System Abnormalities Among Patients with Human T-Lymphotropic Virus Type 1 (HTLV-1)-Associated Disorders

Tomoo Sato, Natsumi Araya, Naoko Yagishita,
Hitoshi Ando and Yoshihisa Yamano
*Department of Rare Diseases Research, Institute of Medical Science,
St. Marianna University School of Medicine,
Japan*

1. Introduction

Human T-cell lymphotropic virus type 1 (HTLV-1) is a human retrovirus that causes persistent infection in the host. While most infected persons remain asymptomatic carriers (ACs), 3–5% develop a T-cell malignancy termed adult T-cell leukemia (ATL) (Uchiyama et al., 1977), and another 0.25–3% develop a chronic progressive inflammatory neurologic disease known as HTLV-1-associated myelopathy/tropical spastic paraparesis (HAM/TSP) (Gessain et al., 1985; Osame et al. 1986). Although HTLV-1-associated disorders have been extensively studied, the exact mechanism by which they are induced by HTLV-1 is not completely understood. The proviral load of HTLV-1 could contribute to the development of these disorders, since the circulating number of HTLV-1-infected T cells in the peripheral blood is associated with the risk of developing HAM/TSP and ATL (Iwanaga et al., 2010; Nagai et al. 1998). However, more detail on the precise immune mechanisms controlling HTLV-1-infected cells is still needed.

HTLV-1 preferentially infects $CD4^+$ T cells, the central regulators of the acquired immune system (Richardson et al., 1990). This is known to induce a variety of abnormalities, such as proliferation, cellular activation, and proinflammatory changes (Boxus et al., 2009; Satou et al., 2010; Yamano et al. 2009). These abnormalities, in turn, may deregulate the balance of the host immune system.

HTLV-1 also causes abnormalities among uninfected immune cells. Patients with HTLV-1-associated disorders demonstrate abnormalities in both the amount and function of CD8+ cytotoxic T lymphocytes (CTL), an important component of host immune response against HTLV-1 (Bangham 2009; Kannagi et al., 2011; Matsuura et al., 2010). Patients with ATL and HAM/TSP may also experience reductions in the amount and efficacy of cellular components of innate immunity, which is vital in regulating the immune response against general viral infections and cancers (Azakami et al., 2009; Matsuura et al., 2010). In this chapter, we have summarized the host immune system abnormalities that are associated with HTLV-1 infection.

2. Abnormality of HTLV-1-infected $CD4^+$ T cells

2.1 $CD4^+CD25^+CCR4^+$ T Cells are a major reservoir of HTLV-1-infected T cells, which increase in HAM/TSP and ATL patients

HTLV-1 mainly infects $CD4^+$ T helper (Th) cells, which play a central role in adaptive immune responses (Richardson et al., 1990). $CD4^+$ Th cells recruit and activate other immune cells, including B cells, CD8 T cells, macrophages, mast cells, neutrophils, eosinophils, and basophils (Zhu et al., 2010). Based on their function, their pattern of cytokine secretion, and their expression of specific transcription factors and chemokine receptors, $CD4^+$ Th cells, differentiated from naïve $CD4^+$ T cells, are classified into 4 major lineages: Th1, Th2, Th17, and T regulatory (Treg) cells. To understand the effects of HTLV-1 infection on the function of CD4 Th cells, it is necessary to know which Th population HTLV-1 infects.

It was recently shown that the chemokine receptor CCR4 is expressed on HTLV-1-infected leukemia cells in ATL patients (Yoshie et al., 2002). CCR4 is selectively expressed on suppressive T cell subsets, such as Treg and Th2 cells, in HTLV-1-seronegative healthy individuals (Yoshie et al., 2001). Using molecular and immunological techniques, we also demonstrated that $CD4^+CD25^+CCR4^+$ T cells were the predominant viral reservoir in both ACs and HAM/TSP patients, and that this T cell subset was increased in HAM/TSP patients (Yamano et al., 2009). Thus, $CD4^+CD25^+CCR4^+$ T cells are a major population of HTLV-1-infected T cells, which increase in number in both HAM/TSP and ATL patients.

The molecular mechanism of HTLV-1 tropism to CCR4 expressing $CD4^+$ T cells was recently uncovered (Hieshima et al., 2008). HTLV-1 Tax, a transcriptional regulator encoded by the HTLV-1 genome, does not induce expression of CCR4, but it does induce expression of CCL22, the ligand for CCR4. Because HTLV-1-infected T cells selectively interact with $CCR4^+CD4^+$ T cells, this results in preferential transmission of HTLV-1 to $CCR4^+CD4^+$ T cells.

2.2 Differences in the fates of $CD4^+CD25^+CCR4^+$ T cells in HAM/TSP and ATL patients

Among $CD4^+$ Th cells, the major reservoir of HTLV-1 is $CD4^+CD25^+CCR4^+$ T cells, including suppressive T cell subsets such as Treg and Th2 under healthy conditions. The exact mechanism by which HTLV-1 induces the deregulation of the host immune system is not completely understood. However, the recent discovery of Treg cells has provided new opportunities and generated increased interest in this issue. In healthy individuals, Treg cells suppress the proliferation of, and cytokine production by, pathogenic T cells, and thereby plays a key role in the maintenance of immune system homeostasis (Sakaguchi et al., 1995). Treg cells can be identified *ex vivo* by the intracellular expression of the transcriptional regulator Foxp3 (Hori et al., 2003), which is critical for the development and function of Treg cells in both mice and humans.

Significant reductions in Foxp3 expression and/or Treg cell function have been observed in several human autoimmune diseases (Sakaguchi et al., 2008), suggesting that defects in Foxp3 expression and/or Treg function may precipitate the loss of immunologic tolerance. Recently, significant reductions in Foxp3 expression and Treg cell function have also been observed in $CD4^+CD25^+$ T cells and/or $CD4^+CD25^+CCR4^+$ T cells from patients with HAM/TSP (Hayashi et al., 2008; Michaelsson et al., 2008; Oh et al., 2006; Ramirez et al., 2010; Yamano et al., 2005). Furthermore, decreased expression levels of the Treg-associated immune suppressive molecules CTLA-4 and GITR were also observed on $CD4^+CD25^+$ T cells in HAM/TSP patients (Ramirez et al., 2010; Yamano et al., 2005). Notably, overexpression of HTLV-1 *tax* can reduce

Foxp3 expression and inhibit the suppressive function of Treg cells (Yamano et al., 2005). Furthermore, because of a Tax-induced defect in TGF-β signaling, HAM/TSP patients experience reductions in Foxp3 expression and impairment of Treg function (Grant et al., 2008). Moreover, a significant reduction in $CD4^+CD25^+Foxp3^+$ Treg cells was demonstrated in HTLV-1-*tax*-expressing transgenic mice, which develop an inflammatory arthropathy (Ohsugi et al., 2011). Thus, HAM/TSP patients display a decreased ratio of $Foxp3^+$ Treg cells within HTLV-1-infected $CD4^+CD25^+CCR4^+$ T cells.

Importantly, a more detailed flow cytometric analysis of Foxp3 expression in $CD4^+CD25^+CCR4^+$ T cells demonstrated that the frequency of "$Foxp3^-$ population" was extraordinary high in HAM/TSP patients (Yamano et al., 2009). Moreover, an analysis of proinflammatory cytokine expression in this $Foxp3^-CD4^+CD25^+CCR4^+$ T cell subset demonstrated that these cells were unique because, in healthy individuals, they produced multiple proinflammatory cytokines such as IL-2, IL-17, and few interferon (IFN)-γ, while $Foxp3^+CD4^+CD25^+CCR4^+$ T cells (Treg cells) did not. Furthermore, HAM/TSP patients were found to exhibit only a few $Foxp3^+CD4^+CD25^+CCR4^+$ T cells that did not produce such cytokines. Rather, these patients had an increased number of $Foxp3^-CD4^+CD25^+CCR4^+$ T cells, which were found to overproduce IFN-γ. Further, given the increase of clinical diseases and severity of HAM/TSP observed in these patients, it appears likely that the frequency of these IFN-γ-producing $Foxp3^-CD4^+CD25^+CCR4^+$ T cells may have a functional consequence (Yamano et al., 2009). Thus, while the $CD4^+CD25^+CCR4^+$ T cell population in healthy patients mainly comprises suppressive T cell subsets such as Treg and Th2, HAM/TSP patients possess an increased proportion of IFN-γ-producing $Foxp3^-CD4^+CD25^+CCR4^+$ T cells, which are rarely encountered in healthy individuals and lead to an overproduction of IFN-γ (Figure 1).

Although Foxp3 expression is decreased by $CD4^+CD25^+$ ($CCR4^+$) T cells in HAM/TSP patients (Hayashi et al., 2008; Michaelsson et al., 2008; Oh et al., 2006; Ramirez et al., 2010; Yamano et al., 2005), it is increased by $CD4^+CD25^+$($CCR4^+$) ATL cells in most ATL patients (Karube et al., 2004; Roncador et al., 2005) (Figure 1). Therefore, it has been hypothesized that ATL cells may be derived from Treg cells (Kohno et al., 2005). Interestingly, some ATL cells exhibit immunosuppressive functions similar to those of Treg cells, which may contribute to the cellular immunodeficiency that has been clinically observed in ATL patients (Chen et al., 2006; Kohno et al., 2005; Matsubar et al., 2006); however, some ATL cells lose this regulatory function (Shimauchi et al., 2008).

2.3 HTLV-1 may induce plasticity of Foxp3+ cells into exFoxp3+ cell

In HTLV-1-seronegative healthy individuals, $CD4^+CD25^+CCR4^+$ T cells mainly include suppressive T cell subsets such as Treg and Th2 (Yoshie et al., 2001). In ATL patients, most of this subset develops leukemogenesis by maintaining the $Foxp3^+$ Treg phenotype (Figure 1). However, as mentioned above, T cells of this subset become Th1-like cells that overproduce IFN-γ in HAM/TSP patients (Figure 1). Since HTLV-1 may preferentially transmit to $CCR4^+CD4^+$ T cells, these findings suggest that HTLV-1 may intracellularly induce T-cell plasticity of Treg cells into IFN-$γ^+$ T cells. Indeed, one recent report indicated that loss of Foxp3 in Treg cells and acquisition of IFN-γ may result in the conversion of suppressor T cells into highly autoaggressive lymphocytes (ex$Foxp3^+$ cells), which can favor the development of autoimmune conditions (Tsuji et al., 2009; Zhou et al., 2009). Importantly, Toulza et al. (2008) demonstrated that the rate of CTL-mediated lysis was negatively correlated with the number of HTLV-1-Tax- CD4+Foxp3+ cells, but not with the number of Tax+ CD4+Foxp3+ cells, suggesting that HTLV-1-infected Treg cells lose their regulatory function, while HTLV-1-uninfected Treg cells contribute substantially to immune control of HTLV-1 infection. Additionally, functional impairment of CD4+Foxp3+ Treg cells was observed in mice that were transgenic mice for the *HTLV-1 bZIP factor* (*HBZ*) gene, which encodes the minus strand of HTLV-1 (Satou et al., 2011). These findings support the hypothesis that HTLV-1 may be one of the exogenous retrovirus genes responsible for immune dysregulation through interference of CD4+CD25+ Treg cell function. This hypothesis is currently under investigation to elucidate the precise molecular mechanisms by which HTLV-1 influences the fate and function of CD4+CD25+CCR4+ T cells, especially Foxp3+ Treg cells.

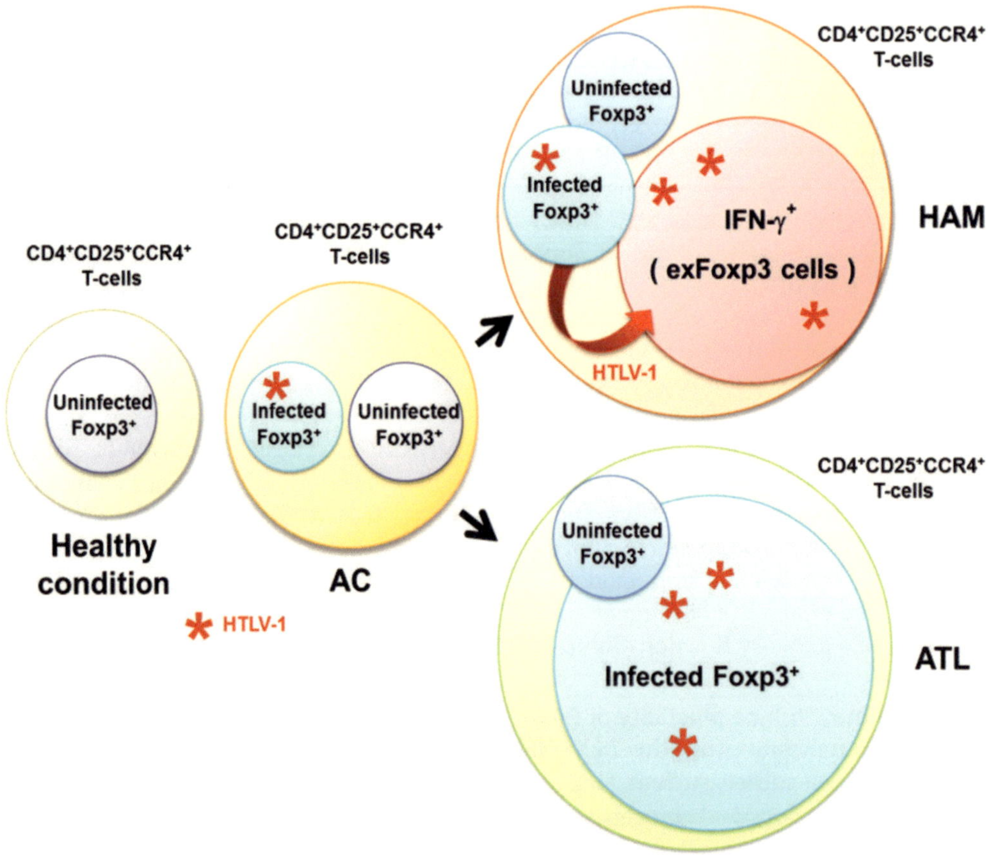

Fig. 1. Cellular components of CD4+CD25+CCR4+ T cells in healthy individuals, asymptomatic carriers, ATL, and HAM/TSP patients.

3. Abnormality of cytotoxic T lymphocyte (CTL) response

CD8+ Cytotoxic T lymphocyte (CTL) responses are an effective host defense system against all virus infections and malignancies. CTLs act by killing autologous cells that express viral or cancer antigen in association with major histocompatibility complex (MHC) class I molecules and by suppressing viral replication and tumor development via IFN-γ secretion. Elucidating the role of HTLV-1–specific CD8+ CTLs has been considered a priority issue in studies of host defense mechanisms involved in HTLV-1 infection (Bangham, 2008; Jacobson, 2002; Kannagi, 2007).

3.1 HTLV-1-specific cytotoxic T lymphocytes

T-cell receptors (TCR) on CTLs recognize peptide fragments derived from viral and tumor antigens that are presented on MHC class I molecules by antigen-presenting cells or virus-infected cells. After TCR binds to the peptide-MHC complex, CTLs are activated and fulfill an effector function. There are 3 main effector mechanisms by which the CD8+ CTL kills virus-infected or tumor cells. One is to release perforin and granzymes. Perforin forms pores in the plasma membrane of the target cells, allowing entry of granzymes; caspases are then activated, leading to apoptosis. Apoptosis may also be induced via a Fas-FasL interaction between CTLs and target cells. Finally, CD8+ cells can produce IFN-γ, which has indirect cytolytic effects by promoting NK cell activity and macrophage activation.
The Tax protein is an immunodominant antigen in HTLV-1 infections. Therefore, CTL activity is predominantly restricted to products of the HTLV-1 Tax gene, although HTLV-1 Env, Pol, Rof, Tof, and HBZ (Elovaara et al., 1993; Hilburn et al., 2011; Macnamara et al., 2010; Pique et al., 2000) could also be target proteins of HTLV-1-specific CTL. In a study that utilized properties of the CTL antigen recognition system, human MHC class I HLA-A2(*0201) tetramers loaded with HTLV-1 Tax peptide were used to detect HTLV-1 Tax specific HLA-A2-restricted CD8+ cells (Bieganowska et al., 1999, Greten et al., 1998). This technique facilitates quantification of the frequency of antigen-specific T cells, as well as direct characterization of these cells. HLA genotype determines which part of the viral protein is presented as an antigen peptide. For HLA-A*0201 and HLA-A*2402, for example, the major epitopes are the Tax 11-19 and Tax 301-309 amino acids, respectively.

3.2 Abnormal CTL response in patients with ATL

An increasing number of studies in patients with HTLV-1-associated disorders have documented an association between the disorders and abnormalities in both the frequency of CTLs and their response to HTLV-1. When peripheral blood mononuclear cells (PBMCs) from HTLV-1 carriers are stimulated with autologous HTLV-1–infected cells *in vitro*, proliferation of HTLV-1-specific CD8+ CTLs is often observed in the presence of IL-2. An increased level of HTLV-1–specific CTL responses occurs in all HAM/TSP patients and in some asymptomatic HTLV-1 carriers; however, HTLV-1–specific CTL responses are rarely induced in PBMC cultures from ATL patients (Jacobson et al., 1990; Kannagi et al., 1984, Parker et al., 1992). HTLV-1–specific CTLs are also present in ATL patients but do not expand sufficiently (Arnulf et al., 2004). Impairment of the HTLV-1 specific CTL response was observed in some individuals during the earlier stages of HTLV-1 infection (AC and smoldering ATL), as well as in advanced ATL patients (Shimizu et al., 2009). This observation suggests that the T-cell insufficiency in ATL patients is present prior to disease onset. In addition, a recent report indicated that, in comparison to ACs, ATL patients have a smaller and less diverse population of HTLV-1 specific CD8+ T cells, as well as lower anti-HTLV-1 CD8+ T cell expression of perforin and granzyme B (Kozako et al., 2006). Thus, the decreased number and functional impairment of CTLs might contribute to the onset and progression of ATL.

Furthermore, Tax-specific CTL responses were strongly activated in some ATL patients who achieved complete remission after hematopoietic stem cell transplantation (HSCT), but were not observed in the same patients before transplantation (Harashima et al., 2004). This suggests that HTLV-1-specific CTLs, including Tax-specific CTLs, play an important role in surveillance against HTLV-1 leukemogenesis.

3.3 Abnormal CTL response in patients with HAM/TSP

One of the most striking features of the adaptive immune system in HAM/TSP patients is the larger number of HTLV-1-specific $CD8^+$ CTLs (Elovaara et al., 1993; Greten et al., 1998; Jacobson et al., 1990; Kubota et al., 2002; Nagai et al., 2001a; Parker et al., 1992). While HTLV-1 specific CTLs are also detectable in the PBMC of ACs (Parker et al., 1992), the magnitude and frequency of these responses are clearly higher in patients with HAM/TSP, particularly in the CSF (Elovaara et al., 1993; Nagai et al. 2001a). In addition, the HTLV-1 proviral load of HAM/TSP patients may be 5- to 16-fold higher than that of ACs (Hashimoto et al., 1998; Kubota et al., 1993; Nagai et al., 1998). While some studies have found a positive correlation between the frequency of HTLV-1-specific $CD8^+$ T cells and HTLV-1 proviral load has been detected in PBMCs from HAM/TSP patients (Kubota et al., 2000, Nagai et al., 2001b, Yamano et al., 2002), this result is not ubiquitous (Wodarz et al., 2001). Thus, the cytolytic activity of CTLs, rather than their frequency, might be impaired in HAM/TSP patients.

There are some methods to measure CTL cytolytic activity. One is the sensitive CD107a mobilization assay, which quantifies the amount of lysosomal membrane protein LAMP-1 (CD107a) present on the CTL surface (CD107a) (Betts et al. 2003). Among studies that have used this method to evaluate CTL function, results are conflicting; while one reported that HTLV-1-specific CTLs of HAM/TSP patients had significantly lower CD107a staining than those of ACs (Sabouri et al., 2008), another study reported the opposite (Abdelbary et al., 2011). Furthermore, higher expression of CD107a/IFN-γ was induced by tax peptide stimulation in the $CD8^+$ T cells of HAM/TSP patients than in those of ACs (Enose-Akahata et al., 2008). Thus, it is not yet clear whether the cytolytic activity of HTLV-1-specific CTL in HAM/TSP patients is insufficient. However, these findings suggest that quantity of HTLV-1-infected cells is not determined by HTLV-1-specific CTL alone; additional factors, such as innate immunity and the proliferative ability of infected cells, must be relevant.

3.4 Pathogenic Role of CTL in HAM/TSP

In HAM/TSP patients, HTLV-1-specific $CD8^+$ CTL levels are extraordinarily high in peripheral blood, and even higher in cerebrospinal fluid (CSF) (Elovaara et al., 1993; Greten et al., 1998; Jacobson et al., 1990; Kubota et al., 2002; Parker et al., 1994; Nagai et al., 2001; Yamano et al., 2002). Immunohistochemical analysis of affected spinal cord lesions in early-stage HAM/TSP patients revealed the presence of infiltrating $CD4^+$ and $CD8^+$ lymphocytes, among which $CD8^+$ cells become increasingly dominant over the duration of the illness (Umehara et al., 1993). The expression of HLA class I antigens (Moore et al., 1989) and the existence of HTLV-1 specific $CD8^+$ CTLs have also been found in such lesions (Levin et al., 1997). In addition, the infiltration of $CD8^+$ CTLs in the affected spinal cord was characterized as positive for TIA-1 that is a marker of CTL (Umehara et al. 1994, Anderson et al. 1990). The number of TIA-1^+ cells was clearly related to the amount of the proviral DNA *in situ*, and the number of infiltrating $CD8^+$ cells appears to correlate with the presence of apoptotic cells.

Tax-specific $CD8^+$ CTL clones secrete various inflammatory cytokines, chemokines, and matrix metalloproteinases (MMP), such as IFN-γ, TNF-α, monocyte inflammatory protein (MIP)-1α, MIP-1β, interleukin(IL)-16, and MMP-9 (Biddison et al., 1997). TNF-α induces cytotoxic damage to endothelial cells, thus decreasing the integrity of the blood-brain barrier. It can also directly injure oligodendrocytes. MIP-1α and 1β can enhance transendothelial migration of lymphocytes into the central nervous system. IL-16 is a chemoattractant for $CD4^+$ cells, which are the major source of IL-2 required by IL-2 non-producer $CD8^+$ cells for proliferation. Therefore, HTLV-1-specific $CD8^+$ CTLs are an important source of proinflammatory soluble mediators that may contribute significantly to the pathogenesis of HAM/TSP. These observations continue to support the hypothesis that HTLV-1-specific $CD8^+$ CTLs are a major contributing factor in the immunopathogenesis of HAM/TSP.

4. Abnormality of innate immunity

Besides CTLs, there are several cell populations in the human immune system that have cytolytic activity against virus-infected cells, including natural killer (NK) cells, natural killer T (NKT) cells, and γδ T cells, which are cellular components of innate immunity. Dendritic cells (DCs) play an important role in the activation of these cell populations and CTLs. There is little evidence suggesting a role for γδ T cells in the pathogenesis of HTLV-1-associated disorders. Thus, this section focuses solely on the roles of DCs, NK cells, and NKT cells in HTLV-1-associated diseases, by comparing with the role of these cells in HIV-1 infection.

4.1 Dendritic cells and HTLV-1

Immature DCs are located in peripheral tissues and can effectively capture antigens, leading to their maturation via the expression of MHC class I/II and co-stimulatory molecules such as CD80, CD86, and CD40. Mature DCs are professional antigen-presenting cells that are uniquely able to prime naïve T cells. There are 2 main subsets of DCs: myeloid DCs (mDCs) and plasmacytoid DCs (pDCs). These cells play important roles in the regulation of innate and adaptive immunity. mDCs can induce the activation of invariant NKT (iNKT) cells via surface expression of the CD1d/glycolipid complex. After antigen capture, pDCs secrete type 1 IFN, which induces the activation of NK cells and promotes the activation of iNKT cells by mDCs.
An *in vitro* study indicated that cell-free HTLV-1 effectively infects DCs, leading to the transmission and transformation of $CD4^+$ T cells (Jones et al. 2008). In addition to suggesting a mechanism for HTLV-1 transmission, this study also indicated that HTLV-1 infection of DCs plays a role in the pathogenesis of HTLV-1-associated disorders. In fact, HTLV-1-infected DCs are observed in the peripheral blood of HTLV-1-infected individuals (Hishizawa et al., 2004; Macatonia et al., 1992), and infected pDCs have an impaired ability to produce type I IFN (Azakami et al., 2009; Hishizawa et al., 2004). In addition, we recently reported that the frequency of mDCs and pDCs is significantly lower in patients with both HAM/TSP and ATL (Azakami et al., 2009). Cumulatively, these studies imply that decreases in the number and functionality of DCs interfere with innate immunity, thus leading to pathogenesis.

4.2 Natural killer cells and HTLV-1

NK cells are major components of the innate immune system and account for 10–15% of PBMCs in normal individuals. They have direct and indirect cytolytic activity against tumor cells and virus-infected cells by producing perforins, granzymes, and IFN-γ. Human NK cells can be divided into 2 subsets on the basis of their cell-surface markers: $CD56^{+}CD16^{+}$ and $CD56^{bright}CD16^{-}$ NK cells. $CD56^{+}CD16^{+}$ NK cells are the major population of NK cells and have natural cytotoxic activity. $CD56^{bright}CD16^{-}$ NK cells are not cytotoxic but have the capacity to produce large amounts of IFN-γ upon activation. The activity of NK cells is regulated by a balance between positive and negative signals from different activating and inhibitory NK receptors. CD94/NKG2 receptor family is expressed on $CD8^{+}$ T cells and γδ T cells as well as NK cells, and is involved in the pathogenesis of HAM/TSP by modulating the activities of those cell populations (Saito et al. 2003, Mosley et al. 2005).

In both HIV-1- and HTLV-1-infected individuals, the number and function of NK cell subsets are impaired (Fortis et al., 2005). Multiple investigators have reported that the numbers of $CD56^{+}CD16^{+}$ NK cells in HAM/TSP and ATL patients are significantly lower than those observed in healthy controls (Azakami et al., 2009; Yu et al., 1991). Furthermore, NK cell activity was also lower in HAM/TSP patients than in healthy controls (Yu et al., 1991). When primary $CD4^{+}$ T cells are infected by HTLV-1, they can escape from NK cell-mediated cytotoxicity; HTLV-1 $p12^{I}$ downregulates the expression of intercellular adhesion molecule-1 (ICAM-1) and -2 on the surface of infected $CD4^{+}$ T cells, resulting in a reduced adherence of NK cells to HTLV-1-infected $CD4^{+}$ T cells (Banerjee et al., 2007).

4.3 Natural killer T cells and HTLV-1

Natural killer T (NKT) cells, a unique T cell subpopulation, constitute a subset of lymphocytes that share the features of innate and adaptive immune cells. Unlike conventional T cells, NKT cells express a TCR that recognizes glycolipids instead of protein antigens. Moreover, these cells share properties and receptors with NK cells. They rapidly produce granzymes and perforins upon stimulation. Among the $CD3^{+}$ T cells in human blood, 10–25% express NK cell surface molecules such as CD161, and these cells are classified as NKT cells. A small population of T cells within this NKT cell subset expresses a highly conserved Vα24Jα18 TCR chain that preferentially associates with Vβ11; these T cells are referred to as iNKT cells. Activation of human iNKT cells requires the presentation of glycolipids such as α-galactosylceramide (α-GalCer) on the MHC class I-like molecule CD1d. α-GalCer induces the rapid production of cytokines and potent antitumor and antipathogen responses by iNKT cells. $CD4^{-}$ iNKT cells preferentially induce the Th1 response and are more important than $CD4^{+}$ iNKT cells in controlling viral infection and cancer (Kim et al., 2002).

HIV-1-infected subjects have fewer iNKT cells in their peripheral blood than healthy donors (Sandberg et al., 2002; van der Vliet et al., 2002). The proliferative potential and INF-γ production of residual iNKT cells are impaired in HIV-1-infected individuals (Moll et al., 2009); likewise, patients with HTLV-1-associated disorders have a decreased frequency of iNKT cells in their peripheral blood (Azakami et al., 2009). Interestingly, in contrast to patterns observed in HIV-1 infections, HTLV-1 infection leads to preferential decreases of $CD4^{-}$ iNKT cells (Azakami et al., 2009). The production of perforin in iNKT cells is impaired in both ACs and HAM/TSP patients (Azakami et al., 2009). In addition, there is an inverse correlation between the frequency of iNKT cells and the HTLV-1 proviral load in the peripheral blood of HTLV-1-infected individuals (Azakami et al., 2009). Notably, *in vitro* stimulation of peripheral blood cells with α-GalCer leads to an increase in the number of iNKT cells and a subsequent decrease in the number of HTLV-1-infected T cells in samples from ACs (Azakami et al., 2009). These results suggest that iNKT cells contribute to the immune defense against HTLV-1, and that iNKT cell depletion plays an important role in the pathogenesis of HAM/TSP and ATL.

5. Conclusion

Advances in our understanding of the immune system enhance studies of virus-host relationships. Although HTLV-1 causes 2 different diseases (ATL and HTM/TSP), $CD4^+CD25^+CCR4^+$ T cells are the common viral reservoir in both disorders. According to recent studies, however, characteristics of $CD4^+CD25^+CCR4^+$ T cells are completely different in the 2 diseases: Foxp3+ leukemic cells are found in ATL patients, while Foxp3- IFN-γ-producing cells are found in HAM/TSP patients. The host immune system plays a crucial role in controlling these HTLV-1-infected cells. HTLV-1-specific CTL is activated in patients with HAM/TSP, but not in those with ATL, indicating that impairment of acquired immunity is not universal. However, both ATL and HAM/TSP patients are known to experience decreases in innate immunity via the functional impairment of DCs, NK cells, and iNKT cells, as well as lower overall population numbers of these cell types. These conditions may contribute to inadequate viral control and play an important role in the pathogenesis of HTLV-1-associated disorders.

6. Acknowledgments

This work was partially supported by a Grant-in-Aid for Scientific Research from the Ministry of Education, Culture, Sports, Science and Technology; the Japanese Ministry of Health, Labor, and Welfare; the Uehara Memorial Foundation; the Nagao Takeshi Nanbyo Foundation; the Kanagawa Nanbyo Foundation; the Mishima Kaiun Memorial Foundation; the Takeda Science Foundation; the ITSUU Laboratory Research Foundation; the Foundation for Total Health Promotion; and the Sankyo Foundation of Life Science.

7. References

Abdelbary, N.H., Abdullah, H.M., Matsuzaki, T., Hayashi, D., Tanaka, Y., Takashima, H., Izumo, S. & Kubota, R. 2011. Reduced Tim-3 expression on human T-lymphotropic virus type I (HTLV-I) Tax-specific cytotoxic T lymphocytes in HTLV-I infection. *Journal of Infectious Diseases*, 203, 7, 948-959

Anderson, P., Nagler-Anderson, C., O'Brien, C., Levine, H., Watkins, S., Slayter, H.S., Blue, M.L. & Schlossman, S.F. 1990. A monoclonal antibody reactive with a 15-kDa cytoplasmic granule-associated protein defines a subpopulation of CD8+ T lymphocytes. *Journal of Immunology*, 144, 2, 574–582

Arnulf, B., Thorel, M., Poirot, Y., Tamouza, R., Boulanger, E., Jaccard, A., Oksenhendler, E., Hermine, O. & Pique, C. 2004. Loss of the ex vivo but not the reinducible CD8+ T-cell response to Tax in human T-cell leukemia virus type 1-infected patients with adult T-cell leukemia/lymphoma. *Leukemia*, 18, 1, 126-132

Asquith, B., Mosley, A.J., Barfield, A., Marshall, S.E., Heaps, A., Goon, P., Hanon, E., Tanaka, Y., Taylor, G.P. & Bangham, C.R. 2005. A functional CD8+ cell assay reveals individual variation in CD8+ cell antiviral efficacy and explains differences in human T-lymphotropic virus type 1 proviral load. *Journal of General Virology*, 86, 5, 1515–23

Azakami, K., Sato, T., Araya, N., Utsunomiya, A., Kubota, R., Suzuki, K., Hasegawa, D., Izumi, T., Fujita, H., Aratani, S., Fujii, R., Yagishita, N., Kamijuku, H., Kanekura, T., Seino, K., Nishioka, K., Nakajima, T. & Yamano, Y. 2009. Severe loss of invariant NKT cells exhibiting anti-HTLV-1 activity in patients with HTLV-1-associated disorders. *Blood*, 114, 15, 3208-3215

Banerjee, P., Feuer, G., Barker, E. 2007. Human T-cell leukemia virus type 1 (HTLV-1) p12I down-modulates ICAM-1 and -2 and reduces adherence of natural killer cells, thereby protecting HTLV-1-infected primary CD4+ T cells from autologous natural killer cell-mediated cytotoxicity despite the reduction of major histocompatibility complex class I molecules on infected cells. *Journal of Virology*, 81, 18 9707-9717

Bangham, C.R. 2008. HTLV-1 infection: role of CTL efficiency. *Blood*, 112, 6, 2176-2177

Bangham, C.R. 2009. CTL quality and the control of human retroviral infections. *European Journal of Immunology*, 39, 7, 1700-1712

Betts, M.R., Brenchley, J.M., Price, D.A., De Rosa, S.C., Douek, D.C., Roederer, M. & Koup, R.A. 2003. Sensitive and viable identification of antigen-specific CD8+ T cells by a flow cytometric assay for degranulation. *Journal of Immunological Methods*, 281, 1-2, 65–78

Biddison, W.E., Kubota, R., Kawanishi, T., Taub, D.D., Cruikshank, W.W., Center, D.M., Connor, E.W., Utz, U. & Jacobson, S. 1997. Human T cell leukemia virus type I (HTLV-I)-specific CD8+ CTL clones from patients with HTLV-I-associated neurologic disease secrete proinflammatory cytokines, chemokines, and matrix metalloproteinase. *Journal of Immunology*, 159, 4, 2018–2025

Bieganowska, K., Hollsberg, P., Buckle, G.J., Lim, D.G., Greten, T.F., Schneck, J., Altman, J.D., Jacobson, S., Ledis, S.L., Hanchard, B., Chin, J., Morgan, O., Roth, P.A. & Hafler, D.A. 1999. Direct analysis of viral-specific CD8+ T cells with soluble HLA-A2/Tax11-19 tetramer complexes in patients with human T cell lymphotropic virus-associated myelopathy. *Journal of Immunology*, 162, 3, 1765–1771.

Boxus, M. & Willems, L. 2009. Mechanisms of HTLV-1 persistence and transformation. *British Journal of Cancer*, 101, 9, 1497-1501

Chen, S., Ishii, N., Ine, S., Ikeda, S., Fujimura, T., Ndhlovu, L.C., Soroosh, P., Tada, K., Harigae, H., Kameoka, J., Noriyuki, K., Sasaki, T. & Sugamura, K. 2006. Regulatory T cell-like activity of Foxp3+ adult T cell leukemia cells. *International Immunology* 18, 2, 269–277

Elovaara, I., Koenig, S., Brewah, A.Y., Woods, R.M., Lehky, T. & Jacobson, S. 1993. High human T cell lymphotropic virus type 1 (HTLV-1)-specific precursor cytotoxic T lymphocyte frequencies in patients with HTLV-1-associated neurological disease. *Journal of Experimental Medicine*, 177, 6, 1567–1573

Enose-Akahata, Y., Oh, U., Grant, C. & Jacobson, S. 2008. Retrovirally induced CTL degranulation mediated by IL-15 expression and infection of mononuclear phagocytes in patients with HTLV-Iassociated neurologic disease. *Blood*, 112, 6, 2400–2410

Fortis, C. & Poli, G. 2005. Dendritic cells and natural killer cells in the pathogenesis of HIV infection. *Immunologic Research*, 33: 1, 1-21

Gessain, A., Barin, F. & Vernant, J.C. 1985. Antibodies to human T-lymphotropic virus type-I in patients with tropical spastic paraparesis. *Lancet*, 2, 8452, 407–410

Goon, P.K., Igakura, T., Hanon, E., Mosley, A.J., Barfield, A., Barnard, A.L., Kaftantzi, L., Tanaka, Y., Taylor, G.P. Weber, J.N. & Bangham, C.R. 2004. Human T cell lymphotropic virus type I (HTLV-I)-specific CD4+ T cells: immunodominance hierarchy and preferential infection with HTLV-I. *Journal of Immunology*, 172, 3, 1735–1743

Grant, C., Oh, U., Yao, K., Yamano, Y. & Jacobson, S. 2008. Dysregulation of TGF-beta signaling and regulatory and effector T-cell function in virus-induced neuroinflammatory disease. *Blood*,111, 12, 5601–5609

Greten, T.F., Slansky, J.E., Kubota, R., Soldan, S.S., Jaffee, E.M., Leist, T.P., Pardoll, D.M., Jacobson, S. & Schneck, J.P. 1998. Direct visualization of antigen-specific T cells: HTLV-1 Tax11-19- specific CD8(+) T cells are activated in peripheral blood and accumulate in cerebrospinal fluid from HAM/TSP patients. Proceedings of the National Academy of Sciences U.S.A., 95, 13, 7568–7573

Harashima, N., Kurihara, K., Utsunomiya, A. Tanosaki, R., Hanabuchi, S., Masuda, M., Ohashi, T., Fukui, F., Hasegawa, A., Masuda, T., Takaue, Y., Okamura, J. & Kannagi, M. 2004. Graft-versus-Tax response in adult T-cell leukemia patients after hematopoietic stem cell transplantation. *Cancer Research*, 64, 391–399

Hashimoto, K., Higuchi, I., Osame, M. & Izumo, S. 1998. Quantitative in situ PCR assay of HTLV-1 infected cells in peripheral blood lymphocytes of patients with ATL, HAM/TSP and asymptomatic carriers. *Journal of the Neurological Sciences*, 159, 1, 67–72

Hayashi, D., Kubota, R., Takenouchi, N., Tanaka, Y., Hirano, R., Takashima, H., Osame, M., Izumo, S. & Arimura, K. 2008. Reduced Foxp3 expression with increased cytomegalovirus-specific CTL in HTLV-I-associated myelopathy. *Journal of Neuroimmunology*, 200, 1-2, 115–124

Hieshima, K., Nagakubo, D., Nakayama, T., Shirakawa, A.K., Jin, Z., & Yoshie, O. 2008. Tax-inducible production of CC chemokine ligand 22 by human T cell leukemia virus type 1 (HTLV-1)-infected T cells promotes preferential transmission of HTLV-1 to CCR4-expressing CD4+ T cells. *Journal of Immuno*logy, 180, 2, 931-9

Hilburn, S., Rowan, A., Demontis, M.A., MacNamara, A., Asquith, B., Bangham, C.R. & Taylor, G.P. 2011. In vivo expression of human T-lymphotropic virus type 1 basic leucine-zipper protein generates specific CD8+ and CD4+ T-lymphocyte responses that correlate with clinical outcome. *Journal of Infectious Diseases*, 203, 4, 529-36

Hishizawa M, Imada K, Kitawaki T, Ueda M, Kadowaki N, Uchiyama T. 2004. Depletion and impaired interferon-alpha-producing capacity of blood plasmacytoid dendritic cells in human T-cell leukaemia virus type I-infected individuals. *British Journal of Haematology*, 125, 5, 568-575

Hori, S., Nomura, T. & Sakaguchi, S. 2003. Control of regulatory T cell development by the transcription factor Foxp3. *Science*, 299, 5609, 1057–1061

Iwanaga, M., Watanabe, T., Utsunomiya, A., Okayama, A., Uchimaru, K., Koh, K.R., Ogata, M., Kikuchi, H., Sagara, Y., Uozumi, K., Mochizuki, M., Tsukasaki, K., Saburi, Y., Yamamura, M., Tanaka, J., Moriuchi, Y., Hino, S., Kamihira, S. & Yamaguchi, K. 2010. Human T-cell leukemia virus type I (HTLV-1) proviral load and disease progression in asymptomatic HTLV-1 carriers: a nationwide prospective study in Japan. *Blood*, 116, 8, 1211-1219

Jacobson, S., Shida, H., McFarlin, D.E., Fauci, A.S. & Koenig, S. 1990. Circulating CD8+ cytotoxic T lymphocytes specific for HTLV-I pX in patients with HTLV-I associated neurological disease. *Nature*, 348, 6298, 245–248

Jacobson, S. 2002. Immunopathogenesis of human T cell lymphotropic virus type I-associated neurologic disease. *Journal of Infectious Diseases*, 186 Suppl, S187–92

Jones, K.S., Petrow-Sadowski, C., Huang, Y.K., Bertolette, D.C. & Ruscetti, F.W. 2008. Cell-free HTLV-1 infects dendritic cells leading to transmission and transformation of CD4(+) T cells. *Nature Medicine*, 14, 4, 429-436

Kannagi, M., Sugamura, K., Kinoshita, K., Uchino, H. & Hinuma, Y. 1984. Specific cytolysis of fresh tumor cells by an autologous killer T cell line derived from an adult T cell leukemia/lymphoma patient. *Journal of Immunology*, 133, 2, 1037-1041.

Kannagi, M., Harada, S., Maruyama, I. Inoko, H., Igarashi, H., Kuwashima, G., Sato, S., Morita, M., Kidokoro, M., Sugimoto, M., Funahashi, S., Osame, M. & Shida, H. 1991. Predominant recognition of human T cell leukemia virus type I (HTLV-I) pX gene products by human CD8+ cytotoxic T cells directed against HTLV- I-infected cells. *International Immunology*, 3, 8, 761–7

Kannagi, M. Immunologic control of human T-cell leukemia virus type I and adult T-cell leukemia. 2007. International Journal of Hematology, 86, 2, 113–117

Kannagi, M., Hasegawa, A., Kinpara, S., Shimizu, Y., Takamori, A. & Utsunomiya, A. 2011. Double control systems for human T-cell leukemia virus type 1 by innate and acquired immunity. *Cancer Science*, 102, 4, 670-6

Karube, K., Ohshima, K., Tsuchiya, T., Yamaguchi, T., Kawano, R., Suzumiya, J., Utsunomiya, A., Harada, M. & Kikuchi, M. 2004. Expression of FoxP3, a key molecule in CD4CD25 regulatory T cells, in adult T-cell leukaemia/lymphoma cells. *British Journal of Haematology*, 126, 1, 81–84

Kim, C.H., Butcher, E.C. & Johnston, B. 2002. Distinct subsets of human Valpha24-invariant NKT cells: cytokine responses and chemokine receptor expression. *Trends in Immunology*, 23, 11, 516-519

Kohno, T., Yamada, Y., Akamatsu, N., Kamihira, S., Imaizumi, Y., Tomonaga, M. & Matsuyama, T. 2005. Possible origin of adult T-cell leukemia/lymphoma cells from human T lymphotropic virus type-1-infected regulatory T cells. *Cancer Science, 96*, 8, 527–533

Kozako, T., Arima, N., Toji, S., Masamoto, I., Akimoto, M., Hamada, H., Che, X.F., Fujiwara, H., Matsushita, K., Tokunaga, M., Haraguchi, K., Uozumi, K., Suzuki, S., Takezaki, T. & Sonoda, S. 2006. Reduced frequency, diversity, and function of human T cell leukemia virus type 1-specific CD8+ T cell in adult T cell leukemia patients. *Journal of Immunology*, 177, 8, 5718–5726

Kubota, R., Fujiyoshi, T., Izumo, S., Yashiki, S., Maruyama, I., Osame, M. & Sonoda, S. 1993. Fluctuation of HTLV-I proviral DNA in peripheral blood mononuclear cells of HTLV-I-associated myelopathy. *Journal of Neuroimmunology*, 42, 2, 147–154

Kubota, R., Nagai, M., Kawanishi, T., Osame, M. & Jacobson, S. 2000. Increased HTLV type 1 tax specific CD8+ cells in HTLV type 1-associated myelopathy/tropical spastic paraparesis: correlation with HTLV type 1 proviral load. *AIDS Research and Human Retroviruses*, 16, 16, 1705–1709

Kubota, R., Soldan, S.S., Martin, R. & Jacobson, S. 2002. Selected cytotoxic T lymphocytes with high specificity for HTLV-I in cerebrospinal fluid from a HAM/TSP patient. Journal of Neurovirology, 8, 1, 53–57

Levin, M.C., Lehky, T.J., Flerlage, A.N., Katz, D., Kingma, D.W., Jaffe, E.S., Heiss, J.D., Patronas, N., McFarland, H.F. & Jacobson, S. 1997. Immunologic analysis of a spinal cord-biopsy specimen from a patient with human T-cell lymphotropic virus type I-associated neurologic disease. *New England Journal of Medicine*, 336, 12, 839–845

Macatonia, S.E., Cruickshank, J.K., Rudge, P. & Knight, S.C. 1992. Dendritic cells from patients with tropical spastic paraparesis are infected with HTLV-1 and stimulate autologous lymphocyte proliferation. *AIDS Research and Human Retroviruses*, 8, 9, 1699-1706

Macnamara, A., Rowan, A., Hilburn, S., Kadolsky, U., Fujiwara, H., Suemori, K., Yasukawa, M., Taylor, G., Bangham, C.R. & Asquith, B. 2010. HLA class I binding of HBZ determines outcome in HTLV-1 infection. *PLoS Pathogens*, 6, 9, e1001117

Matsubar, Y., Hori, T., Morita, R., Sakaguchi, S. & Uchiyama, T. 2006. Delineation of immunoregulatory properties of adult T-cell leukemia cells. *International Journal of Hematology*, 84, 1, 63–69

Matsuura, E., Yamano, Y. & Jacobson, S. 2010. Neuroimmunity of HTLV-I Infection. *Journal of Neuroimmune Pharmacology*, 5, 3, 310-25

Michaëlsson, J., Barbosa, H.M., Jordan, K.A., Chapman, J.M., Brunialti, M.K., Neto, W.K., Nukui, Y., Sabino, E.C., Chieia, M.A., Oliveira, A.S.B., Nixon, D.F. & Kallas, E.G. 2008. The frequency of CD127low expressing CD4+CD25high T regulatory cells is inversely correlated with human T lymphotrophic virus type-1 (HTLV-1) proviral load in HTLV-1-infection and HTLV-1-associated myelopathy/tropical spastic paraparesis. *BMC Immunology*, 9, 41

Moll, M., Kuylenstierna, C., Gonzalez, V.D., Andersson, S.K., Bosnjak, L., Sönnerborg, A., Quigley, M.F. & Sandberg, J.K. 2009.Severe functional impairment and elevated PD-1 expression in CD1d-restricted NKT cells retained during chronic HIV-1 infection. *European Journal of Immunology*, 39, 3, 902-911

Mosley, A.J., Asquith, B. & Bangham, C.R. 2005. Cell-mediated immune response to human T-lymphotropic virus type I. *Viral Immunology*, 18, 2, 293-305

Nagai, M., Usuku, K., Matsumoto, W., Kodama, D., Takenouchi, N., Moritoyo, T., Hashiguchi, S., Ichinose, M., Bangham, C.R., Izumo, S. & Osame, M. 1998. Analysis of HTLV-I proviral load in 202 HAM/TSP patients and 243 asymptomatic HTLV-I carriers: high proviral load strongly predisposes to HAM/TSP. *Journal of Neurovirology*, 4, 6, 586-593

Nagai, M., Kubota, R., Greten, T.F., Schneck, J.P., Leist, T.P. & Jacobson, S. 2001a. Increased activated human T cell lymphotropic virus type I (HTLV-I) Tax11-19-specific memory and effector CD8+ cells in patients with HTLV-I-associated myelopathy/tropical spastic paraparesis: correlation with HTLV-I provirus load. *Journal of Infectious Diseases*, 183, 2, 197–205

Nagai, M., Yamano, Y., Brennan, M.B., Mora, C.A. & Jacobson, S. 2001b. Increased HTLV-I proviral load and preferential expansion of HTLV-I Tax-specific CD8+ T cells in cerebrospinal fluid from patients with HAM/TSP. *Annals of Neurology*, 50, 6, 807-812

Oh, U., Grant, C., Griffith, C., Fugo, K., Takenouchi, N. & Jacobson, S. 2006. Reduced Foxp3 protein expression is associated with inflammatory disease during human t lymphotropic virus type 1 Infection. *Journal of Infectious Diseases*, 193, 11, 1557–1566

Ohsugi, T. & Kumasaka, 2011. T. Low CD4/CD8 T-cell ratio associated with inflammatory arthropathy in human T-cell leukemia virus type I Tax transgenic mice. *PLoS One*, 6, 4, e18518

Osame, M., Usuku, K., Izumo, S., Ijichi, N., Amitani, H., Igata, A., Matsumoto, M. & Tara, M. 1986. HTLV-I associated myelopathy, a new clinical entity. *Lancet* 1, 8488, 1031–1032

Parker, C.E., Daenke, S., Nightingale, S. & Bangham, C.R. 1992. Activated, HTLV-1-specific cytotoxic T-lymphocytes are found in healthy seropositives as well as in patients with tropical spastic paraparesis. *Virology*. 188, 2, 628-636

Pique, C., Ureta-Vidal, A., Gessain, A., Chancerel, B., Gout, O., Tamouza, R., Agis, F. & Dokhélar, M.C. Evidence for the chronic in vivo production of human T cell leukemia virus type I Rof and Tof proteins from cytotoxic T lymphocytes directed against viral peptides. 2000. *Journal of Experimental Medicine*, 191, 3, 567–72

Ramirez, J.M., Brembilla, N.C., Sorg, O., Chicheportiche, R., Matthes, T., Dayer, J.M., Saurat, J.H., Roosnek, E., & Chizzolini, C. 2010. Activation of the aryl hydrocarbon receptor reveals distinct requirements for IL-22 and IL-17 production by human T helper cells. *European Journal of Immunology*, 40, 9, 2450–2459

Richardson, J.H., Edwards, A.J., Cruickshank, J.K., Rudge, P. & Dalgleish, A.G. In vivo cellular tropism of human T-cell leukemia virus type 1. 1990. *Journal of Virology*, 64, 11, 5682–5687

Roncador, G., Garcia, J.F., Maestre, L., Lucas, E., Menarguez, J., Ohshima, K., Nakamura, S., Banham, A.H., Piris, M.A. FOXP3, a selective marker for a subset of adult T-cell leukaemia/lymphoma. *Leukemia*, 19, 12, 2247–2253

Sabouri, A.H., Usuku, K., Hayashi, D., Izumo, S., Ohara, Y., Osame, M. & Saito, M. 2008 Impaired function of human T-lymphotropic virus type 1 (HTLV-1)-specific CD8+ T cells in HTLV-1-associated neurologic disease. *Blood*, 112, 6, 2411–2420

Saito, M., Braud, V.M., Goon, P., Hanon, E., Taylor, G.P., Saito, A., Eiraku, N., Tanaka, Y., Usuku, K., Weber, J.N., Osame, M. & Bangham, C.R. 2003. Low frequency of CD94/NKG2A+ T lymphocytes in patients with HTLV-1-associated myelopathy/tropical spastic paraparesis, but not in asymptomatic carriers. *Blood*, 102, 2, 577-584

Sakaguchi, S., Sakaguchi, N., Asano, M., Itoh, M. & Toda, M. 1995. Immunologic self-tolerance maintained by activated T cells expressing IL-2 receptor alpha-chains (CD25). Breakdown of a single mechanism of self-tolerance causes various autoimmune diseases. *Journal of Immunology*, 155, 3, 1151–1164

Sakaguchi, S., Yamaguchi, T., Nomura, T., & Ono, M. 2008. Regulatory T cells and immune tolerance. *Cell*, 133, 5, 775–787

Sandberg, J.K., Fast, N.M., Palacios, E.H., Fennelly, G., Dobroszycki, J., Palumbo, P., Wiznia, A., Grant, R.M., Bhardwaj, N., Rosenberg, M.G. & Nixon, D.F. 2002. Selective loss of innate CD4(+) V alpha 24 natural killer T cells in human immunodeficiency virus infection. *Journal of Virology*, 76, 15, 7528-7534

Sato, T., Araya, N. & Yamano, Y. 2011. Human T-lymphotropic virus type 1 (HTLV-1) and innate immunity. *Inflammation and Regeneration*, 31, 1, 110-115

Satou, Y & Matsuoka, M. 2010. HTLV-1 and the host immune system: how the virus disrupts immune regulation, leading to HTLV-1 associated diseases. *Journal of Clinical and Experimental Hematopathology*. 50, 1, 1-8

Satou, Y., Yasunaga, J., Zhao, T., Yoshida, M., Miyazato, P., Takai, K., Shimizu, K., Ohshima, K., Green, P.L., Ohkura, N., Yamaguchi, T., Ono, M., Sakaguchi, S. & Matsuoka, M. 2011. HTLV-1 bZIP factor induces T-cell lymphoma and systemic inflammation in vivo. *PLoS Pathogens,* 7, 2, e1001274

Shimauchi, T., Kabashima, K. & Tokura, Y. 2008. Adult T-cell leukemia/lymphoma cells from blood and skin tumors express cytotoxic T lymphocyte-associated antigen-4 and Foxp3 but lack suppressor activity toward autologous CD8+ T cells. *Cancer Science,* 99, 1, 98–106

Shimizu, Y., Takamori, A., Utsunomiya, A., Kurimura, M., Yamano, Y., Hishizawa, M., Hasegawa, A., Kondo, F., Kurihara, K., Harashima, N., Watanabe, T., Okamura, J., Masuda, T. & Kannagi, M. 2009. Impaired Tax-specific T-cell responses with insufficient control of HTLV-1 in a subgroup of individuals at asymptomatic and smoldering stages. *Cancer Science,* 100, 3, 481–489

Toulza, F., Heaps, A., Tanaka, Y., Taylor, G.P. & Bangham, C.R. 2008. High frequency of CD4+FoxP3+ cells in HTLV-1 infection: inverse correlation with HTLV-1-specific CTL response. *Blood* 111, 10, 5047–5053

Tsuji, M., Komatsu, N., Kawamoto, S., Suzuki, K., Kanagawa, O., Honjo, T., Hori, S. & Fagarasan, S. 2009. Preferential generation of follicular B helper T cells from Foxp3+ T cells in gut Peyer's patches. *Science* 323, 5920, 1488–1492

Uchiyama, T., Yodoi, J., Sagawa, K., Takatsuki, K. & Uchino, H. Adult T-cell leukemia: clinical and hematologic features of 16 cases. 1977. *Blood,* 50, 3, 481-92

Umehara, F., Izumo, S., Nakagawa, M., Ronquillo, A.T., Takahashi, K., Matsumuro, K., Sato, E. & Osame M. 1993. Immunocytochemical analysis of the cellular infiltrate in the spinal cord lesions in HTLV-Iassociated myelopathy. *Journal of Neuropathology and Experimental Neurology,* 52, 4, 424–430

Umehara, F., Nakamura, A., Izumo, S., Kubota, R., Ijichi, S., Kashio, N., Hashimoto, K., Usuku, K., Sato, E. & Osame, M. 1994. Apoptosis of T lymphocytes in the spinal cord lesions in HTLV-I-associated myelopathy: a possible mechanism to control viral infection in the central nervous system. *Journal of Neuropathology and Experimental Neurology,* 53, 6, 617–624

van der Vliet, H.J., von Blomberg, B.M., Hazenberg, M.D., Nishi, N., Otto, S.A., van Benthem, B.H., Prins, M., Claessen, F.A., van den Eertwegh, A.J., Giaccone, G., Miedema, F., Scheper, R.J. & Pinedo, H.M. 2002. Selective decrease in circulating V alpha 24+V beta 11+ NKT cells during HIV type 1 infection. *Journal of Immunology,* 168, 3, 1490-1495

Wodarz, D., Nowak, M.A. & Bangham, C.R. 1999. The dynamics of HTLV-I and the CTL response. *Immunology Today,* 20, 5, 220–227

Wodarz, D., Hall, S.E., Usuku, K., Osame, M., Ogg, G.S., McMichael, A.J., Nowak, M.A. & Bangham, C.R.M.. 2001. Cytotoxic T-cell abundance and virus load in human immunodeficiency virus type 1 and human T-cell leukaemia virus type 1. Proceedings of the Royal Society of London B, 268, 1473, 1215–21Yamano, Y., Nagai, M., Brennan, M. Mora, C.A., Soldan, S.S., Tomaru, U., Takenouchi, N., Izumo, S., Osame, M. & Jacobson, S. 2002. Correlation of human T-cell lymphotropic virus type 1 (HTLV-1) mRNA with proviral DNA load, virusspecific CD8(+) T cells, and disease severity in HTLV-1-associated myelopathy (HAM/TSP). *Blood* 99, 1, 88–94

Yamano, Y., Takenouchi, N., Li, H.C., Tomaru, U., Yao, K., Grant, C.W., Maric, D.A. & Jacobson, S. 2005. Virus-induced dysfunction of CD4+CD25+ T cells in patients with HTLV-I-associated neuroimmunological disease. *Journal of Clinical Investigations*, 115, 5, 1361–1368

Yamano, Y., Araya, N., Sato, T., Utsunomiya, A., Azakami, K., Hasegawa, D., Izumi, T., Fujita, H., Aratani, S., Yagishita, N., Fujii, R., Nishioka, K., Jacobson, S. & Nakajima, T. 2009. Abnormally high levels of virus-infected IFN-gamma+ CCR4+ CD4+ CD25+ T cells in a retrovirus-associated neuroinflammatory disorder. *PLoS One, 4*, 8, e6517

Yu, F., Itoyama, Y., Fujihara, K. & Goto, I. 1991. Natural killer (NK) cells in HTLV-I-associated myelopathy/tropical spastic paraparesis-decrease in NK cell subset populations and activity in HTLV-I seropositive individuals. Journal of Neuroimmunology, 33, 2, 121-128

Yoshie, O., Imai, T. & Nomiyama, H. 2001. Chemokines in immunity. *Advances in Immunology*, 78, 57–110

Yoshie, O., Fujisawa, R., Nakayama, T., Harasawa, H., Tago, H., Izawa, D., Hieshima, K., Tatsumi, Y., Matsushima, K., Hasegawa, H., Kanamaru, A., Kamihira, S. & Yamada, Y. 2002. Frequent expression of CCR4 in adult T-cell leukemia and human T-cell leukemia virus type 1-transformed T cells. *Blood*, 99, 5, 1505–11

Zhou, X., Bailey-Bucktrout, S.L., Jeker, L.T., Penaranda, C., Martinez-Llordella, M., Ashby, M., Nakayama, M., Rosenthal, W. & Bluestone, J.A. 2009. Instability of the transcription factor Foxp3 leads to the generation of pathogenic memory T cells in vivo. *Nature Immunology*, 10, 9, 1000–1007

Zhu, J. & Paul, W.E. 2010. Heterogeneity and plasticity of T helper cells. Cell Research, 20, 1, 4-12

5

Constitutive Activation of the JAK/STAT and Toll-Like Receptor Signaling Pathways in Adult T-Cell Leukemia/Lymphoma

Takehiro Higashi, Takefumi Katsuragi, Atsushi Iwashige,
Hiroaki Morimoto and Junichi Tsukada
Cancer Chemotherapy Center and Hematology
University of Occupational and Environmental Health, Kitakyushu
Japan

1. Introduction

Adult T-cell leukemia/lymphoma (ATLL) caused by the retrovirus human T-cell leukemia virus type 1 (HTLV-1) infection is one of aggressive mature CD4+ T-cell neoplasms with a marked expansion of leukemic cells during the acute phase. ATLL is endemic in several regions of the world, especially in southwest Japan, the Caribbean basin, and parts of Central Africa. ATLL is divided into four clinical subtypes: acute, chronic, smoldering, and lymphoma type, based on the number of leukemic cells in peripheral blood, serum lactic acid dehydrogenase level, tumor lesions in various organs, and clinical course. The acute and lymphoma types still have an extremely poor prognosis, despite the advance in chemotherapy. Chemotherapy for ATLL has limited efficacy with median survivals of approximate one year.

The HTLV-1 genome encodes not only structural proteins, but also non-structural proteins such as Tax, Rex, p13, p12, p30, p21Rex and HTLV-1 bZIP factor (HBZ). The functional analysis of the viral proteins such as Tax has shed light on the pathogenesis of ATLL. Tax is a crucial viral protein encoded by the pX region, which can induce viral replication and a variety of cellular genes associated with cytokine production, inhibition of apoptosis and cell cycle dysregulation (Arima 1999, Azimi 1998, Geleziunas 1998, Kanno 1994, Mori 1996b). Tax-induced gene regulation, which is linked to malignant transformation of HTLV-1-infected T-cells, has been shown to be mediated by CREB/ATF, NF-κB and SRF pathways. Constitutive activation of NF-κB is one of common features of HTLV-1-transformed T-cells and ATLL leukemic cells, since inhibition of NF-κB activity reduces cell growth and induces apoptosis of cells, suggesting a central role of NF-κB in their proliferation and survival. Moreover, Tax binds to the upstream kinase, the mitogen-activated protein kinase/ERK kinase kinase-1 and enhance its kinase activity (Harhaj 1999, Huang 2002, Jin 1999). Nevertheless, ATLL develops in a period 40 to 60 years after initial infection, indicating that the development of ATLL requires a multistep oncogenic process including accumulation of genetic mutations. HTLV-1 infection alone is not sufficient to induce neoplastic transformation of infected cells. In fact, viral gene expression is at extremely low levels in primary ATLL cells (Franchini 1984). Thus, the mechanism which develops ATLL still remains unclear.

The general subject of signaling pathways in ATLL cells and HTLV-1-transformed cells has been covered by many excellent original reports and reviews. In this review, authors focus on recent advances of two signaling pathways in ATLL cells and HTLV-1–transformed T-cells; the JAK (Janus kinase)-STAT (signal transducer and activator of transcription) and TLR (Toll-like receptor) signaling pathways.

2. Constitutive activation of the JAK-STAT signaling pathway in ATLL cells and HTLV-1-transformed T-cells

STAT proteins play important roles in regulating cellular response to a variety of cytokines. STATs are latent cytosolic transcriptional factors that are activated by tyrosine phosphorylation in response to cytokines. The four mammalian members of the JAK family (Jak1, Jak2, Jak3, and Tyk2) are non-receptor tyrosine kinases functioning as signal transducers, that control activation of STATs. Jaks associate constitutively with cytokine receptors, and promote signals by phosphorylating tyrosine residues of activated receptors to allow the recruitment and activation of STAT proteins. STATs can form homo- or heterodimers in which amino acid sequence containing a phospho-tyrosine residue in one partner binds to the SH2 domain in the other vice versa, leading to nuclear translocation of STAT dimers and their participation in transcriptional regulation of various cytokine responsive genes (Darnell 1997, Ihle 2001, Leonard 1998).

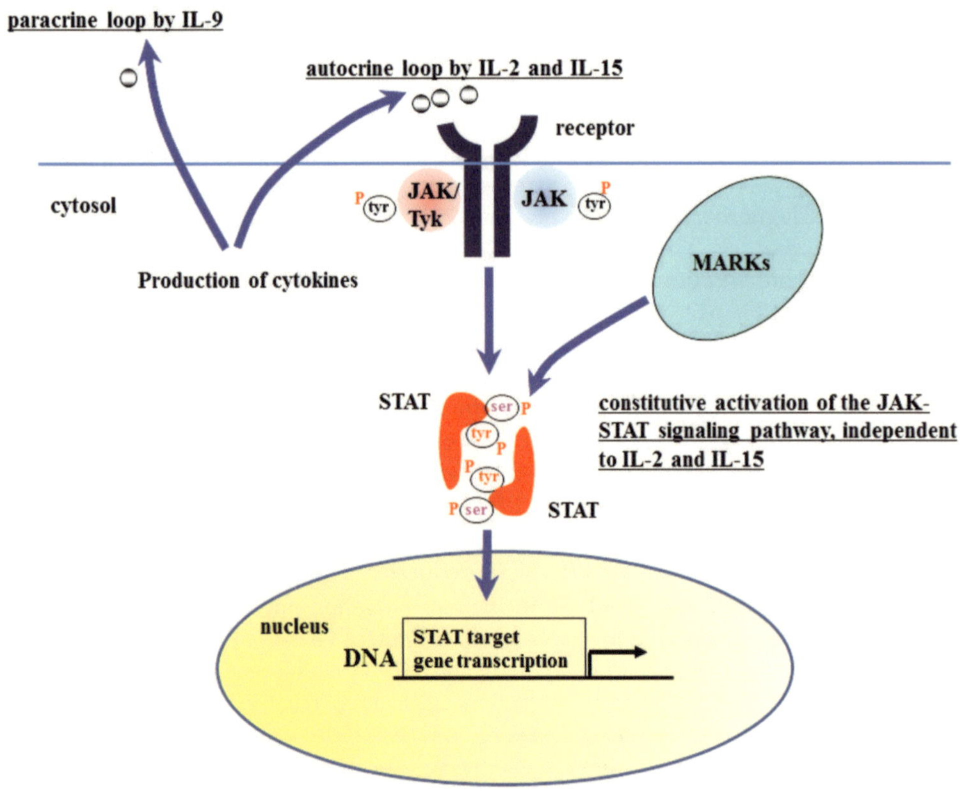

Fig. 1. The JAK-STAT signaling pathway in ATLL cells and HTLV-1-transformed T-cells.

Recent reports have emphasized the significance of STATs in oncogenesis (Akira 1997) and leukemogenesis (Bowman 2000, Lin 2000, Levy 2000, Coffer 2000, Akira 1997). Many oncoproteins can activate STATs. In contrast to the normal cellular response, which shows rapid and transient activation of STATs, aberrant activation of JAK-STAT signaling contributes to malignant transformation. The v-abl oncogene of the Abelson murine leukemia virus (A-MuLV) induces JAK-STAT signaling, involving Jak1 and Jak3 (Danial 1995). Interestingly, constitutive expression of a dominant-active STAT3 induces neoplastic transformation (Bromberg 1999). STAT1 and STAT5 are active in BCR-ABL-positive leukemias (Carlesso 1996, Shuai 1996, Frank 1996) and STAT1, STAT3 and STAT5 are constitutively activated in acute leukemia blasts (Gouilleux-Gruart 1996, Weber-Nordt 1996, Xia 1998, Spiekermann 2001). A constitutively active form of STAT3 can transform cells (Bromberg 1999). Constitutive activation of Jaks and STATs has been observed in murine pre-B lymphocytes transformed with the A-MuLV(Danial 1995), human B cells transformed with Epstein-Barr virus (Gouilleux-Gruart 1996) and murine erythroleukemia induced by spleen focus-forming virus (Ohashi 1995). Primary acute leukemia cells also show constitutive activation of STATs (Gouilleux-Gruart 1996, Weber-Nordt 1996, Xia 1998, Spiekermann 2001). Moreover, constitutive STAT3 activation in acute myeloid leukemia blasts has been reported to be associated with short disease-free survival, showing a prognostic significance for STAT3 (Benekli 2002).

HLTV-1 infects and immortalizes primary human T-cells. In early stage, the viral regulatory proteins Tax and Rex are involved in the up-regulation of IL-2 and IL-2R. In some ATL cases, IL-2 and IL-15 can induce growth of ATLL cells (Arima 1996, Maeda 1987, Yamada 1998) (Fig. 1). Phosphorylation of STAT3 and STAT5 in ATL cells is induced by IL-2, IL-15 and IL-21 (Ueda 2005). A paracrine growth loop that involves Tax-induced IL-9 production in ATL cells and expression of IL-9 receptor α on monocytes has been also observed (Chen 2008).

However, constitutive activation of the JAK-STAT pathway is generally correlated with IL-2 independence. Transformation of T-cells by HTLV-1 is associated with constitutive activation of the JAK-STAT pathway (Migone 1995, Xu 1995) (Fig1). Migone *et al.* (Migone 1995) demonstrated activation of Jak1, Jak3, STAT3 and STAT5 correlated with the transition from an IL-2-dependent to an IL-2-independent phase in HTLV-1-transformed cells. Spontaneous phosphorylation of Jak2 and Jak3 has also been observed in T-cells transformed with HTLV-1 (Xu 1995). Leukemia cells obtained from ATL patients also showed constitutive activation of STATs (Takemoto 1997, Tsukada 2000). Takemoto *et al.*(Takemoto 1997) observed constitutive activation of STAT1, STAT3 and STAT5 in leukemic cells of ATL patients, and demonstrated the association of leukemic cell proliferation with constitutive JAK-STAT activity.

In addition, no gain-of-function mutations of the Jak1 and Jak3 in primary ATLL cells has been detected (Kameda 2010). These data are contrast to the results obtained from acute T-lymphoblastic leukemia (T-ALL). Flex *et al.* demonstrated that *JAK1* gene mutations occur in ALL and are more frequently observed among adult individuals with involvement of the T cell lineage (Flex 2008). The mutations promote gain of kinase function, and are associated with poor response to therapy and overall prognosis.

2.1 Unique function of the Jak-STAT signaling pathway in HTLV-1-infected T-cells

HTLV-1 infection up-regulates expression of the suppressor of cytokine signaling 1 (SOCS1). HTLV-1-induced SOCS1 inhibits the type I IFN antiviral response against HTLV-1 by targeting IRF3 for SOCS1-induced proteasome degradation (Oliere 2010). As an adaptor, SOCS1 brings target proteins to the elongin B/C-Cullin E3 ligase complex for ubiquitination. It may represent an immune evasion strategy and survival advantage to HTLV-1-infected cells. HTLV-1 inhibits IFNα-induced phosphorylation of STAT2 and Tyk2 (Feng 2008). Zhang *et al.* further indicate that Tax interferes with IFN-α-induced JAK-STAT signaling by completion with STAT2 for CBP/p300 binding (Zhang 2008) (Fig2).

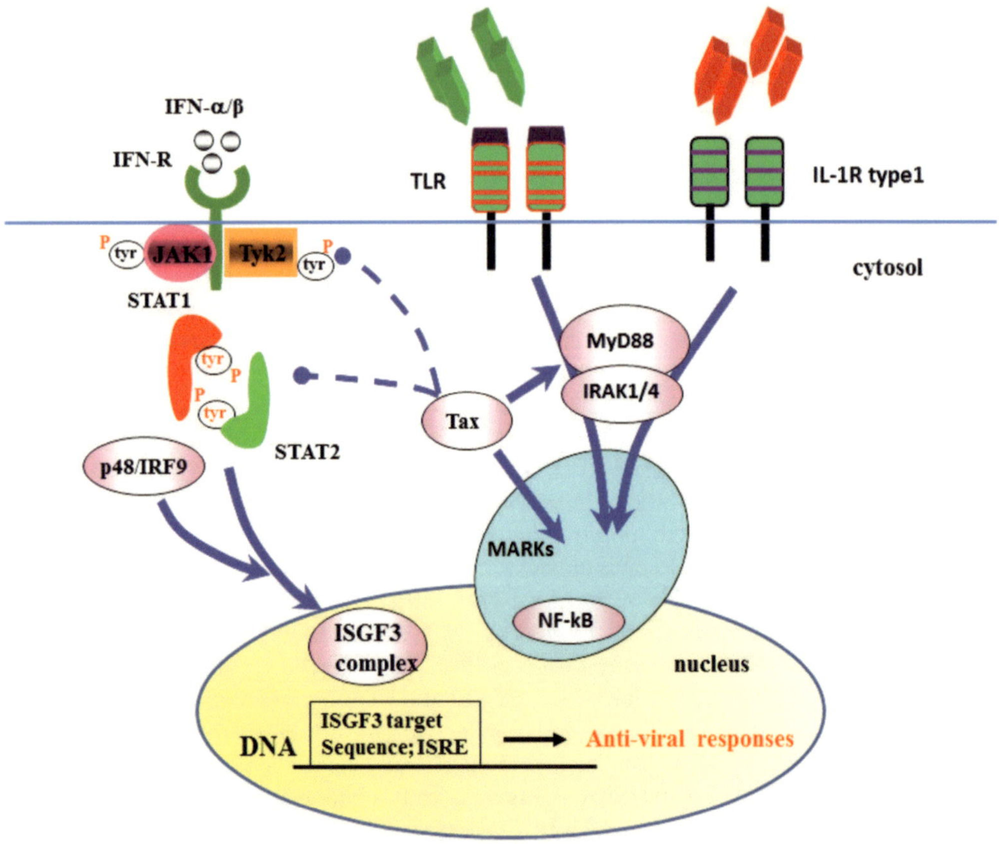

Fig. 2. Constitutive association of MyD88 with IRAK in HTLV-1-transformed T-cells.

The viral p12 protein from the pX open reading frame I (ORFI) activates Jak1/3 and STAT5, and decrease the IL-2-requirement for T-cell proliferation *via* binding to the cytoplasmic domain of IL-2Rβ chain (Nicot 2001). Although the IL-2-Jak-STAT pathway is not associated with viral gene expression, viral RNA encapsidation, the maturation of the viral particle, cell-cell adherence or Gag polarization, p12 enhances viral transmission through activation of the IL-2-Jak-STAT pathway (Taylor 2009).

2.1.1 Inhibition of the JAK-STAT signaling pathway in ATLL cells and HTLV-1-transformed T-cells; therapeutic approach

Several recent studies reported inhibition of constitutive activation of the JAK-STAT signaling pathway in ATLL cells and HTLV-1-transformed T-cells. Src-related kinase Lyn co-immunopreciptates with Jak3 in HTLV-1-transformed cell lines HUT102, MT2, MS9 and MS68. Phosphorylation of STAT5 and STAT3 are inhibited by cell treatment with the Src kinase inhibitor PP2 or by ectopic expression of a dominant negative Lyn kinase protein (Shuh 2011). Dequelin, a naturally occurring retinoid shows anti-proliferative effect on HTLV-1-transformed cells, MT-2 and KUT-1 in part through the down-regulation of survivin and constitutive phosphorylation of STAT3. In contrast, STAT5 phosphorylation is not affected by Deguelin (Ito 2010). roscovitine, an inhibitor of cyclin-dependent kinases (CDKs) inhibits STAT5 activity required for the survival of MT-2 cells. A dominant negative STAT5 expression induces apoptosis and reduces the abundance of an anti-apoptotic protein XIAP in MT-2 cells. In ChIP assay, interaction of STAT5, but not STAT1 with the XIAP promoter has been observed. Interaction of STAT5 and PDGFα receptor is also prevented by roscovitine (Mohapatra 2003). Curcumin (diferuloylmethane), a naturally occurring yellow pigment isolated from the rhizomes of the plant *Curcuma longa*, induces apoptosis and anti-proliferative response in HTLV-1-transformed cells; MT-2, HUT102 and SLB-1. These responses are associated with inhibition of constitutive phosphorylation of Jak3, Tyk2, STAT3 and STAT5. Additionally, AP-1, especially JunD and NF-κB activity in HTLV-1-transfromed T-cells and primary ATLL cells are also inhibited by curcumin (Tomita 2006a, Tomita 2006b).

In a clinical study, Berkowitz et al. reported a single institute open-label phase II trial of intravenous daclizumab, a humanized monoclonal antibody that binds specifically to the alpha (CD25) subunit of the high-affinity IL-2R in ATLL patients. No responses were observed in aggressive acute or lymphoma type of ATLL. Partial responses were observed in 36% of patients with chronic and smoldering ATLL (Berkowitz JL 2010).

In addition, Tasocitinib (CP-690,550), a potent and selective Jak3 inhibitor is an orally active immunosuppressant undergoing clinical trials for the treatment of autoimmune diseases and transplant rejection. It is interesting to note that Tasocitinib (CP-690,550) inhibits proliferation of peripheral blood mononuclear cells (PBMCs) from patients with chronic and smoldering form of ATLL or with HAM/TSP that manifest constitutive Jak3/STAT5 activation. This agent prolongs the survival of transgenic mice bearing human CD8 T-cell leukemia with IL-15/IL-15R autocrine growth loop required for leukemia cell survival (Ju 2011). These results suggest clinical effect of CP-690,550 on chronic and smoldering ATLL.

2.1.2 Constitutive tyrosine and serine phosphorylation of STAT4 in T-cells transformed with HTLV-1

STAT4 is a crucial mediator of IL-12-stimulated gene regulation (Jacobson 1995, Bacon 1995b). In fact, the development of type-1 helper T (Th1) cells and production of IFN-γ in response to IL-12 are disrupted in STAT4-deficient mice (Thierfelder 1996, Kaplan 1996). STAT4 is phosphorylated on tyrosine by Jak2 and Tyk2 (Bacon 1995a, Cho 1996). Moreover, IL-12 activates the p38/MKK6 signaling pathway that in turn phosphorylates STAT4 on serine (Visconti 2000). Activation of p38 and its upstream activator MKK6 is an important step for IL-12-induced STAT4 transcriptional activity (Visconti 2000, Zhang 2000). In fact, previous studies indicated that IFN-γ production is blocked by a p38 inhibitor (Zhang 2000, Rincon 1998). Transgenic mice expressing a dominant-negative p38 showed impaired Th1 differentiation (Rincon 1998). The expression of STAT4 is observed in limited types of tissues such as testis, spleen, lung, bone marrow, thymus and muscle (Zhong 1994, Yamamoto 1994). Several T-cell lines including EL4 and DA2 contain no

STAT4 transcripts (Yamamoto 1994). However, our study showed that tyrosine-phosphorylated STAT4 was detected in HTLV-1-transformed cell lines. In addition, STAT4 protein was constitutively phosphorylated on serine as well as on tyrosine in HTLV-1-transformed cell lines (Higashi 2005).

The relevance of phosphorylation of serine in STAT4 has been recently reported. Serine phosphorylation of STAT4 is dispensable for nuclear translocation or DNA binding of STAT4, but is indispensable for its maximal transcriptional activity (Visconti 2000). Serine phosphorylation of STAT4 is required for IL-12-induced IFN-γ production and IL-12-mediated Th1 development, but not for IL-12-induced cell proliferation (Morinobu 2002). Furthermore, they have shown that serine phosphorylation of STAT4 is partially dependent on precedent tyrosine phosphorylation of STAT4, whereas tyrosine phosphorylation of STAT4 can be seen even in the absence of serine phosphorylation. In contrast, it has been shown that in leukemic cells from chronic lymphocytic leukemia patients, STAT1 and STAT3 are constitutively phosphorylated on serine, but not on tyrosine residue (Frank 1997). In the other leukemias such as AML and ALL, serine phosphorylation of the STATs was occasionally seen (Frank 1997, Hayakawa 1998). Thus, STATs may have selective effects on gene expression of leukemia cells in a manner dependent upon serine phosphorylation. We observed that IFN-γ, but not IL-12 or IFN-α was produced in HTLV-1-transformed cells.

2.1.3 Constitutive association of MyD88 to IRAK in HTLV-1 -transformed cells

Aberrant cytokine gene expression is a hallmark of ATLL cells (Franchini 1995, Grossman 1997, Kanno 1994, Mori 1999, Mori 1996a, Mori 1996b, Siekevitz 1987, Yamada 1996). The cytokine gene promoters possess enhancer elements for NF-κB and/or C/EBPβ (NF-IL6) (Azimi 1998, Faggioli 1996, Mercurio 1997, Perkins 1997, Schmitz 1995, Washizu 1998). C/EBPβ (NF-IL6), β isoform of CCAAT/enhancer (C/EBP) family of basic-leucine zipper (bZIP) transcription factors (Tsukada 2011) was originally identified as a nuclear factor that binds to IL-1-responsive element in the *IL6* gene (Akira 1990). Moreover, inhibition of NF-kB activity results in enhanced apoptosis and growth suppression of primary ATLL cells and HTLV-1-transformed T-cells, indicating a central role for NF-κB in their survival and proliferation. Antisense oligonucleotides to RelA/p65 inhibit Tax-transformed tumor cell growth (Kitajima 1992). Sodium salicylate and cyclopentenone prostaglandins suppress proliferation of Tax-transgenic mouse spleen cells (Portis 2001). Bay-7082, an inhibitor of IκB phosphorylation induces apoptosis of HTLV-1-transformed T-cell lines and primary ATLL cells *via* reduced expression of the anti-apoptotic gene BCL-XL (Mori 2002). *Ex vivo* treatment of PBMCs with dehydroxymethylepoxyquinomicin selectively purges HTLV-1-infected cells without toxicity to normal cells in HTLV-1 carriers (Watanabe 2005). More recently, activation of the classical pathway of NF-κB by the HBZ has been reported (Zhao 2009). HBZ does not affect the alternative pathway of NF-κB, but induces polyubiquitination and degradation of p65. Yasunaga *et al.* demonstrated that ubiquitin-specific peptidase USP20 deubiquitinates TRAF6 and Tax and suppresses Tax-induced NF-κB activation (Yasunaga 2011). Several agents such as Bidens pilosa, a plant found in tropical and subtropical regions (Nakama 2011) and hippuristanol, an eukaryotic translation initiation inhibitor from the coral Isis hippuris (Tsumuraya 2011) also show inhibitory effect on ATLL cells through suppression of NF-κB activity. On the other hand, pan-aurora kinase inhibitor has been shown to have anti-proliferative effect on HTLV-1-transformed T-cells and primary ATLL cells through the suppression of NF-κB activity (Tomita 2009). However, the same study group reported that AZD1152, a selective inhibitor for Aurora B kinase had no effect on NF-κB activity in MT-4 and HUT102 cells (Tomita 2010).

The TLR comprise a subfamily within the larger superfamily of interleukin (IL) receptors, based on similarity within their cytoplasmic regions (Dunne 2003, Matsushima 2007, McGettrick 2007, Takeda 2003) The extracellular region of the IL-1 receptors (IL-1Rs) possesses three immunoglobulin-like domains, those of TLRs are characterized by the presence of 16-28 leucine-rich repeats. Engagement of IL-1R or TLR with their cognate ligands causes an adaptor protein MyD88 to be recruited to the receptor complex, which, in turn, promotes its association with the IL-1R–associated kinase (IRAK) *via* an interaction between the respective death domains of each molecule. This is followed by auto-phosphorylation of IRAK that results in dissociation from the receptor complex and its subsequent interaction with tumor-necrosis-factor (TNF) receptor–associated factor-6 (TRAF-6). Emanating from TRAF-6, two signaling pathways diverge, one eventually leading to NF-κB activation, and another to mitogen-activated protein (MAP) kinase activation (Takeuchi 2007).

In this regard, our study demonstrated an alternative mechanism of NF-κB activation through the TLR signaling cascade including MyD88 and IRAK in HTLV-1--transformed T-cells and ATLL cells (Fig. 2). MyD88 and IRAK1 are constitutively active in HTLV-1-transformed T-cells, but not in HTLV-1-negative T-cells (Mizobe 2007). MyD88, originally isolated as a myeloid differentiation primary response gene product, possesses its C-terminal domain, which is highly homologous to the cytoplasmic regions of the TLR family of proteins (Dunne 2003, Takeda 2003). However, unlike members of the TLR family, MyD88 contains no transmembrane domain. MyD88 acts an adaptor molecule of most TLRs and receptors for IL-1 and IL-18 to recruit IRAK to the TLR complex, thereby regulating activation of various transcription factors involved in inflammatory responses, such as NF-κB and C/EBPβ (NF-IL6) (Akira 2003a, Akira 2001, Akira 2003b, Boch 2003, Burns 1998, Dunne 2003, Jefferies 2001, Muzio 2000, O'Neill 2003, Takeda 2003).

Expression of a dominant negative MyD88 (MyD88dn) lacking its death domain (DD), MyD88dn induces apoptosis and anti-proliferative response in HTLV-1-transformed T-cells. In HTLV-1-transformed T-cells, MyD88dn protein expression inhibits constitutive activation of C/EBPβ (NF-IL6) and NF-κB, and proinflamatory cytokine gene promoters such as IL-1α, IFN-γ and TNF-α. Furthermore, Tax synergistically activates NF-κB with MyD88 (Mizobe 2007). The synergy may suggest ligand-independent activation of MyD88 in HTLV-1-transformed cells (Fig. 2). However, NF-κB activation has been observed even in ATLL cells lacking detectable Tax expression. The mechanism for activation of NF-κB in ATLL cells is not still clear. A recent study reported contribution of elevated CD30 expression to constitutive activation of NF-κB in ATLL cells (Higuchi 2005). In this regard, the non-canonical pathway for NF-κB activation, induced by B-cell activation factor (Claudio 2002, Kayagaki 2002), lymphotoxin-β (Dejardin 2002, Saitoh 2002), CD40 (Coope 2002), TNF-like weak inducer of apoptosis (Saitoh 2003) or CD30 (Higuchi 2005) may be also involved in constitutive NF-κB activation in ATLL cells (Hironaka 2004).

In addition, MT-2 cells express TLR-1, 6 and 10 mRNA. Several recent reports have indicated unique expression profiles of TLRs on different subsets of T-cells. Gelman *et al.* (Gelman 2004) reported that TLR-3, -5 and -9 are expressed selectively on activated human $CD4^+$ T cells, and that treatment of activated human $CD4^+$ T-cells, with dsRNA synthetic analogs, poly(I:C) and CpGoligodeoxynucleotides (CpG DNA), directly enhance their survival without affecting proliferation. A TLR-5 ligand flagellin and a TLR7/8 ligand R-848 promotes proliferation and to upregulate production of IFN-γ, IL-8 and IL-10, but not IL-4, in human CD4+ T-cells (Caron 2005). In particular, engagement of TLR-5 with flagellin enhances the suppressive capacity and FOXP3 expression in Treg cells (Crellin 2005). Direct modulation of Treg function by TLR2 ligands has been also reported (Oberg 2010). On the other hand, IRF-5 (P68) with a mutation of Ala to Pro at amino acid 68 (G202C; position relative to translation start codon) suppresses TLR-mediated IL-6 and IL-12p40 induction. The mutation has been identified in peripheral blood of ATLL patients (Yang 2009).

A more recent report has emphasized the significance of MyD88 in the pathogenesis and therapeutic approach for lymphoma. Ngo *et al.* identified a single leucine-to-proline substitution at amino acid position 265 of MyD88 protein (L265P) in 29% of activated B-cell (ABC) subtype of diffuse large B-cell lymphoma (DLBCL) biopsy samples. This mutation occurs at an evolutionally invariant residue in the hydrophobic core and is rare or absent in the other DLBCL subtypes. They further demonstrated that in ABC DLBCL with L265P mutation, MyD88 L265P rescued the cell after MyD88 knockdown, but wild-type MyD88 was ineffective, showing that the L265P is a gain-of-function mutation and ABC DLBCL with L265P mutation depends upon the MyD88 signaling pathway. A selective small molecule inhibitor of IRAK1 and IRAK4 killed the ABC DLBCL cells. Moreover, in ABC DLBCL cell lines, MyD88 knockdown diminishes the secretion of IL-6 and IL-10 and phosphorylation of STAT3 (Ngo 2011).

3. Conclusion

Investigations have led to the demonstration of the several regulatory mechanisms presented in this review. Recent reports have provided detailed insight into the crucial functional roles of JAK-STAT and MyD88-TLR in ATLL. An important goal of such approaches would be the identification of unique targets for clinical intervention. The fact that the two signaling pathway are attractive targets for leukemia therapies further argues the importance of constitutive activation of these factors in ATLL cells.

4. References

Akira, S (1997) IL-6-regulated transcription factors. *Int J Biochem Cell Biol,* 29, 12, 1401-18.

Akira, S (2003) Toll-like receptor signaling. *J Biol Chem,* 278, 40, 38105-8, 0021-9258.

Akira, S, Isshiki, H, Sugita, T, Tanabe, O, Kinoshita, S, Nishio, Y, Nakajima, T, Hirano, T & Kishimoto, T (1990) A nuclear factor for IL-6 expression (NF-IL6) is a member of a C/EBP family. *EMBO J,* 9, 6, 1897-906, 0261-4189.

Akira, S, Takeda, K & Kaisho, T (2001) Toll-like receptors: critical proteins linking innate and acquired immunity. *Nat Immunol,* 2, 8, 675-80, 1529-2908.

Akira, S, Yamamoto, M & Takeda, K (2003) Role of adapters in Toll-like receptor signalling. *Biochem Soc Trans,* 31, Pt 3, 637-42, 0300-5127.

Arima, N, Hidaka, S, Fujiwara, H, Matsushita, K, Ohtsubo, H, Arimura, K, Kukita, T, Fukumori, J & Tanaka, H (1996) Relation of autonomous and interleukin-2-responsive growth of leukemic cells to survival in adult T-cell leukemia. *Blood,* 87, 7, 2900-4, 0006-4971.

Arima, N, Matsushita, K, Obata, H, Ohtsubo, H, Fujiwara, H, Arimura, K, Kukita, T, Suruga, Y, Wakamatsu, S, Hidaka, S & Tei, C (1999) NF-κB involvement in the activation of primary adult T-cell leukemia cells and its clinical implications. *Exp Hematol*, 27, 7, 1168-75, 0301-472X.

Azimi, N, Brown, K, Bamford, RN, Tagaya, Y, Siebenlist, U & Waldmann, TA (1998) Human T cell lymphotropic virus type I Tax protein trans-activates interleukin 15 gene transcription through an NF-κB site. *Proc Natl Acad Sci U S A*, 95, 5, 2452-7, 0027-8424

Bacon, CM, McVicar, DW, Ortaldo, JR, Rees, RC, O'Shea, JJ & Johnston, JA (1995a) Interleukin 12 (IL-12) induces tyrosine phosphorylation of JAK2 and TYK2: differential use of Janus family tyrosine kinases by IL-2 and IL-12. *J Exp Med*, 181, 1, 399-404.

Bacon, CM, Petricoin, EF, 3rd, Ortaldo, JR, Rees, RC, Larner, AC, Johnston, JA & O'Shea, JJ (1995b) Interleukin 12 induces tyrosine phosphorylation and activation of STAT4 in human lymphocytes. *Proc Natl Acad Sci U S A*, 92, 16, 7307-11.

Benekli, M, Xia, Z, Donohue, KA, Ford, LA, Pixley, LA, Baer, MR, Baumann, H & Wetzler, M (2002) Constitutive activity of signal transducer and activator of transcription 3 protein in acute myeloid leukemia blasts is associated with short disease-free survival. *Blood*, 99, 1, 252-7.

Berkowitz JL, JJ, Stewart DM, Fioravanti S, Jaffe ES, Fleisher TA, Urquhart N,Wharfe JH, Waldmann TA, Morris JC (2010) Phase II trial of daclizumab in human T-cell lymphotropic virus type-1 (HTLV-1)-associated adult T-cell leukemia/lymphoma (ATL). *J Clin Oncol*, 28, 15s, suppl; abstr 8043.

Boch, JA, Yoshida, Y, Koyama, Y, Wara-Aswapati, N, Peng, H, Unlu, S & Auron, PE (2003) Characterization of a cascade of protein interactions initiated at the IL-1 receptor. *Biochem Biophys Res Commun*, 303, 2, 525-31, 0006-291X.

Bowman, T, Garcia, R, Turkson, J & Jove, R (2000) STATs in oncogenesis. *Oncogene*, 19, 21, 2474-88.

Bromberg, JF, Wrzeszczynska, MH, Devgan, G, Zhao, Y, Pestell, RG, Albanese, C & Darnell, JE, Jr. (1999) Stat3 as an oncogene. *Cell*, 98, 3, 295-303.

Burns, K, Martinon, F, Esslinger, C, Pahl, H, Schneider, P, Bodmer, JL, Di Marco, F, French, L & Tschopp, J (1998) MyD88, an adapter protein involved in interleukin-1 signaling. *J Biol Chem*, 273, 20, 12203-9, 0021-9258..

Carlesso, N, Frank, DA & Griffin, JD (1996) Tyrosyl phosphorylation and DNA binding activity of signal transducers and activators of transcription (STAT) proteins in hematopoietic cell lines transformed by Bcr/Abl. *J Exp Med*, 183, 3, 811-20.

Caron, G, Duluc, D, Fremaux, I, Jeannin, P, David, C, Gascan, H & Delneste, Y (2005) Direct stimulation of human T cells via TLR5 and TLR7/8: flagellin and R-848 up-regulate proliferation and IFN-γ production by memory CD4+ T cells. *J Immunol*, 175, 3, 1551-7, 0022-1767..

Chen, J, Petrus, M, Bryant, BR, Phuc Nguyen, V, Stamer, M, Goldman, CK, Bamford, R, Morris, JC, Janik, JE & Waldmann, TA (2008) Induction of the IL-9 gene by HTLV-I Tax stimulates the spontaneous proliferation of primary adult T-cell leukemia cells by a paracrine mechanism. *Blood*, 111, 10, 5163-72, 1528-0020.

Cho, SS, Bacon, CM, Sudarshan, C, Rees, RC, Finbloom, D, Pine, R & O'Shea, JJ (1996) Activation of STAT4 by IL-12 and IFN-α: evidence for the involvement of ligand-induced tyrosine and serine phosphorylation. *J Immunol*, 157, 11, 4781-9.

Claudio, E, Brown, K, Park, S, Wang, H & Siebenlist, U (2002) BAFF-induced NEMO-independent processing of NF-κB2 in maturing B cells. *Nat Immunol,* 3, 10, 958-65, 1529-2908.

Coffer, PJ, Koenderman, L & de Groot, RP (2000) The role of STATs in myeloid differentiation and leukemia. *Oncogene,* 19, 21, 2511-22.

Coope, HJ, Atkinson, PG, Huhse, B, Belich, M, Janzen, J, Holman, MJ, Klaus, GG, Johnston, LH & Ley, SC (2002) CD40 regulates the processing of NF-κB2 p100 to p52. *EMBO J,* 21, 20, 5375-85, 0261-4189.

Crellin, NK, Garcia, RV, Hadisfar, O, Allan, SE, Steiner, TS & Levings, MK (2005) Human CD4+ T cells express TLR5 and its ligand flagellin enhances the suppressive capacity and expression of FOXP3 in CD4+CD25+ T regulatory cells. *J Immunol,* 175, 12, 8051-9, 0022-1767.

Danial, NN, Pernis, A & Rothman, PB (1995) Jak-STAT signaling induced by the v-abl oncogene. *Science,* 269, 5232, 1875-7.

Darnell, JE, Jr. (1997) STATs and gene regulation. *Science,* 277, 5332, 1630-5.

Dejardin, E, Droin, NM, Delhase, M, Haas, E, Cao, Y, Makris, C, Li, ZW, Karin, M, Ware, CF & Green, DR (2002) The lymphotoxin-beta receptor induces different patterns of gene expression via two NF-κB pathways. *Immunity,* 17, 4, 525-35, 1074-7613.

Dunne, A & O'Neill, LA (2003) The interleukin-1 receptor/Toll-like receptor superfamily: signal transduction during inflammation and host defense. *Sci STKE,* 2003, 171, re3, 1525-8882.

Faggioli, L, Costanzo, C, Merola, M, Bianchini, E, Furia, A, Carsana, A & Palmieri, M (1996) Nuclear factor κB (NF-κB), nuclear factor interleukin-6 (NFIL-6 or C/EBPβ) and nuclear factor interleukin-6β (NFIL6-β or C/EBPδ) are not sufficient to activate the endogenous interleukin-6 gene in the human breast carcinoma cell line MCF-7. Comparative analysis with MDA-MB-231 cells, an interleukin-6-expressing human breast carcinoma cell line. *Eur J Biochem,* 239, 3, 624-31, 0014-2956.

Feng, X & Ratner, L (2008) Human T-cell leukemia virus type 1 blunts signaling by interferon α. *Virology,* 374, 1, 210-6, 0042-6822.

Flex, E, Petrangeli, V, Stella, L, Chiaretti, S, Hornakova, T, Knoops, L, Ariola, C, Fodale, V, Clappier, E, Paoloni, F, Martinelli, S, Fragale, A, Sanchez, M, Tavolaro, S, Messina, M, Cazzaniga, G, Camera, A, Pizzolo, G, Tornesello, A, Vignetti, M, Battistini, A, Cave, H, Gelb, BD, Renauld, JC, Biondi, A, Constantinescu, SN, Foa, R & Tartaglia, M (2008) Somatically acquired JAK1 mutations in adult acute lymphoblastic leukemia. *J Exp Med,* 205, 4, 751-8, 1540-9538.

Franchini, G (1995) Molecular mechanisms of human T-cell leukemia/lymphotropic virus type I infection. *Blood,* 86, 10, 3619-39, 0006-4971.

Franchini, G, Wong-Staal, F & Gallo, RC (1984) Human T-cell leukemia virus (HTLV-I) transcripts in fresh and cultured cells of patients with adult T-cell leukemia. *Proc Natl Acad Sci U S A,* 81, 19, 6207-11, 0027-8424.

Frank, DA, Mahajan, S & Ritz, J (1997) B lymphocytes from patients with chronic lymphocytic leukemia contain signal transducer and activator of transcription (STAT) 1 and STAT3 constitutively phosphorylated on serine residues. *J Clin Invest,* 100, 12, 3140-8.

Frank, DA & Varticovski, L (1996) BCR/abl leads to the constitutive activation of Stat proteins, and shares an epitope with tyrosine phosphorylated Stats. *Leukemia,* 10, 11, 1724-30.

Geleziunas, R, Ferrell, S, Lin, X, Mu, Y, Cunningham, ET, Jr., Grant, M, Connelly, MA, Hambor, JE, Marcu, KB & Greene, WC (1998) Human T-cell leukemia virus type 1 Tax induction of NF-κB involves activation of the IκB kinaseα (IKKα) and IKKβ cellular kinases. *Mol Cell Biol,* 18, 9, 5157-65, 0270-7306.

Gelman, AE, Zhang, J, Choi, Y & Turka, LA (2004) Toll-like receptor ligands directly promote activated CD4+ T cell survival. *J Immunol,* 172, 10, 6065-73, 0022-1767.

Gouilleux-Gruart, V, Gouilleux, F, Desaint, C, Claisse, JF, Capiod, JC, Delobel, J, Weber-Nordt, R, Dusanter-Fourt, I, Dreyfus, F, Groner, B & Prin, L (1996) STAT-related transcription factors are constitutively activated in peripheral blood cells from acute leukemia patients. *Blood,* 87, 5, 1692-7.

Grossman, WJ & Ratner, L (1997) Cytokine expression and tumorigenicity of large granular lymphocytic leukemia cells from mice transgenic for the tax gene of human T-cell leukemia virus type I. *Blood,* 90, 2, 783-94, 0006-4971.

Harhaj, EW & Sun, SC (1999) IKKγ serves as a docking subunit of the IκB kinase (IKK) and mediates interaction of IKK with the human T-cell leukemia virus Tax protein. *J Biol Chem,* 274, 33, 22911-4, 0021-9258.

Hayakawa, F, Towatari, M, Iida, H, Wakao, H, Kiyoi, H, Naoe, T & Saito, H (1998) Differential constitutive activation between STAT-related proteins and MAP kinase in primary acute myelogenous leukaemia. *Br J Haematol,* 101, 3, 521-8.

Higashi, T, Tsukada, J, Yoshida, Y, Mizobe, T, Mouri, F, Minami, Y, Morimoto, H & Tanaka, Y (2005) Constitutive tyrosine and serine phosphorylation of STAT4 in T-cells transformed with HTLV-I. *Genes Cells,* 10, 12, 1153-62, 1356-9597.

Higuchi, M, Matsuda, T, Mori, N, Yamada, Y, Horie, R, Watanabe, T, Takahashi, M, Oie, M & Fujii, M (2005) Elevated expression of CD30 in adult T-cell leukemia cell lines: possible role in constitutive NF-κB activation. *Retrovirology,* 2, 29, 1742-4690.

Hironaka, N, Mochida, K, Mori, N, Maeda, M, Yamamoto, N & Yamaoka, S (2004) Tax-independent constitutive IκB kinase activation in adult T-cell leukemia cells. *Neoplasia,* 6, 3, 266-78, 1522-8002.

Huang, GJ, Zhang, ZQ & Jin, DY (2002) Stimulation of IKK-γ oligomerization by the human T-cell leukemia virus oncoprotein Tax. *FEBS Lett,* 531, 3, 494-8, 0014-5793.

Ihle, JN (2001) The Stat family in cytokine signaling. *Curr Opin Cell Biol,* 13, 2, 211-7.

Ito, S, Oyake, T, Murai, K & Ishida, Y (2010) Deguelin suppresses cell proliferation via the inhibition of survivin expression and STAT3 phosphorylation in HTLV-1-transformed T cells. *Leuk Res,* 34, 3, 352-7, 1873-5835.

Jacobson, NG, Szabo, SJ, Weber-Nordt, RM, Zhong, Z, Schreiber, RD, Darnell, JE, Jr. & Murphy, KM (1995) Interleukin 12 signaling in T helper type 1 (Th1) cells involves tyrosine phosphorylation of signal transducer and activator of transcription (Stat)3 and Stat4. *J Exp Med,* 181, 5, 1755-62.

Jefferies, C, Bowie, A, Brady, G, Cooke, EL, Li, X & O'Neill, LA (2001) Transactivation by the p65 subunit of NF-κB in response to interleukin-1 (IL-1) involves MyD88, IL-1 receptor-associated kinase 1, TRAF-6, and Rac1. *Mol Cell Biol,* 21, 14, 4544-52, 0270-7306.

Jin, DY, Giordano, V, Kibler, KV, Nakano, H & Jeang, KT (1999) Role of adapter function in oncoprotein-mediated activation of NF-κB. Human T-cell leukemia virus type I Tax interacts directly with IκB kinase γ. *J Biol Chem,* 274, 25, 17402-5, 0021-9258.

Ju, W, Zhang, M, Jiang, JK, Thomas, CJ, Oh, U, Bryant, BR, Chen, J, Sato, N, Tagaya, Y, Morris, JC, Janik, JE, Jacobson, S & Waldmann, TA (2011) CP-690,550, a therapeutic agent, inhibits cytokine-mediated Jak3 activation and proliferation of T cells from patients with ATL and HAM/TSP. *Blood,* 117, 6, 1938-46, 1528-0020.

Kameda, T, Shide, K, Shimoda, HK, Hidaka, T, Kubuki, Y, Katayose, K, Taniguchi, Y, Sekine, M, Kamiunntenn, A, Maeda, K, Nagata, K, Matsunaga, T & Shimoda, K (2010) Absence of gain-of-function JAK1 and JAK3 mutations in adult T cell leukemia/lymphoma. *Int J Hematol,* 92, 2, 320-5, 1865-3774.

Kanno, T, Brown, K, Franzoso, G & Siebenlist, U (1994) Kinetic analysis of human T-cell leukemia virus type I Tax-mediated activation of NF-κB. *Mol Cell Biol,* 14, 10, 6443-51, 0270-7306.

Kaplan, MH, Sun, YL, Hoey, T & Grusby, MJ (1996) Impaired IL-12 responses and enhanced development of Th2 cells in Stat4-deficient mice. *Nature,* 382, 6587, 174-7.

Kayagaki, N, Yan, M, Seshasayee, D, Wang, H, Lee, W, French, DM, Grewal, IS, Cochran, AG, Gordon, NC, Yin, J, Starovasnik, MA & Dixit, VM (2002) BAFF/BLyS receptor 3 binds the B cell survival factor BAFF ligand through a discrete surface loop and promotes processing of NF-κB2. *Immunity,* 17, 4, 515-24, 1074-7613.

Kitajima, I, Shinohara, T, Bilakovics, J, Brown, DA, Xu, X & Nerenberg, M (1992) Ablation of transplanted HTLV-I Tax-transformed tumors in mice by antisense inhibition of NF-κB. *Science,* 258, 5089, 1792-5, 0036-8075.

Leonard, WJ & O'Shea, JJ (1998) Jaks and STATs: biological implications. *Annu Rev Immunol,* 16, 293-322.

Levy, DE & Gilliland, DG (2000) Divergent roles of STAT1 and STAT5 in malignancy as revealed by gene disruptions in mice. *Oncogene,* 19, 21, 2505-10.

Lin, TS, Mahajan, S & Frank, DA (2000) STAT signaling in the pathogenesis and treatment of leukemias. *Oncogene,* 19, 21, 2496-504.

Maeda, M, Arima, N, Daitoku, Y, Kashihara, M, Okamoto, H, Uchiyama, T, Shirono, K, Matsuoka, M, Hattori, T, Takatsuki, K & et al. (1987) Evidence for the interleukin-2 dependent expansion of leukemic cells in adult T cell leukemia. *Blood,* 70, 5, 1407-11, 0006-4971.

Matsushima, N, Tanaka, T, Enkhbayar, P, Mikami, T, Taga, M, Yamada, K & Kuroki, Y (2007) Comparative sequence analysis of leucine-rich repeats (LRRs) within vertebrate toll-like receptors. *BMC Genomics,* 8, 124, 1471-2164.

McGettrick, AF & O'Neill, LA (2007) Toll-like receptors: key activators of leucocytes and regulator of haematopoiesis. *Br J Haematol,* 139, 2, 185-93, 0007-1048.

Mercurio, F, Zhu, H, Murray, BW, Shevchenko, A, Bennett, BL, Li, J, Young, DB, Barbosa, M, Mann, M, Manning, A & Rao, A (1997) IKK-1 and IKK-2: cytokine-activated IκB kinases essential for NF-κB activation. *Science,* 278, 5339, 860-6, 0036-8075.

Migone, TS, Lin, JX, Cereseto, A, Mulloy, JC, O'Shea, JJ, Franchini, G & Leonard, WJ (1995) Constitutively activated Jak-STAT pathway in T cells transformed with HTLV-I. *Science,* 269, 5220, 79-81.

Mizobe, T, Tsukada, J, Higashi, T, Mouri, F, Matsuura, A, Tanikawa, R, Minami, Y, Yoshida, Y & Tanaka, Y (2007) Constitutive association of MyD88 to IRAK in HTLV-I-transformed T cells. *Exp Hematol,* 35, 12, 1812-22, 0301-472X.

Mohapatra, S, Chu, B, Wei, S, Djeu, J, Epling-Burnette, PK, Loughran, T, Jove, R & Pledger, WJ (2003) Roscovitine inhibits STAT5 activity and induces apoptosis in the human leukemia virus type 1-transformed cell line MT-2. *Cancer Res,* 63, 23, 8523-30, 0008-5472.

Mori, N, Fujii, M, Ikeda, S, Yamada, Y, Tomonaga, M, Ballard, DW & Yamamoto, N (1999) Constitutive activation of NF-κB in primary adult T-cell leukemia cells. *Blood,* 93, 7, 2360-8, 0006-4971.

Mori, N, Gill, PS, Mougdil, T, Murakami, S, Eto, S & Prager, D (1996) Interleukin-10 gene expression in adult T-cell leukemia. *Blood,* 88, 3, 1035-45, 0006-4971.

Mori, N & Prager, D (1996) Transactivation of the interleukin-1alpha promoter by human T-cell leukemia virus type I and type II Tax proteins. *Blood,* 87, 8, 3410-7, 0006-4971.

Mori, N, Yamada, Y, Ikeda, S, Yamasaki, Y, Tsukasaki, K, Tanaka, Y, Tomonaga, M, Yamamoto, N & Fujii, M (2002) Bay 11-7082 inhibits transcription factor NF-κB and induces apoptosis of HTLV-I-infected T-cell lines and primary adult T-cell leukemia cells. *Blood,* 100, 5, 1828-34, 0006-4971.

Morinobu, A, Gadina, M, Strober, W, Visconti, R, Fornace, A, Montagna, C, Feldman, GM, Nishikomori, R & O'Shea, JJ (2002) STAT4 serine phosphorylation is critical for IL-12-induced IFN-γ production but not for cell proliferation. *Proc Natl Acad Sci U S A,* 99, 19, 12281-6.

Muzio, M, Polentarutti, N, Bosisio, D, Manoj Kumar, PP & Mantovani, A (2000) Toll-like receptor family and signalling pathway. *Biochem Soc Trans,* 28, 5, 563-6, 0300-5127.

Nakama, S, Ishikawa, C, Nakachi, S & Mori, N (2011) Anti-adult T-cell leukemia effects of Bidens pilosa. *Int J Oncol,* 38, 4, 1163-73, 1791-2423.

Ngo, VN, Young, RM, Schmitz, R, Jhavar, S, Xiao, W, Lim, KH, Kohlhammer, H, Xu, W, Yang, Y, Zhao, H, Shaffer, AL, Romesser, P, Wright, G, Powell, J, Rosenwald, A, Muller-Hermelink, HK, Ott, G, Gascoyne, RD, Connors, JM, Rimsza, LM, Campo, E, Jaffe, ES, Delabie, J, Smeland, EB, Fisher, RI, Braziel, RM, Tubbs, RR, Cook, JR, Weisenburger, DD, Chan, WC & Staudt, LM (2011) Oncogenically active MYD88 mutations in human lymphoma. *Nature,* 470, 7332, 115-9, 1476-4687 .

Nicot, C, Mulloy, JC, Ferrari, MG, Johnson, JM, Fu, K, Fukumoto, R, Trovato, R, Fullen, J, Leonard, WJ & Franchini, G (2001) HTLV-1 p12(I) protein enhances STAT5 activation and decreases the interleukin-2 requirement for proliferation of primary human peripheral blood mononuclear cells. *Blood,* 98, 3, 823-9, 0006-4971.

O'Neill, LA (2003) The role of MyD88-like adapters in Toll-like receptor signal transduction. *Biochem Soc Trans,* 31, Pt 3, 643-7, 0300-5127.

Oberg, HH, Ly, TT, Ussat, S, Meyer, T, Kabelitz, D & Wesch, D (2010) Differential but direct abolishment of human regulatory T cell suppressive capacity by various TLR2 ligands. *J Immunol,* 184, 9, 4733-40, 1550-6606.

Ohashi, T, Masuda, M & Ruscetti, SK (1995) Induction of sequence-specific DNA-binding factors by erythropoietin and the spleen focus-forming virus. *Blood,* 85, 6, 1454-62.

Oliere, S, Hernandez, E, Lezin, A, Arguello, M, Douville, R, Nguyen, TL, Olindo, S, Panelatti, G, Kazanji, M, Wilkinson, P, Sekaly, RP, Cesaire, R & Hiscott, J (2010)

HTLV-1 evades type I interferon antiviral signaling by inducing the suppressor of cytokine signaling 1 (SOCS1). *PLoS Pathog,* 6, 11, e1001177, 1553-7374.

Perkins, ND (1997) Achieving transcriptional specificity with NF-κB. *Int J Biochem Cell Biol,* 29, 12, 1433-48, 1357-2725.

Portis, T, Harding, JC & Ratner, L (2001) The contribution of NF-κB activity to spontaneous proliferation and resistance to apoptosis in human T-cell leukemia virus type 1 Tax-induced tumors. *Blood,* 98, 4, 1200-8, 0006-4971.

Rincon, M, Enslen, H, Raingeaud, J, Recht, M, Zapton, T, Su, MS, Penix, LA, Davis, RJ & Flavell, RA (1998) Interferon-γ expression by Th1 effector T cells mediated by the p38 MAP kinase signaling pathway. *Embo J,* 17, 10, 2817-29.

Saitoh, T, Nakano, H, Yamamoto, N & Yamaoka, S (2002) Lymphotoxin-beta receptor mediates NEMO-independent NF-κB activation. *FEBS Lett,* 532, 1-2, 45-51, 0014-5793.

Saitoh, T, Nakayama, M, Nakano, H, Yagita, H, Yamamoto, N & Yamaoka, S (2003) TWEAK induces NF-κB2 p100 processing and long lasting NF-κB activation. *J Biol Chem,* 278, 38, 36005-12, 0021-9258.

Schmitz, ML & Baeuerle, PA (1995) Multi-step activation of NF-κB/Rel transcription factors. *Immunobiology,* 193, 2-4, 116-27, 0171-2985.

Shuai, K, Halpern, J, ten Hoeve, J, Rao, X & Sawyers, CL (1996) Constitutive activation of STAT5 by the BCR-ABL oncogene in chronic myelogenous leukemia. *Oncogene,* 13, 2, 247-54.

Shuh, M, Morse, BA, Heidecker, G & Derse, D (2011) Association of SRC-related kinase lyn with the interleukin-2 receptor and its role in maintaining constitutive phosphorylation of Jak/STAT in human T-cell leukemia virus type 1-transformed T cells. *J Virol,* 85, 9, 4623-7, 1098-5514 .

Siekevitz, M, Feinberg, MB, Holbrook, N, Wong-Staal, F & Greene, WC (1987) Activation of interleukin 2 and interleukin 2 receptor (Tac) promoter expression by the trans-activator (tat) gene product of human T-cell leukemia virus, type I. *Proc Natl Acad Sci U S A,* 84, 15, 5389-93, 0027-8424.

Spiekermann, K, Biethahn, S, Wilde, S, Hiddemann, W & Alves, F (2001) Constitutive activation of STAT transcription factors in acute myelogenous leukemia. *Eur J Haematol,* 67, 2, 63-71.

Takeda, K, Kaisho, T & Akira, S (2003) Toll-like receptors. *Annu Rev Immunol,* 21, 335-76, 0732-0582.

Takemoto, S, Mulloy, JC, Cereseto, A, Migone, TS, Patel, BK, Matsuoka, M, Yamaguchi, K, Takatsuki, K, Kamihira, S, White, JD, Leonard, WJ, Waldmann, T & Franchini, G (1997) Proliferation of adult T cell leukemia/lymphoma cells is associated with the constitutive activation of JAK/STAT proteins. *Proc Natl Acad Sci U S A,* 94, 25, 13897-902.

Takeuchi, O & Akira, S (2007) Signaling pathways activated by microorganisms. *Curr Opin Cell Biol,* 19, 2, 185-91, 0955-0674.

Taylor, JM, Brown, M, Nejmeddine, M, Kim, KJ, Ratner, L, Lairmore, M & Nicot, C (2009) Novel role for interleukin-2 receptor-Jak signaling in retrovirus transmission. *J Virol,* 83, 22, 11467-76, 1098-5514 .

Thierfelder, WE, van Deursen, JM, Yamamoto, K, Tripp, RA, Sarawar, SR, Carson, RT, Sangster, MY, Vignali, DA, Doherty, PC, Grosveld, GC & Ihle, JN (1996)

Requirement for Stat4 in interleukin-12-mediated responses of natural killer and T cells. *Nature,* 382, 6587, 171-4.

Tomita, M, Kawakami, H, Uchihara, JN, Okudaira, T, Masuda, M, Takasu, N, Matsuda, T, Ohta, T, Tanaka, Y & Mori, N (2006a) Curcumin suppresses constitutive activation of AP-1 by downregulation of JunD protein in HTLV-1-infected T-cell lines. *Leuk Res,* 30, 3, 313-21, 0145-2126.

Tomita, M, Kawakami, H, Uchihara, JN, Okudaira, T, Masuda, M, Takasu, N, Matsuda, T, Ohta, T, Tanaka, Y, Ohshiro, K & Mori, N (2006b) Curcumin (diferuloylmethane) inhibits constitutive active NF-κB, leading to suppression of cell growth of human T-cell leukemia virus type I-infected T-cell lines and primary adult T-cell leukemia cells. *Int J Cancer,* 118, 3, 765-72, 0020-7136.

Tomita, M, Tanaka, Y & Mori, N (2010) Aurora kinase inhibitor AZD1152 negatively affects the growth and survival of HTLV-1-infected T lymphocytes in vitro. *Int J Cancer,* 127, 7, 1584-94, 1097-0215 .

Tomita, M, Toyota, M, Ishikawa, C, Nakazato, T, Okudaira, T, Matsuda, T, Uchihara, JN, Taira, N, Ohshiro, K, Senba, M, Tanaka, Y, Ohshima, K, Saya, H, Tokino, T & Mori, N (2009) Overexpression of Aurora A by loss of CHFR gene expression increases the growth and survival of HTLV-1-infected T cells through enhanced NF-κB activity. *Int J Cancer,* 124, 11, 2607-15, 1097-0215.

Tsukada, J, Toda, Y, Misago, M, Tanaka, Y, Auron, PE & Eto, S (2000) Constitutive activation of LIL-Stat in adult T-cell leukemia cells. *Blood,* 95, 8, 2715-8.

Tsukada, J, Yoshida, Y, Kominato, Y & Auron, PE (2011) The CCAAT/enhancer (C/EBP) family of basic-leucine zipper (bZIP) transcription factors is a multifaceted highly-regulated system for gene regulation. *Cytokine,* 54, 1, 6-19, 1096-0023.

Tsumuraya, T, Ishikawa, C, Machijima, Y, Nakachi, S, Senba, M, Tanaka, J & Mori, N (2011) Effects of hippuristanol, an inhibitor of eIF4A, on adult T-cell leukemia. *Biochem Pharmacol,* 81, 6, 713-22, 1873-2968.

Ueda, M, Imada, K, Imura, A, Koga, H, Hishizawa, M & Uchiyama, T (2005) Expression of functional interleukin-21 receptor on adult T-cell leukaemia cells. *Br J Haematol,* 128, 2, 169-76, 0007-1048 .

Visconti, R, Gadina, M, Chiariello, M, Chen, EH, Stancato, LF, Gutkind, JS & O'Shea, JJ (2000) Importance of the MKK6/p38 pathway for interleukin-12-induced STAT4 serine phosphorylation and transcriptional activity. *Blood,* 96, 5, 1844-52.

Washizu, J, Nishimura, H, Nakamura, N, Nimura, Y & Yoshikai, Y (1998) The NF-κB binding site is essential for transcriptional activation of the IL-15 gene. *Immunogenetics,* 48, 1, 1-7, 0093-7711 .

Watanabe, M, Ohsugi, T, Shoda, M, Ishida, T, Aizawa, S, Maruyama-Nagai, M, Utsunomiya, A, Koga, S, Yamada, Y, Kamihira, S, Okayama, A, Kikuchi, H, Uozumi, K, Yamaguchi, K, Higashihara, M, Umezawa, K, Watanabe, T & Horie, R (2005) Dual targeting of transformed and untransformed HTLV-1-infected T cells by DHMEQ, a potent and selective inhibitor of NF-κB, as a strategy for chemoprevention and therapy of adult T-cell leukemia. *Blood,* 106, 7, 2462-71, 0006-4971.

Weber-Nordt, RM, Egen, C, Wehinger, J, Ludwig, W, Gouilleux-Gruart, V, Mertelsmann, R & Finke, J (1996) Constitutive activation of STAT proteins in primary lymphoid and myeloid leukemia cells and in Epstein-Barr virus (EBV)-related lymphoma cell lines. *Blood,* 88, 3, 809-16.

Xia, Z, Baer, MR, Block, AW, Baumann, H & Wetzler, M (1998) Expression of signal transducers and activators of transcription proteins in acute myeloid leukemia blasts. *Cancer Res,* 58, 14, 3173-80.

Xu, X, Kang, SH, Heidenreich, O, Okerholm, M, O'Shea, JJ & Nerenberg, MI (1995) Constitutive activation of different Jak tyrosine kinases in human T cell leukemia virus type 1 (HTLV-1) tax protein or virus-transformed cells. *J Clin Invest,* 96, 3, 1548-55.

Yamada, Y, Ohmoto, Y, Hata, T, Yamamura, M, Murata, K, Tsukasaki, K, Kohno, T, Chen, Y, Kamihira, S & Tomonaga, M (1996) Features of the cytokines secreted by adult T cell leukemia (ATL) cells. *Leuk Lymphoma,* 21, 5-6, 443-7, 1042-8194.

Yamada, Y, Sugawara, K, Hata, T, Tsuruta, K, Moriuchi, R, Maeda, T, Atogami, S, Murata, K, Fujimoto, K, Kohno, T, Tsukasaki, K, Tomonaga, M, Hirakata, Y & Kamihira, S (1998) Interleukin-15 (IL-15) can replace the IL-2 signal in IL-2-dependent adult T-cell leukemia (ATL) cell lines: expression of IL-15 receptor alpha on ATL cells. *Blood,* 91, 11, 4265-72, 0006-4971.

Yamamoto, K, Quelle, FW, Thierfelder, WE, Kreider, BL, Gilbert, DJ, Jenkins, NA, Copeland, NG, Silvennoinen, O & Ihle, JN (1994) Stat4, a novel γ interferon activation site-binding protein expressed in early myeloid differentiation. *Mol Cell Biol,* 14, 7, 4342-9.

Yang, L, Zhao, T, Shi, X, Nakhaei, P, Wang, Y, Sun, Q, Hiscott, J & Lin, R (2009) Functional analysis of a dominant negative mutation of interferon regulatory factor 5. *PLoS One,* 4, 5, e5500, 1932-6203 .

Yasunaga, J, Lin, FC, Lu, X & Jeang, KT (2011) Ubiquitin-specific peptidase 20 (USP20) targets TRAF6 and HTLV-1 Tax to negatively regulate NF-{κ}B signaling. *J Virol,* 1098-5514.

Zhang, J, Yamada, O, Kawagishi, K, Araki, H, Yamaoka, S, Hattori, T & Shimotohno, K (2008) Human T-cell leukemia virus type 1 Tax modulates interferon-alpha signal transduction through competitive usage of the coactivator CBP/p300. *Virology,* 379, 2, 306-13, 1096-0341.

Zhang, S & Kaplan, MH (2000) The p38 mitogen-activated protein kinase is required for IL-12-induced IFN-γ expression. *J Immunol,* 165, 3, 1374-80.

Zhao, T, Yasunaga, J, Satou, Y, Nakao, M, Takahashi, M, Fujii, M & Matsuoka, M (2009) Human T-cell leukemia virus type 1 bZIP factor selectively suppresses the classical pathway of NF-κB. *Blood,* 113, 12, 2755-64, 1528-0020.

Zhong, Z, Wen, Z & Darnell, JE, Jr. (1994) Stat3 and Stat4: members of the family of signal transducers and activators of transcription. *Proc Natl Acad Sci U S A,* 91, 11, 4806-10.

6

Ikaros in T-Cell Leukemia

Sinisa Dovat[1] and Kimberly J. Payne[2]
[1]*Pennsylvania State University College of Medicine*
[2]*Loma Linda University*
United States of America

1. Introduction

Although extensive clinical data have established that the loss of Ikaros tumor suppressor activity *via* genetic inactivation is a major contributor to leukemogenesis leading to B-cell ALL, less is known about the role of Ikaros in T-cell leukemia. The T-cell malignancies observed in Ikaros-deficient mice suggest that Ikaros is likely to function as a tumor suppressor in T-cells. In human, multiple studies have identified genetic inactivation of Ikaros (deletion or mutation) to be associated with ~5% of T-ALL cases. Additional studies provide evidence that the functional inactivation of Ikaros due to defects in signal pathways that normally regulate Ikaros activity is likely to be a critical factor in the development of T-cell malignancies. These studies provide a rationale for new chemotherapeutic strategies in the treatment of T-cell leukemia. In this chapter, we summarize the newest advances that shed light on the role of Ikaros in T-cell leukemia.

2. Structure and function of Ikaros

The *Ikaros* gene, discovered independently by K. Georgopoulos and S. Smale, encodes multiple Ikaros protein isoforms *via* alternate splicing (Lo et al. 1991; Georgopoulos et al. 1992; Hahm et al. 1994). The structure of Ikaros protein reveals several known structural motifs corresponding to distinct functional domains as described below.

2.1 Molecular structure of Ikaros

2.1.1 DNA-binding domain

The N-terminal region of the Ikaros protein contains four zinc finger motifs (Fig. 1). Three of these exhibit a typical C2H2 structure with two cysteines and two histidines covalently bound to a zinc atom, while the fourth zinc finger has a CCHC structure. The four N terminal zinc fingers in the Ikaros protein function in DNA binding. Point mutational analysis revealed that zinc fingers #2 and #3 are essential for the DNA-binding function of Ikaros, as well as its localization to pericentromeric heterochromatin (see 2.2.1). Based on DNA-se footprint analysis, it has been suggested that the first zinc finger contributes to DNA binding specificity. The role of the fourth zinc finger in DNA-binding remains unknown, although it has been noted that Ikaros isoforms that lack the fourth zinc finger exhibit a unique expression pattern during hematopoiesis (Payne et al. 2003). Recently, a point mutation in a single allele of the fourth zinc finger has been associated with primary immunodeficiency and pancytopenia in humans (Goldman, et al. In press.).

2.1.2 Dimerization domain

The C-terminal region of the Ikaros protein contains two zinc finger motifs (Fig. 1). These zinc fingers do not bind DNA, but mediate protein-protein interactions with other Ikaros isoforms, and/or with Ikaros family proteins (Helios, Aiolos, etc.) that share the same motif (Sun et al. 1996). Every described Ikaros isoform contains the two C terminal zinc fingers, thus allowing for the formation of diverse Ikaros dimers with the potential for unique and specific functions. Ikaros binds DNA as a dimer, which underscores the importance of this domain for Ikaros function.

2.1.3 Bipartite activation-repression domain

All of the Ikaros proteins share a bipartite activation domain, that is adjacent to the two C-terminal zinc fingers (Fig. 1). This domain is responsible for stimulating basal levels of transcription of Ikaros target genes (Sun et al. 1996; Georgopoulos et al. 1997). Within the bipartite activation domain, there are two distinct stretches of amino acids - acidic and hydrophobic. It has been established that acidic amino acids are responsible for transcriptional activation, while the hydrophobic amino acids do not exhibit such an effect (Sun et al. 1996). However, the presence of the hydrophobic amino acids next to the acidic stretch increases their transcriptional activation activity, suggesting that the hydrophobic residues have a functional role in transcriptional regulation (Sun et al. 1996; Georgopoulos et al. 1997).

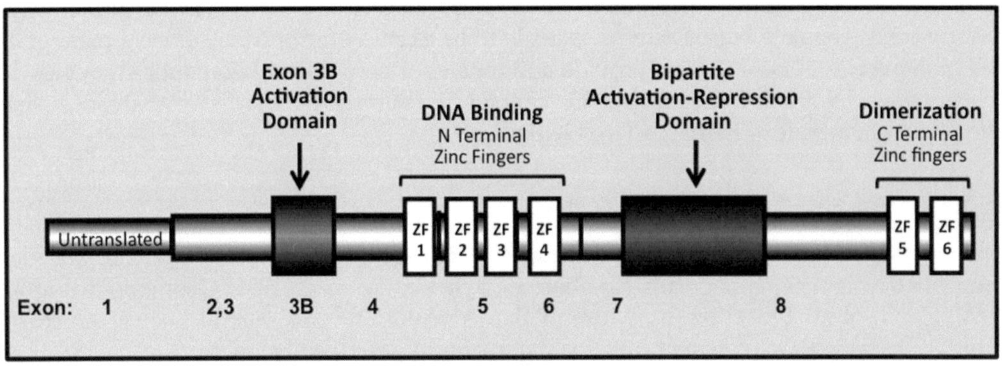

Fig. 1. Major structural features of the Ikaros protein. The *Ikaros* gene (*Ikzf1)* includes eight coding exons. Exon 1 is untranslated and was not identified in initial reports. Current Genbank sequences do not identify Exon 3B which encodes the 20 amino acid activation domain.

2.1.4 Exon 3B activation domain

Exon 3B of the *Ikaros* gene encodes a short, 20-amino acid stretch in the N region of the Ikaros protein (Fig. 1). This domain has been described (Hahm et al. 1994; Sun et al. 1999; Payne et al. 2001) and functionally analyzed in human Ikaros (Ronni et al. 2007). This domain has been shown to take part in determining the DNA-binding specificity of the Ikaros protein complex and in regulating the expression of Ikaros target genes (Ronni et al. 2007).

We would like to emphasize that there are functionally significant domains of the Ikaros protein that are as yet unidentified. It is known that Ikaros can act as a transcriptional repressor and that it has a role in chromatin remodeling (see 2.2.2). However, the structures and/or particular amino acids within the Ikaros protein that are responsible for these functions remain unknown. Further studies are needed to provide more detailed maps of the functional domains within the Ikaros protein.

2.2 Ikaros function in regulating gene expression

2.2.1 Ikaros regulates gene expression *via* chromatin remodeling

Ikaros has been shown to regulate transcription by binding DNA at the upstream regulatory elements of its target genes (Georgopoulos et al. 1992; Ernst et al. 1993; Hahm et al. 1994; Molnar and Georgopoulos 1994). Thus, DNA binding is essential for Ikaros function. While Ikaros can directly activate or repress its target genes, subsequent experiments established that Ikaros function as a regulator of gene expression occurs *via* its role in chromatin remodeling. Studies by A. Fisher's group demonstrated that Ikaros is abundantly localized in pericentromeric heterochromatin in cells (Brown et al. 1997). In pericentromeric regions, transcriptionally inactive genes have been shown to selectively associate with Ikaros foci, while transcriptionally active genes do not (Brown et al. 1997). The expression status of several genes that are differentially expressed during T and B cell maturation correlate with their association with Ikaros. Mutations in Ikaros binding sites interferes with the developmentally-regulated shut-down of the λ5 gene (Sabbattini et al. 2001), as well as the gene that encodes TdT *(dntt)* (Trinh et al. 2001) during lymphoid differentiation. These data further support a role for Ikaros in gene silencing *via* chromatin remodeling. Experiments by Georgopoulos' group also demonstrated that Ikaros regulates expression of its target genes by recruiting them to pericentromeric heterochromatin, but that recruitment to pericentromeric heterochromatin can lead to activation of the target genes (Koipally et al. 2002). Studies in human T-cells revealed that Ikaros binding to human pericentromeric heterochromatin is regulated in a complex way by the association of different Ikaros isoforms. A model has been proposed whereby Ikaros regulates expression of its target genes by recruiting them to pericentromeric heterochromatin leading to either their activation or repression, and that switching from repression to activation depends on the presence of particular Ikaros isoforms in the Ikaros DNA-binding complex (Ronni et al. 2007; Kim et al. 2009). **Thus, the current hypothesis is that Ikaros binds the upstream region of target genes and aids in their recruitment to pericentromeric heterochromatin, resulting in repression or activation of the target gene (Brown et al. 1997; Liberg et al. 2003).**

2.2.2 Molecular mechanisms of chromatin remodeling and gene regulation by Ikaros

Ikaros associates with histone deacetylase (HDAC)-containing complexes (NuRD and Sin3A and Sin3B) (Koipally et al. 1999). Ikaros directly interacts with the NuRD complex ATPase, Mi-2β, and with Sin3A and Sin3B through both its N-terminal and C-terminal regions (Kim et al. 1999; Koipally et al. 1999). The histone deacetylase complex acts as a transcriptional repressor *via* chromatin remodeling. It has been hypothesized that Ikaros recruits histone deacetylase complex to the upstream regulatory elements of its target genes resulting in **chromatin remodeling and repression** of the target genes (Brown et al. 1997; Liberg et al. 2003).

Ikaros has been shown to interact with the CtBP corepressor *in vivo*. This interaction with CtBP is achieved through amino acids at the N-terminal region of Ikaros (Koipally and Georgopoulos 2000). The Ikaros-CtBP complex acts as a transcriptional repressor. This repression is HDAC-independent, and represents **an additional means by which Ikaros represses transcription** of its target genes (Koipally and Georgopoulos 2000).

Ikaros also associates with Brg-1, a catalytic subunit of the SWI/SNF nucleosome remodeling complex that acts as an activator of gene expression (Kim et al. 1999; O'Neill et al. 2000). It has been hypothesized that Ikaros recruits the SWI/SNF nucleosome remodeling complex to the upstream regions of its target genes (in a similar fashion to the NuRD complex) resulting in **chromatin remodeling and activation** of its target genes. **Thus, Ikaros can act as either an activator or a repressor of its target genes, depending on whether it associates with the NuRD, the CtBP or the SWI/SNF complex.**

3. Ikaros in T-cell development

The role of Ikaros in normal T-cell development is demonstrated by evidence that Ikaros regulates the expression of key genes in T-cell differentiation and by the impaired T-cell differentiation observed in Ikaros-defficient mice.

3.1 Ikaros regulates genes critical for the development of T-cells (*TdT*)

The role of Ikaros in regulating expression of the gene encoding terminal deoxynucleotide transferase (*TdT*) during thymocyte differentiation has been extensively studied (Ernst et al. 1993; Ernst et al. 1996; Trinh et al. 2001; Su et al. 2005). Ikaros has been shown to bind *in vivo* to the D' upstream regulatory element of the *TdT* (*dntt*) gene. This region contains a perfect Ikaros consensus DNA-binding site, and mutational analysis has demonstrated that the presence of this sequence is essential for Ikaros binding to the upstream regulatory element of the *TdT* gene. This same region contains a consensus binding site that is bound *in vivo* by Elf-1, a member of the Ets family of transcription factors. The binding of Elf-1 and Ikaros have been shown to be mutually exclusive. Ikaros binding to the *TdT* upstream regulatory element leads to repositioning of the *TdT* gene to pericentromeric heterochromatin and to repression of *TdT* transcription. Elf-1, in contrast, acts as positive regulator of *TdT* expression. Thus, Ikaros and Elf-1 compete for occupancy of the same upstream control region during thymocyte development and have the opposite effect on *TdT* expression (Trinh et al. 2001). In CD4+CD8+ thymocytes, the upstream region of *TdT* is occupied by Elf-1 leading to expression of the *TdT* gene. During the induction of T-cell differentiation, Ikaros displaces Elf-1 from binding the upstream regulatory element of *TdT*, resulting in the loss of *TdT* expression. The absence of Ikaros results in failure to repress *TdT* expression during thymocyte differentiation leading to impaired T-cell development. The exact molecular mechanisms by which Ikaros displaces Elf-1 during thymocyte differentiation remains to be determined, although there is compelling evidence that the reversible phosphorylation of Ikaros (see 6.1 and 6.2 below) is responsible for this regulation.

3.2 Ikaros regulation of CD4, CD8, and IL-2 expression

During T-cell development, Ikaros has been demonstrated to bind to the regulatory element of the CD8α gene *in vivo* by chromatin immunoprecipitation (ChIP) assay. Ikaros has been hypothesized to positively regulate expression of the CD8α gene during thymocyte differentiation (Harker et al. 2002). This has been supported by evidence that Ikaros-defficient mice have decreased numbers of CD8+ T-cells (see 3.3 below).

Studies by Georgopoulos' group demonstrated that Ikaros binds *in vivo* to a silencer that is located in the first intron of the *Cd4* gene resulting in the suppression of *Cd4* transcription. Further analysis revealed that Ikaros can bind concommitantly with the Mi-2β chromatin remodeler leading to suppression of the Cd4 silencer and upregulation of *Cd4* gene expression. The Ikaros-Mi2β complex aids in recruitment of histone acetyl transferases. Thus Ikaros appeaars to be able to both activate or repress expression of *Cd4 via* chromatin remodeling (Naito et al. 2007).

In mature CD4+ cells, Ikaros was shown to bind *in vivo* to the upstream regulatory element of the *IL-2* gene. Further analysis demonstrated that Ikaros represses expression of the *IL-2* gene in mature CD4+ cells *via* chromatin remodeling. This established Ikaros as a regulator of anergy induction in CD4+ T-cells (Thomas et al. 2007).

3.3 T-cell development in Ikaros-defficient mice

Studies of Ikaros-deficient mice established Ikaros as a master regulator of T-cell development and identified several biological functions of Ikaros:

1. Thymocytes that lack Ikaros expression progress from the double negative (DN) CD4–CD8– to the double positive (DP) CD4+CD8+ stage in the absence of β selection (Wang et al. 1996). The proliferative response of thymocytes following TCR β ligation is ~9 fold higher in thymocytes from Ikaros null mice, compared to the wild-type. Thus, Ikaros has been identified as a key regulator of the β selection checkpoint in T-cell differentiation and a regulator of thymocyte expansion following β selection (Winandy et al. 1999).
2. Thymocytes from Ikaros-deficient mice downregulate CD8 to become CD4 single positive (SP) thymocytes without positive selection signals that are normally required for differentiation from the DP to the SP stage (Winandy et al. 1999; Urban and Winandy 2004). Ikaros has also been shown to regulate negative selection that occurs during the DP stage (Urban and Winandy 2004). T-cell production in these mice is skewed toward the production of CD4 T-cells. Thus, Ikaros functions as a regulator that controls the TCR selection checkpoint in T-cell development, as well as a regulator of CD4 versus CD8 T-cell fate decisions (Wang et al. 1996; Winandy et al. 1999; Urban and Winandy 2004).
3. Ikaros-deficient T-cells from all three Ikaros knock-out mice strains possess a lower activation threshold than normal T-cells and enter the cell cycle at an accelerated pace (Avitahl et al. 1999; Winandy et al. 1999). Thus, Ikaros sets the activation threshold in mature T-cells and regulates cell cycle progression.

4. Ikaros and T-cell leukemia

4.1 Ikaros-deficient mice develop T-cell leukemia

The Ikaros-defficient mouse described above clearly established that Ikaros has an essential role in T-cell development. Subsequent analysis of heterozygous Ikaros-defficient mice revealed that Ikaros has tumor suppressor activity. Between the second and third month of age, these mice display an aberration in thymic differentiation with an accumulation of triple-positive thymocytes that have intermediate expression levels of CD4, CD8, and the TCR complex (Winandy et al. 1995). At the same time, a polyclonal expansion of mature T lymphocytes occurs in the spleen of these mice. Proliferation assays established that thymocytes from heterozygous Ikaros-defficient mice have hyperproliferative potential, and that they can proliferate in the absence of TCR stimulation. It is worth noting that these changes precede the malignant transformation of thymocytes described below (Winandy et al. 1995).

After 3 month of age, all of the Ikaros-defficient heterozygous mice develop T-cell leukemia and lymphoma (Winandy et al. 1995). This is manifested by severe generalized lymphadenopathy and splenomegaly, along with an increased number of malignant lymphoblasts in the peripheral blood. Flow cytometry analysis of malignant lymphoblasts established that they are monoclonal in origin, and that malignancy arises in the thymus. The expression analysis of maliganT-cells revealed that the wild type Ikaros copy was lost in these cells, thus they have a loss of Ikaros heterozygosity (Winandy et al. 1995).

An additional Ikaros-defficient biological model provided evidence for the loss of Ikaros tumor suppressor activity in T-cell leukemia. This *Ikaros*-targeted mouse ($IK^{L/L}$) had the β-galactosidase (βgal) reporter gene inserted in-frame into exon 2 that is present in all known Ikaros isoforms. These mice produce very low levels of Ikaros proteins (Kirstetter et al. 2002; Dumortier et al. 2003; Dumortier et al. 2006). The $IK^{L/L}$ mice exhibit T lineage defects that are identical to those reported in Ikaros null mice including a lowered threshold to activation stimuli and the invariable development of thymic tumors.

These findings strongly suggested that Ikaros acts as a tumor suppressor for T-cell leukemia. They also provide support for the hypothesis that Ikaros regulates normal thymocyte differentiation, and controls the proliferation of thymocytes and mature T-cells in response to TCR signaling.

Further studies directly addressed the question of whether normal Ikaros function is essential and sufficient to induce tumor suppression of T-cell leukemia. The re-introduction of Ikaros *via* retroviral insertion into T leukemia cells that were derived from Ikaros-defficient mice resulted in their cessation of growth (Kathrein et al. 2005). Expression of Ikaros in T-cell leukemia induced T-cell differentiation that was characterized by increased expression of CD4, CD69, CD5, and TCR. These data suggested that Ikaros tumor suppressor activity involves positive regulation of normal thymocyte differentiation, and that a potential mechanism for malignant transformation of Ikaros-defficient thymocytes involves failure of T-cell differentiation.

The induction of T-cell differentiatiom following re-introduction of Ikaros was accompanied by induction of cell cycle arrest at the G0/G1 stage of the cell cycle (Kathrein et al. 2005). The exact mechanism by which Ikaros induces cell cycle arrest remains unknown, although it has been observed that the induction of Ikaros expression in leukemia cells correlates with the increased expression of the cell cycle-dependent kinase inhibitor $p27^{kip1}$ (Kathrein et al. 2005). One possibility is that Ikaros affects global chromatin remodeling, since restoration of Ikaros activity in T-cell leukemia correlates with a global increase in histone H3 acetylation (Kathrein et al. 2005).

These complementary studies established Ikaros as a *bona fide* tumor suppressor in T-cell leukemia and demonstrate that the lack of Ikaros is the major causative factor of T-cell malignancy in Ikaros-deficient mice.

4.2 Ikaros deficiency in human T-cell leukemia

Since the discovery of the *Ikaros* gene and the identification of its function as a master regulator of lymphocyte differentiation and a tumor suppressor in mice, a number of studies have examined human leukemia samples to determine if an alteration of Ikaros' function is associated with the development of hematopoietic malignancies in humans. Increased expression of dominant-negative Ikaros isoforms has been associated with a variety of hematopoietic malignancies in humans. These include childhood ALL (Kuiper et al. 2007; Mullighan et al. 2007; Mullighan et al. 2008; Dovat and Payne 2010; Marcais et al.), adult B cell ALL (Nakase et al. 2000), myelodysplastic syndrome (Crescenzi et al. 2004), AML (Yagi et al. 2002), and adult and juvenile CML (Nakayama et al. 1999). Deletion of an Ikaros allele was detected in over 80% of BCR-ABL1 ALL and the deletion or mutation of Ikaros has been identified as a poor prognostic marker for childhood ALL (Mullighan et al. 2007; Mullighan et al. 2008; Martinelli et al. 2009; Martinelli et al. 2009; Martinelli et al. 2009; Mullighan et al. 2009). These data established Ikaros as a major tumor suppressor in human leukemia. The most compelling data supporting the tumor suppressor activity of Ikaros in human hematopoietic malignancies was established for B-cell ALL.

In T-cell ALL, the initial studies produced somewhat conflicting data. The first report described expression of dominant-negative Ikaros isoforms (using Western blot and RT-PCR) in all 18 pediatric T-cell ALL patients that were studied (Sun et al. 1999), suggesting a strong correlation of the loss of Ikaros function with the development of T-cell ALL. However, subsequent studies on a total of 14 patients with T-cell ALL (both adult and pediatric) did not detect the presence of dominant-negative Ikaros isoforms (using Western blot and RT-PCR) in T-cell ALL (Nakase et al. 2000; Ruiz et al. 2004), although one study detected an association of the expression of a dominant-negative isoform of the Ikaros-family member - Helios with T-cell ALL (Nakase et al. 2002).

More comprehensive studies that utilized high-resolution CGH-arrays in a total of 81 patients, detected deletion of one copy of Ikaros in 5% of T-cell ALL patients (Kuiper et al. 2007; Maser et al. 2007; Mullighan et al. 2008). The most recent study of 25 cases of human T-cell ALL, that combined Western blot, CGH-array analysis, and sequencing of Ikaros cDNA following RT-PCR, provided a more complete view of the relation of Ikaros and T-cell ALL. This study detected one patient (4%) in which one Ikaros allele had been deleted, while the Ikaros protein produced by the other intact allele exhibited a loss of nuclear localization with an abnormal localization in the cytoplasmic structure (Marcais et al. 2010). This study provided the first definitive functional evidence of the complete loss of Ikaros function and T-cell ALL in humans.

In summary, studies in human T-cell ALL have demonstrated that genetic inactivation of the *Ikaros* gene by deletion or mutation does occur in human T-cell ALL in at least 5% of cases. Although Ikaros deletion is not as frequent an event in T-cell ALL when compared to B-cell ALL (30%) or BCR-ABL1 ALL (80%), it is a notable cause of T-cell ALL, and needs to be tested in newly diagnosed patients with this disease. The prognostic significance of Ikaros deletion in T-cell ALL remains to be determined. Studies also suggest that functional inactivation of Ikaros plays a significant role in T-cell ALL, although the mechanisms by which Ikaros function is impaired in T-cell ALL is still unknown. Recent findings discussed below provide insights into signal transduction pathways that potentially affect Ikaros tumor suppressor function in T-cell ALL.

5. Mechanisms of Ikaros tumor suppressor activity

The mechanisms of Ikaros tumor suppressor activity are not well understood. One major obstacle is the paucity of known Ikaros target genes. The best evidence for the mechanisms of tumor suppression by Ikaros in T-cell ALL comes from studies that identified the role of Ikaros in the Notch pathway.

5.1 Ikaros-mediated repression of the downstream effectors of the Notch pathway (Deltex and Hes1)

The Notch pathway is essential for normal T-cell differentiation. However, activation of the Notch 1 gene has been found in over 50% of T-ALLs (Weng et al. 2004) and T-ALL leukemia cells often express the Notch target genes Hes-1 and pTα (Chiaramonte et al. 2005). The intracelular domain of Notch^{IC} forms a complex with the Notch transcription factor RBP-Jk/CSL and the cofactor Mastermind. This complex activates expression of Notch pathway target genes. Studies by S. Chen's group demonstrated that the Notch pathway is activated in the T-cell leukemia that develops in Ikaros-defficient mice (Dumortier et al. 2006). Additional analysis showed that Ikaros directly downregulates a Notch target gene, Hes-1. Ikaros directly competes with CSL for binding to the upstream regulator element of Hes-1 (Kleinmann et al. 2008). Since CSL acts as a stimulator of transcription, and Ikaros represses transcription of Hes-1, Ikaros counteracts the pro-oncogenic Notch signaling in T-cell ALL. Repression of Hes-1 by Ikaros likely involves chromatin remodeling since Ikaros binding to the upstream regulatory region of Hes-1 leads to a decrease in histone H3 acetylation (Kathrein et al. 2008), and Ikaros-defficient mice have reduced trimethylation of histone H3 at the K27 residue (Kleinmann et al. 2008).

A link between Ikaros deficiency and Notch activation in T-cell ALL had been suggested by Beverly and Capobianco (Beverly and Capobianco 2003). They found synergism between Notch activation and the inactivation of Ikaros in T-cell leukemogenesis. Sequence analysis of the consensus binding sequence for CSL and Ikaros revealed remarkable similarities and the authors hypothesized that Ikaros may interfere with CSL binding and Notch signaling (Beverly and Capobianco 2003).

Additional experiments showed that Ikaros represses another target gene of the Notch signaling pathway - Deltex1 (Kathrein et al. 2008). Similarly to the regulation of Hes-1, Ikaros competes with CSL for binding to the upstream regulatory region of Deltex1 and represses expression of Deltex1 by chromatin remodeling. Ikaros binding to the upstream region of Deltex1 also results in decreased histone H3 acetylation (Kathrein et al. 2008).

These data strongly suggest that one of the mechanisms by which Ikaros suppresses leukemogenesis in T-cells involves inhibition of the Notch signal transduction pathway.

5.2 Additional mechanisms of Ikaros tumor suppressor activity in T-cell ALL

One possible explanation for why the lack of Ikaros function leads to leukemia is the fact that Ikaros regulates expression of several genes that are essential for normal T-cell development (section 3 above). Often, malignant transformation is characterized by a failure (or arrest) of normal differentiation. Thus, the absence of Ikaros activity and its subsequent impact on T-cell differentiation is likely to be an important step toward the development of leukemia.

It has been demonstrated that Ikaros can negatively regulate cell cycle progression at the G1/S transition (Gomez-del Arco et al. 2004), thus the absence of Ikaros would impair the G1/S check point in the regulation of the cell cycle.

Several reports suggested that Ikaros downregulates $Bcl\text{-}x_L$ expression (Yagi et al. 2002; Ezzat et al. 2006; Kano et al. 2008). Thus, Ikaros might regulate apoptosis, and the lack of

Ikaros activity would have an oncogenic effect similar to the overexpression of Bcl2 in chronic lymphocytic leukemia (CLL). This would also lead to the development of leukemia that is more highly resistance to chemotherapy.
In summary, multiple mechanisms including the loss of Notch pathway inhibition, blocked T-cell differentiation and impaired cell cycle control are likely to play a role in the T-cell leukemogenesis that occurs with the loss of Ikaros activity. However, the specific mechanisms by which Ikaros exerts its tumor suppressor activity remain largely unknown. Identification of additional genes that are regulated by Ikaros will provide more insight on this important process.

6. Regulation of Ikaros' function in T-cell leukemia

6.1 Phosphorylation of Ikaros by CK2 kinase inactivates the Ikaros protein

Despite the fact that Ikaros plays a critical role in regulating T-cell proliferation and differentiation, the level of Ikaros expression remains high throughout the cell cycle and during lymphocyte differentiation. This suggests that Ikaros function is regulated by posttranslational modifications. The role of phosphorylation in regulating Ikaros function has been studied the most extensively. Studies that identified mitosis-specific hyperphopshorylation of Ikaros at an evolutionarily conserved linker sequence, provided evidence that the cell cycle-specific phosphorylation of Ikaros regulates its DNA-binding ability and nuclear localization during mitosis (Dovat et al. 2002). This provided the first evidence that phosphorylation can regulate Ikaros function in cells.
Subsequent studies demonstrated that Ikaros is a direct substrate of Casein Kinase II (CK2) and that CK2-mediated phosphorylation regulates multiple functions of Ikaros in normal and leukemia cells:
Experiments performed by Georgopoulos' group identified several amino acids located in the C-terminal region of the Ikaros protein that are directly phoshorylated by CK2. Mutational analysis of phosphoacceptor sites revealed that CK2-mediated phosphorylation regulates Ikaros' ability to control cell cycle progression during the G1/S transition.
Studies by Dovat's group identified additional phosphorylation sites in the N-terminal region of the Ikaros protein that are phosphorylated by CK2 (Gurel et al. 2008). Experiments with Ikaros phosphomimetic mutants (that mimic constitutive phosphorylation) and phosphoresistant mutants (that mimic constitutive dephosphorylation) revealed that CK2-mediated phosphorylation of two amino acids located in the N-terminal region of Ikaros controls two essential functions of Ikaros: 1) Ikaros' DNA-binding activity and 2) Ikaros' subcellular localization to pericentromeric heterochromatin (Gurel et al. 2008). Increased phosphorylation of Ikaros by CK2 results in severely decreased DNA-binding affinity and the loss of pericentromeric localization, thus **CK2-mediated phosphorylation leads to inactivation of Ikaros function** (Gurel et al. 2008).

6.2 CK2-mediated phosphorylation controls Ikaros function in T-cell differentiation

The significance of CK2-mediated phosphorylation for normal T-cell development was underscored by the discovery that Ikaraos in CD4+CD8+ thymocytes is phosphorylated at multiple sites by CK2 (Gurel et al. 2008). As described above, in thymocytes, Ikaros binds to the upstream regulatory region of its target gene, *TdT,* leading to repression of *TdT* transcription. Phosphorylation of Ikaros in CD4+CD8+ thymocytes by CK2 decreases its

DNA-binding affinity toward the upstream regulatory element of *TdT*, which results in occupancy of this region by the transcription factor Elf-1 and expression of *TdT*. During induction of thymocyte differentiation, Ikaros undergoes dephosphorylation at amino acids #13 and #294 (Gurel et al. 2008). Differentiation-specific dephosphorylation of Ikaros results in its increased DNA-binding affinity toward the upstream regulatory element of *TdT*, displacement of Elf-1, and repression of *TdT* transcription. These data demonstrate that the regulation of Ikaros phosphorylation by CK2 plays an important role in T-cell differentiation and suggest that increased activity of CK2 kinase in thymocytes would lead to impaired T-cell development due to interference with normal Ikaros function.

6.3 CK2-mediated phosphorylation leads to ubiquitination and degradation of the Ikaros protein

Further functional analysis of Ikaros phosphorylation revealed that CK2-mediated phosphorylation occurs at PEST sequences in the Ikaros protein. PEST sequences are comprised of a region that is rich in Proline (P), Gluamate (E), Serine (S) and Threonine (T). It has been demonstrated that phosophorylation of the serines or threonines located within the PEST sequence typically results in increased degradation of the respective protein. Ikaros contains two PEST sequences that are phosphorylated *in vivo* by CK2 (Popescu et al. 2009). Phosphorylation at PEST sequences leads to decreased half-life and increased degradation of Ikaros, resulting in a low level of Ikaros protein in cells. Hyperphoshorylated Ikaros undergoes polyubiquitination, which leads to its degradation *via* the ubiquitin/ proteasome pathway (Popescu et al. 2009).

6.4 Dephosphorylation of Ikaros by PP1 opposes CK2-mediated phosphorylation

The discovery that Ikaros is a direct substrate for Protein Phosphatase 1 (PP1) (Popescu et al. 2009), a well-known tumor suppressor protein, provided additional evidence that phosphorylation plays an extremely important role in the regulation of Ikaros activity in normal hematopoiesis and in leukemia. Ikaros interacts with PP1 directly by binding *via* a PP1 consensus recognition motif that is located near the C-terminal zinc fingers. Dephosphorylation of Ikaros by PP1 is essential for preservation of Ikaros DNA-binding activity and subcelular localization to pericentromeric heterochromatin (Popescu et al. 2009). Mutated Ikaros protein that is unable to interact with PP1 undergoes accelerated degradation *via* the ubiquitin pathway. This results in a 5- to 10-fold decrease in the level of Ikaros protein in cells, when compared to wild type Ikaros (Popescu et al. 2009). Thus, PP1-mediated dephosphorylation of Ikaros counteracts the effect of CK2-mediated phosphorylation of Ikaros. This provides evidence that two major signal transduction pathways – one involving CK2 and the other PP1 – converge on the Ikaros protein (Fig. 2).
These pathways exert opposite effects on Ikaros function and thus regulate T-cell differentiation and proliferation.

Both CK2 and PP1 proteins are known to play a critical role in malignant transformation. Increased expression of CK2 during T-cell differentiation results in the development of T-cell leukemia in mice (Seldin and Leder 1995). Furthermore, CK2 activity is elevated in many other types of human malignancies (Phan-Dinh-Tuy et al. 1985; Pinna 1997; Roig et al. 1999; Kim et al. 2007). The activity of CK2 and PP1 is closely tied to the ability of cells to proliferate, and thus the balance of their function is essential to prevent malignant transformation. Both CK2 and PP1 exerts strong effects on multiple functions of Ikaros – its role in T-cell differentiation, ability to regulate cell cycle progression, DNA-binding affinity, chromatin remodeling capability (by controlling its subcellular localization to pericentromeric heterochromatin), regulation of gene expression, and protein stability. This suggests that the pro-oncogenic activity of CK2 involves inactivation of the *Ikaros* gene, while the tumor suppressor activity of PP1 is mediated by preserving the tumor suppressor function of Ikaros. These data also strongly suggest that in leukemia cells that have increased activity of CK2, but no deletion/mutation in the *Ikaros* gene, the Ikaros protein that is present is unlikely to be a functionally active Ikaros protein with tumor suppressor activity. Instead, recent discoveries suggest that the functional inactivation of Ikaros by CK2-mediated hyperphopshorylation might be one important mechanism leading to T-cell leukemia. This provides new insight into the role of Ikaros, CK2, and PP1 in T-cell leukemia, and identifies CK2 kinase as a potential target for novel chemotherapy for T-cell ALL.

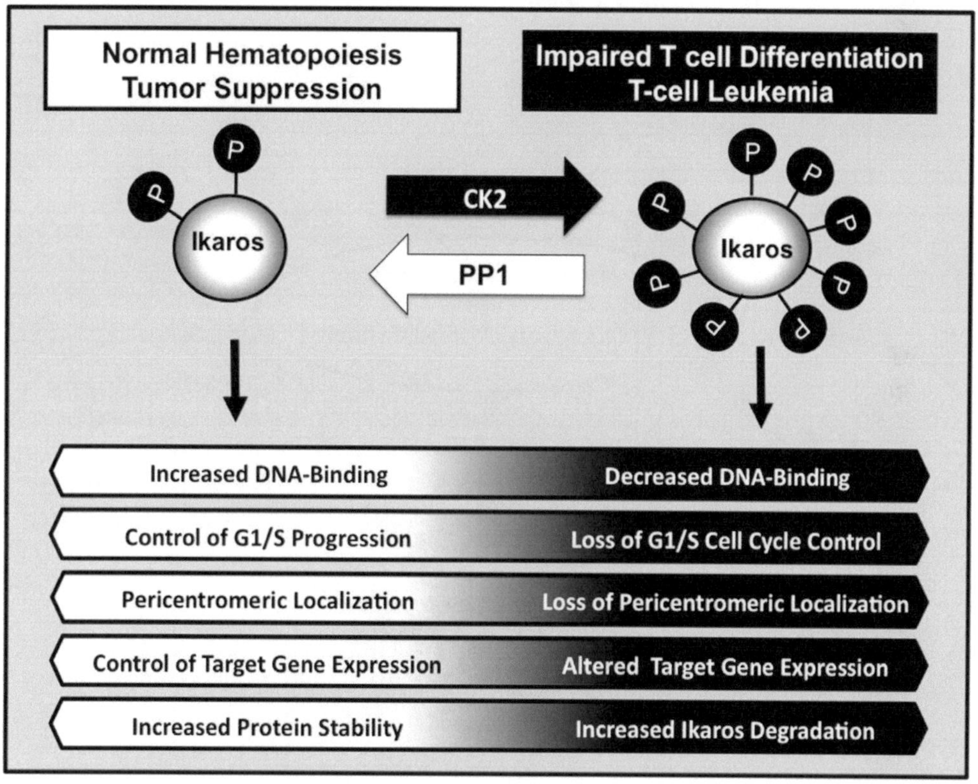

Fig. 2. CK2 kinase-mediated hyperphosphorylation results in functional inactivation of Ikaros and T-cell ALL. Hyperphosphorylation of Ikaros by CK2 kinase leads to the loss of Ikaros' ability to bind DNA, control cell cycle progression, regulate chromatin remodelling, regulate gene expression and to increased degradation of the Ikaros protein. The loss of Ikaros tumor suppressor function leads to the development of T-cell ALL.

7. Conclusion: The role of Ikaros in T-cell leukemia – overall hypothesis

Numerous clinical and experimental studies established the absence of Ikaros activity as a causative and/or contributory factor to the development of T-cell ALL. While genetic inactivation of Ikaros is evident in about 5% of T-cell ALL, recent evidence suggests that the functional inactivation of Ikaros by CK2 kinase-mediated phosphorylation is an important factor for the development of T-cell ALL. **With regard to Ikaros activity, we propose that there are three types of T-cell leukemia (Fig. 3):**

4. T-cell leukemia with the presence of genetic inactivation (deletion or mutation) of at least one Ikaros allele - responsible for ~5% of T-cell leukemia.
5. T-cell leukemia with functional inactivation of the Ikaros protein in leukemia cells due to overexpression of CK2 kinase.
6. T-cell leukemia with intact Ikaros function, but with defects in other genes and proteins that regulate T-cell proliferation and differentiation.

The prognostic and therapeutic significance of these three types of T-cell leukemia will be the subject of intense investigation in the future.

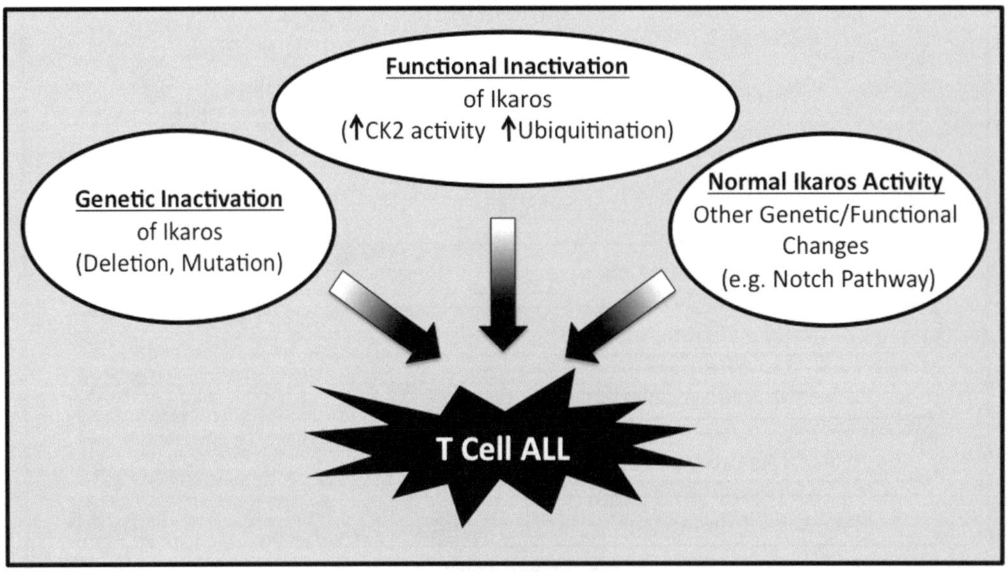

Fig. 3. Three types of T-cell leukemia with regards to Ikaros activity. Genetic and functional inactivation of Ikaros, in addition to changes in previously identified pathways, lead to T-cell leukemogenesis.

8. Acknowledgements

This work was supported in part by an R01 HL095120 grant, a St. Baldrick's Foundation Career Development Award, the Four Diamonds Fund of the Pennsylvania State University College of Medicine, and the John Wawrynovic Leukemia Research Scholar Endowment (SD). This work was supported by the Department of Pathology and Human Anatomy and the Center for Health Dispartities and Molecular Medicine, Loma Linda University School of Medicine (to KJP) and by a Grant for Research and School Partnerships from Loma Linda University (to KJP).

9. References

Avitahl, N., S. Winandy, C. Friedrich, B. Jones, Y. Ge and K. Georgopoulos (1999). Ikaros sets thresholds for T-cell activation and regulates chromosome propagation, Immunity 10(3): 333-343.

Beverly, L. J. and A. J. Capobianco (2003). Perturbation of Ikaros isoform selection by MLV integration is a cooperative event in Notch(IC)-induced T-cell leukemogenesis, Cancer Cell 3(6): 551-564.

Brown, K. E., S. S. Guest, S. T. Smale, K. Hahm, M. Merkenschlager and A. G. Fisher (1997). Association of transcriptionally silent genes with Ikaros complexes at centromeric heterochromatin, Cell 91(6): 845-854.

Chiaramonte, R., A. Basile, E. Tassi, E. Calzavara, V. Cecchinato, V. Rossi, A. Biondi and P. Comi (2005). A wide role for NOTCH1 signaling in acute leukemia, Cancer Lett 219(1): 113-120.

Crescenzi, B., R. La Starza, S. Romoli, D. Beacci, C. Matteucci, G. Barba, A. Aventin, P. Marynen, S. Ciolli, C. Nozzoli, M. F. Martelli and C. Mecucci (2004). Submicroscopic deletions in 5q- associated malignancies, Haematologica 89(3):281-285.

Dovat, S. and K. J. Payne (2010). Tumor suppression in T-cell leukemia--the role of Ikaros, Leuk Res 34(4): 416-417.

Dovat, S., T. Ronni, D. Russell, R. Ferrini, B. S. Cobb and S. T. Smale (2002). A common mechanism for mitotic inactivation of C2H2 zinc finger DNA-binding domains, Genes Dev 16(23): 2985-2990.

Dumortier, A., R. Jeannet, P. Kirstetter, E. Kleinmann, M. Sellars, N. R. dos Santos, C. Thibault, J. Barths, J. Ghysdael, J. A. Punt, P. Kastner and S. Chan (2006). Notch activation is an early and critical event during T-Cell leukemogenesis in Ikaros-deficient mice, Mol Cell Biol 26(1): 209-220.

Dumortier, A., P. Kirstetter, P. Kastner and S. Chan (2003). Ikaros regulates neutrophil differentiation, Blood 101(6): 2219-2226.

Ernst, P., K. Hahm and S. T. Smale (1993). Both LyF-1 and an Ets protein interact with a critical promoter element in the murine terminal transferase gene, Mol Cell Biol 13(5): 2982-2992.

Ernst, P., K. Hahm, L. Trinh, J. N. Davis, M. F. Roussel, C. W. Turck and S. T. Smale (1996). A potential role for Elf-1 in terminal transferase gene regulation, Mol Cell Biol 16(11): 6121-6131.

Ezzat, S., X. Zhu, S. Loeper, S. Fischer and S. L. Asa (2006). Tumor-derived Ikaros 6 acetylates the Bcl-XL promoter to up-regulate a survival signal in pituitary cells, Mol Endocrinol 20(11): 2976-2986.

Georgopoulos, K., D. D. Moore and B. Derfler (1992). Ikaros, an early lymphoid-specific transcription factor and a putative mediator for T-cell commitment, Science 258(5083): 808-812.

Georgopoulos, K., S. Winandy and N. Avitahl (1997). The role of the Ikaros gene in lymphocyte development and homeostasis, Annu Rev Immunol 15: 155-176.

Gomez-del Arco, P., K. Maki and K. Georgopoulos (2004). Phosphorylation controls Ikaros's ability to negatively regulate the G(1)-S transition, Mol Cell Biol 24(7): 2797-2807.

Gurel, Z., T. Ronni, S. Ho, J. Kuchar, K. J. Payne, C. W. Turk and S. Dovat (2008). Recruitment of ikaros to pericentromeric heterochromatin is regulated by phosphorylation, J Biol Chem 283(13): 8291-8300.

Hahm, K., P. Ernst, K. Lo, G. S. Kim, C. Turck and S. T. Smale (1994). The lymphoid transcription factor LyF-1 is encoded by specific, alternatively spliced mRNAs derived from the Ikaros gene, Mol Cell Biol 14(11): 7111-7123.

Harker, N., T. Naito, M. Cortes, A. Hostert, S. Hirschberg, M. Tolaini, K. Roderick, K. Georgopoulos and D. Kioussis (2002). The CD8alpha gene locus is regulated by the Ikaros family of proteins, Mol Cell 10(6): 1403-1415.

Kano, G., A. Morimoto, M. Takanashi, S. Hibi, T. Sugimoto, T. Inaba, T. Yagi and S. Imashuku (2008). Ikaros dominant negative isoform (Ik6) induces IL-3-independent survival of murine pro-B lymphocytes by activating JAK-STAT and up-regulating Bcl-xl levels, Leuk Lymphoma 49(5): 965-973.

Kathrein, K. L., S. Chari and S. Winandy (2008). Ikaros directly represses the notch target gene Hes1 in a leukemia T-cell line: implications for CD4 regulation, J Biol Chem 283(16): 10476-10484.

Kathrein, K. L., R. Lorenz, A. M. Innes, E. Griffiths and S. Winandy (2005). Ikaros induces quiescence and T-cell differentiation in a leukemia cell line, Mol Cell Biol 25(5): 1645-1654.

Kim, J., S. Sif, B. Jones, A. Jackson, J. Koipally, E. Heller, S. Winandy, A. Viel, A. Sawyer, T. Ikeda, R. Kingston and K. Georgopoulos (1999). Ikaros DNA-binding proteins direct formation of chromatin remodeling complexes in lymphocytes, Immunity 10(3): 345-355.

Kim, J. H., T. Ebersole, N. Kouprina, V. N. Noskov, J. Ohzeki, H. Masumoto, B. Mravinac, B. A. Sullivan, A. Pavlicek, S. Dovat, S. D. Pack, Y. W. Kwon, P. T. Flanagan, D. Loukinov, V. Lobanenkov, et al. (2009). Human gamma-satellite DNA maintains open chromatin structure and protects a transgene from epigenetic silencing, Genome Res 19(4): 533-544.

Kim, J. S., J. I. Eom, J. W. Cheong, A. J. Choi, J. K. Lee, W. I. Yang and Y. H. Min (2007). Protein kinase CK2alpha as an unfavorable prognostic marker and novel therapeutic target in acute myeloid leukemia, Clin Cancer Res 13(3): 1019-1028.

Kirstetter, P., M. Thomas, A. Dierich, P. Kastner and S. Chan (2002). Ikaros is critical for B cell differentiation and function, Eur J Immunol 32(3): 720-730.

Kleinmann, E., A. S. Geimer Le Lay, M. Sellars, P. Kastner and S. Chan (2008). Ikaros represses the transcriptional response to Notch signaling in T-cell development, Mol Cell Biol 28(24): 7465-7475.

Koipally, J. and K. Georgopoulos (2000). Ikaros interactions with CtBP reveal a repression mechanism that is independent of histone deacetylase activity, J Biol Chem 275(26): 19594-19602.

Koipally, J., E. J. Heller, J. R. Seavitt and K. Georgopoulos (2002). Unconventional potentiation of gene expression by ikaros, J Biol Chem 277(15): 13007-13015.

Koipally, J., A. Renold, J. Kim and K. Georgopoulos (1999). Repression by Ikaros and Aiolos is mediated through histone deacetylase complexes, Embo J 18(11): 3090-3100.

Kuiper, R. P., E. F. Schoenmakers, S. V. van Reijmersdal, J. Y. Hehir-Kwa, A. G. van Kessel, F. N. van Leeuwen and P. M. Hoogerbrugge (2007). High-resolution genomic profiling of childhood ALL reveals novel recurrent genetic lesions affecting pathways involved in lymphocyte differentiation and cell cycle progression, Leukemia 21(6): 1258-1266.

Liberg, D., S. T. Smale and M. Merkenschlager (2003). Upstream of Ikaros, Trends Immunol 24(11): 567-570.

Lo, K., N. R. Landau and S. T. Smale (1991). LyF-1, a transcriptional regulator that interactswith a novel class of promoters for lymphocyte-specific genes, Mollecular Cellular Biology 11: 5229-5243.

Marcais, A., R. Jeannet, L. Hernandez, J. Soulier, F. Sigaux, S. Chan and P. Kastner (2010). Genetic inactivation of Ikaros is a rare event in human T-ALL, Leuk Res 34(4): 426-429.

Martinelli, G., I. Iacobucci, C. Papayannidis and S. Soverini (2009). New targets for Ph+ leukaemia therapy, Best Pract Res Clin Haematol 22(3): 445-454.

Martinelli, G., I. Iacobucci, S. Soverini, P. P. Piccaluga, D. Cilloni and F. Pane (2009). New mechanisms of resistance in Philadelphia chromosome acute lymphoblastic leukemia, Expert Rev Hematol 2(3): 297-303.

Martinelli, G., I. Iacobucci, C. T. Storlazzi, M. Vignetti, F. Paoloni, D. Cilloni, S. Soverini, A. Vitale, S. Chiaretti, G. Cimino, C. Papayannidis, S. Paolini, L. Elia, P. Fazi, G. Meloni, et al. (2009). IKZF1 (Ikaros) deletions in BCR-ABL1-positive acute lymphoblastic leukemia are associated with short disease-free survival and high rate of cumulative incidence of relapse: a GIMEMA AL WP report, J Clin Oncol 27(31): 5202-5207.

Maser, R. S., B. Choudhury, P. J. Campbell, B. Feng, K. K. Wong, A. Protopopov, J. O'Neil, A. Gutierrez, E. Ivanova, I. Perna, E. Lin, V. Mani, S. Jiang, K. McNamara, S. Zaghlul, et al. (2007). Chromosomally unstable mouse tumours have genomic alterations similar to diverse human cancers, Nature 447(7147): 966-971.

Molnar, A. and K. Georgopoulos (1994). The Ikaros gene encodes a family of functionally diverse zinc finger DNA-binding proteins, Mol Cell Biol 14(12): 8292-8303.

Mullighan, C. G., S. Goorha, I. Radtke, C. B. Miller, E. Coustan-Smith, J. D. Dalton, K. Girtman, S. Mathew, J. Ma, S. B. Pounds, X. Su, C. H. Pui, M. V. Relling, W. E. Evans, S. A. Shurtleff, et al. (2007). Genome-wide analysis of genetic alterations in acute lymphoblastic leukaemia, Nature 446(7137): 758-764.

Mullighan, C. G., C. B. Miller, I. Radtke, L. A. Phillips, J. Dalton, J. Ma, D. White, T. P. Hughes, M. M. Le Beau, C. H. Pui, M. V. Relling, S. A. Shurtleff and J. R. Downing (2008). BCR-ABL1 lymphoblastic leukaemia is characterized by the deletion of Ikaros, Nature 453(7191): 110-114.

Mullighan, C. G., X. Su, J. Zhang, I. Radtke, L. A. Phillips, C. B. Miller, J. Ma, W. Liu, C. Cheng, B. A. Schulman, R. C. Harvey, I. M. Chen, R. J. Clifford, W. L. Carroll, G. Reaman, et al. (2009). Deletion of IKZF1 and prognosis in acute lymphoblastic leukemia, N Engl J Med 360(5): 470-480.

Naito, T., P. Gomez-Del Arco, C. J. Williams and K. Georgopoulos (2007). Antagonistic interactions between Ikaros and the chromatin remodeler Mi-2beta determine silencer activity and Cd4 gene expression, Immunity 27(5): 723-734.

Nakase, K., F. Ishimaru, N. Avitahl, H. Dansako, K. Matsuo, K. Fujii, N. Sezaki, H. Nakayama, T. Yano, S. Fukuda, K. Imajoh, M. Takeuchi, A. Miyata, M. Hara, M. Yasukawa, et al. (2000). Dominant negative isoform of the Ikaros gene in patients with adult B- cell acute lymphoblastic leukemia, Cancer Res 60(15): 4062-4065.

Nakase, K., F. Ishimaru, K. Fujii, T. Tabayashi, T. Kozuka, N. Sezaki, Y. Matsuo and M. Harada (2002). Overexpression of novel short isoforms of Helios in a patient with T- cell acute lymphoblastic leukemia, Exp Hematol 30(4): 313-317.

Nakayama, H., F. Ishimaru, N. Avitahl, N. Sezaki, N. Fujii, K. Nakase, Y. Ninomiya, A. Harashima, J. Minowada, J. Tsuchiyama, K. Imajoh, T. Tsubota, S. Fukuda, T. Sezaki, K. Kojima, et al. (1999). Decreases in Ikaros activity correlate with blast crisis in patients with chronic myelogenous leukemia, Cancer Res 59(16): 3931-3934.

O'Neill, D. W., S. S. Schoetz, R. A. Lopez, M. Castle, L. Rabinowitz, E. Shor, D. Krawchuk, M. G. Goll, M. Renz, H. P. Seelig, S. Han, R. H. Seong, S. D. Park, T. Agalioti, N. Munshi, et al. (2000). An ikaros-containing chromatin-remodeling complex in adult-type erythroid cells, Mol Cell Biol 20(20): 7572-7582.

Payne, K. J., G. Huang, E. Sahakian, J. Y. Zhu, N. S. Barteneva, L. W. Barsky, M. A. Payne and G. M. Crooks (2003). Ikaros isoform x is selectively expressed in myeloid differentiation, J Immunol 170(6): 3091-3098.

Payne, K. J., J. H. Nicolas, J. Y. Zhu, L. W. Barsky and G. M. Crooks (2001). Cutting edge: predominant expression of a novel Ikaros isoform in normal human hemopoiesis, J Immunol 167(4): 1867-1870.

Phan-Dinh-Tuy, F., J. Henry, C. Boucheix, J. Y. Perrot, C. Rosenfeld and A. Kahn (1985). Protein kinases in human leukemic cells, Am J Hematol 19(3): 209-218.

Pinna, L. A. (1997). Protein kinase CK2, Int J Biochem Cell Biol 29(4): 551-554.

Popescu, M., Z. Gurel, T. Ronni, C. Song, K. Y. Hung, K. J. Payne and S. Dovat (2009). Ikaros stability and pericentromeric localization are regulated by protein phosphatase 1, J Biol Chem 284(20): 13869-13880.

Roig, J., A. Krehan, D. Colomer, W. Pyerin, E. Itarte and M. Plana (1999). Multiple forms of protein kinase CK2 present in leukemic cells: in vitro study of its origin by proteolysis, Mol Cell Biochem 191(1-2): 229-234.

Ronni, T., K. J. Payne, S. Ho, M. N. Bradley, G. Dorsam and S. Dovat (2007). Human Ikaros function in activated T-cells is regulated by coordinated expression of its largest isoforms, J Biol Chem 282(4): 2538-2547.

Ruiz, A., J. Jiang, H. Kempski and H. J. Brady (2004). Overexpression of the Ikaros 6 isoform is restricted to t(4;11) acute lymphoblastic leukaemia in children and infants and has a role in B-cell survival, Br J Haematol 125(1): 31-37.

Sabbattini, P., M. Lundgren, A. Georgiou, C. Chow, G. Warnes and N. Dillon (2001). Binding of Ikaros to the lambda5 promoter silences transcription through a mechanism that does not require heterochromatin formation, Embo J 20(11): 2812-2822.

Seldin, D. C. and P. Leder (1995). Casein kinase II alpha transgene-induced murine lymphoma: relation to theileriosis in cattle, Science 267(5199): 894-897.

Su, R. C., R. Sridharan and S. T. Smale (2005). Assembly of silent chromatin during thymocyte development, Semin Immunol 17(2): 129-140.

Sun, L., M. L. Crotty, M. Sensel, H. Sather, C. Navara, J. Nachman, P. G. Steinherz, P. S. Gaynon, N. Seibel, C. Mao, A. Vassilev, G. H. Reaman and F. M. Uckun (1999). Expression of dominant-negative Ikaros isoforms in T-cell acute lymphoblastic leukemia, Clin Cancer Res 5(8): 2112-2120.

Sun, L., A. Liu and K. Georgopoulos (1996). Zinc finger-mediated protein interactions modulate Ikaros activity, a molecular control of lymphocyte development, Embo J 15(19): 5358-5369.

Thomas, R. M., N. Chunder, C. Chen, S. E. Umetsu, S. Winandy and A. D. Wells (2007). Ikaros enforces the costimulatory requirement for IL2 gene expression and is required for anergy induction in CD4+ T lymphocytes, J Immunol 179(11):7305-7315.

Trinh, L. A., R. Ferrini, B. S. Cobb, A. S. Weinmann, K. Hahm, P. Ernst, I. P. Garraway, M. Merkenschlager and S. T. Smale (2001). Down-regulation of TdT transcription in $CD4^{+}CD8^{+}$ thymocytes by Ikaros proteins in direct competition with an Ets activator, Genes and Development 15: 1817-1832.

Urban, J. A. and S. Winandy (2004). Ikaros null mice display defects in T-cell selection and CD4 versus CD8 lineage decisions, J Immunol 173(7): 4470-4478.

Wang, J. H., A. Nichogiannopoulou, L. Wu, L. Sun, A. H. Sharpe, M. Bigby and K. Georgopoulos (1996). Selective defects in the development of the fetal and adult lymphoid system in mice with an Ikaros null mutation, Immunity 5(6): 537-549.

Weng, A. P., A. A. Ferrando, W. Lee, J. P. t. Morris, L. B. Silverman, C. Sanchez-Irizarry, S. C. Blacklow, A. T. Look and J. C. Aster (2004). Activating mutations of NOTCH1 in human T-cell acute lymphoblastic leukemia, Science 306(5694): 269-271.

Winandy, S., L. Wu, J. H. Wang and K. Georgopoulos (1999). Pre-T-cell receptor (TCR) and TCR-controlled checkpoints in T-cell differentiation are set by Ikaros, J Exp Med 190(8): 1039-1048.

Winandy, S., P. Wu and K. Georgopoulos (1995). A dominant mutation in the Ikaros gene leads to rapid development of leukemia and lymphoma, Cell 83(2): 289-299.

Yagi, T., S. Hibi, M. Takanashi, G. Kano, Y. Tabata, T. Imamura, T. Inaba, A. Morimoto, S. Todo and S. Imashuku (2002). High frequency of Ikaros isoform 6 expression in acute myelomonocytic and monocytic leukemias: implications for up-regulation of the antiapoptotic protein Bcl-XL in leukemogenesis, Blood 99(4): 1350-1355.

7

p16^{INK4A} – Connecting Cell Cycle Control to Cell Death Regulation in Human Leukemia

Petra Obexer[1,3], Judith Hagenbuchner[1,3]
Markus Holzner[3] and Michael J. Ausserlechner[2,3]
[1]*Department of Pediatrics IV and*
[2]*Department of Pediatrics II and*
[3]*Tyrolean Cancer Research Institute*
Medical University Innsbruck
Austria

1. Introduction

To expand without limitation cancerous cells have to acquire the ability to proliferate without external or internal restrictions. Whereas almost all normal cells within a body will not proliferate without external mitogenic stimuli cancer cells gain defects in growth factor signaling control that mimic external stimulation and thus allow them to divide. However, this unrestricted proliferation also activates an internal barrier to transformation, i.e. it induces the expression of so called cell cycle brakes that stop unrestricted growth at the very basal level of the cell cycle. These cell cycle inhibitors prevent increased cycling by controlling the activity of cyclin/CDK holoenzyms which are the central promoters of cell cycle progression. These cell cycle inhibitors or "brakes" are divided into two families, the INK4 inhibitors and the Cip/Kip inhibitor family. In this chapter we will mainly focus on the INK4 inhibitor protein p16INK4A which is encoded by the INK4A gene locus.

Inactivation of the INK4A gene locus occurs frequently in primary tumor cells of T-cell acute lymphoblastic leukemia (T-ALL), suggesting a critical role of this locus in disease development. Its deletion predicts relapse in childhood acute lymphoblastic leukemia (ALL). Interestingly, this gene locus also represents a main barrier to the generation of induced progenitor stem (iPS) cells and evidence has been provided that downregulation of p16INK4A is associated with enhanced self-renewal and proliferative capacity of hematopoietic stem cells. This suggests that the inactivation of this tumor suppressor in immature pre-cancerous cells might allow them to overcome replicative senescence. Importantly, p16INK4A exerts its effects not only on cell cycle control but changes cell death sensitivity of T-ALL cells by affecting glucocorticoid sensitivity, death receptor-mediated- and intrinsic programmed cell death pathways that are controlled at the level of BCL2 proteins. These effects of p16INK4A on the cell death machinery in ALL cells support the notion that loss of the INK4A gene locus has a two-sided effect during the development of ALL, on one hand it allows unrestricted proliferation of ALL progenitor cells and on the other hand this deletion rescues leukemic cells from cell death. Thus, the effects of p16INK4A in hematopoietic cells and during leukemia development seem to be much more than "just inhibiting cyclin-dependent kinases".

2. Stop or go: A general overview on cell cycle entry

Proliferating eukaryotic cells pass through a complex cell division cycle that is divided into four phases: the gap-phase before DNA replication (G1-phase), the phase of DNA synthesis (S-phase), the gap after DNA synthesis (G2-phase) and mitosis (M-phase). Whereas the length of DNA-synthesis, G2 and M-phase are relatively constant within different cell types, the greatest variation is observed in the duration of G1. Highly proliferative cells pass through this phase within a few hours; differentiated cells, on the other hand, may stay in this cell cycle stage for months, years, or even life time. This situation of final differentiation is called G0. The G0/G1 cell cycle state is usually considered as the time window, in which a cell decides whether to proliferate or to arrest.
Progression through the cell cycle is governed by a family of serine-threonine kinases called cyclin-dependent kinases (CDKs) that associate with different cyclins in distinct phases of the cell cycle (Murray and Hunt 1993; Sherr and Roberts 2004). Whereas the cellular concentration of CDK proteins does not vary significantly during cell cycle, the levels of cyclins undergo dramatic changes during the different phases. They reach characteristic peak levels in specific cell cycle phases and are degraded in other phases.
When quiescent cells re-enter the cell cycle, D-type and E-type cyclins are synthesized sequentially during the G1 interval; both types are rate-limiting for S-phase entry (Quelle et al, 1993). Cyclin Ds assemble with CDK4 (Matsushime et al, 1992) and CDK6 (Meyerson and Harlow 1994) and these complexes are activated by phosphorylation via the so called cyclin activating kinase (Murray and Hunt 1993). Critical substrates of G1 cyclin/CDK complexes are the retinoblastoma gene product pRB and its family members p107 and p130, which are transcriptional repressors that are bound to transcription factors essential for S-phase entry (Cobrinik 2005; Grana et al, 1998). Upon phosphorylation on distinct sites by both, cyclin D/CDK4/6 and cyclin E/CDK2 complexes pRB and its family members lose their function as transcriptional repressors thereby activating the transcription of genes essential for S-phase progression. The activity of CDK4, CDK6 and CDK2 is regulated by mitogenic hormones and by binding of CDK inhibitors (CDKI) of the INK4A family, like p16INK4A, and of the Cip/Kip family, i.e. p21Cip1, p27Kip1 and p57Kip2 (Sherr and Roberts 1999; Ekholm and Reed 2000) (see Figure 1).

3. The strange case of INK4A: One gene locus that codes for two unrelated tumor suppressors

The INK4A gene locus on chromosome 9p21 codes for the two functionally fully unrelated tumor suppressor genes p16INK4A and ARF (known as p14ARF in human and p19ARF in mouse). As outlined above, p16INK4A/CDKN2A was originally identified as a cyclin-dependent kinase inhibitor that, like its family members p15INK4B, p18INK4C and p19INK4D, binds to the kinase subunits CDK4 and CDK6 of D-type cyclins. Cyclin D1, D2 and D3 govern the decision of cell cycle entry from quiescent G0 state. In contrast to other cyclins the activity of cyclin Ds/CDK4 and CDK6 holoenzymes is controlled by various survival signaling pathways e.g. by Ras/Raf signaling, by the PI3K/PKB pathway or by the Wnt signaling pathway which are frequently perturbed in cancer cells thereby leading to aberrant cell cycle entry and cell proliferation. p16INK4A and other inhibitors of the INK4-family (INK4 means "inhibitor of kinase 4") thereby represent a main barrier to increased proliferation of cells with defects in growth factor signaling control. Human tumor cells that lack functional pRB, either by mutation or due to viral proteins that target and inactivate pRB, usually show high levels of p16INK4A (Aagaard et al, 1995). In such cells CDK4 and CDK6 do not interact with D-type cyclins but form stable, long half-life, binary complexes with p16INK4A (Parry et al, 1995) demonstrating that the cell cycle inhibitory effect of p16INK4A depends on the functionality of the tumor suppressor pRB.

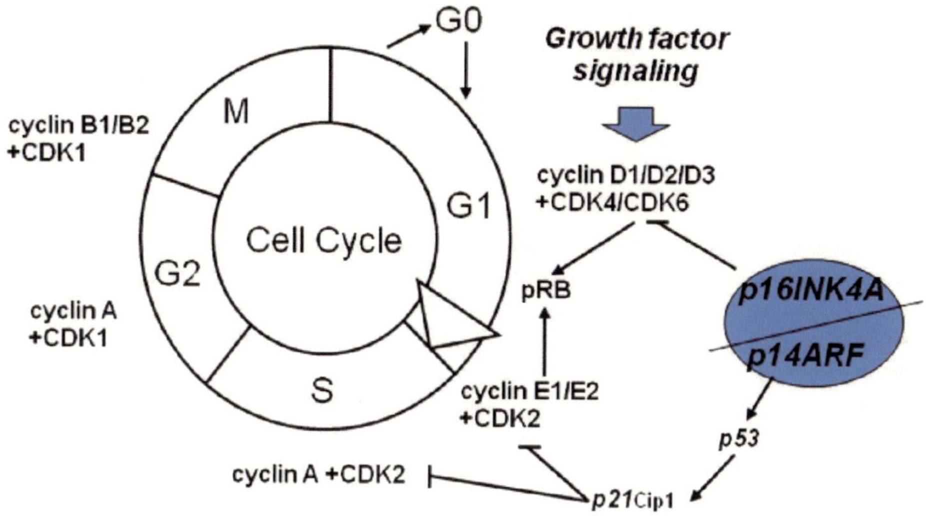

Fig. 1. Dynamic accumulation and assembly of cyclin/CDK complexes in different phases of the cell cycle. Schematic presentation of the cell cycle with emphasis on the G1/S checkpoint regulation by CDK inhibitors, detailed explanation in the text.

However nature has found an elegant way of redundancy to compensate for the loss of p16INK4A function in pRB-deficient tumors by an alternative protein. Adjacent to the INK4A gene locus on chromosome 9p21 an additional promoter region exists that produces a transcript which includes exon 2 and exon 3 of p16INK4A but has an alternate exon 1 (exon1β) (Figure 2). Since the exon 2 is translated in an alternative reading frame (ARF) the resulting protein is completely unrelated to the gene product of INK4A although it shares parts of the mRNA sequence (Quelle et al, 1995). p16INK4A and ARF have no similarities in amino acid composition and are two completely different proteins with distinct functions - but both act as efficient tumor suppressors (Figure 2). This is demonstrated by the fact that mice that are deficient for either ARF or p16INK4A have increased susceptibility to spontaneous or carcinogen-induced cancers (Sharpless et al, 2001; Kamijo et al, 1997). p16INK4A-deficient mice show a much less spontaneous tumor rate than ARF null mice. p16INK4A ablation leads to spontaneous sarcomas and lymphomas within 17 months (Sharpless et al, 2001), whereas the onset of spontaneous sarcomas, carcinomas and lymphomas in ARF-null mice is already observed at the age of 9 months (Kamijo et al, 1997). However, it is difficult to compare results from ARF null mice with the situation in human cells since human (p14ARF) and mouse p19ARF share only about 50% sequence homology. In addition there are apparent regulatory and functional differences between human and mouse ARF. Whereas in senescent mouse fibroblasts p19ARF accumulates and is critical for senescence-induced growth arrest, the human p14ARF seems not involved and is dispensable for this process (Sharpless et al, 2004). In human cells, the senescence process is

mainly controlled by the unrelated twin p16INK4A and the relevance of p14ARF seems also limited for other processes such as prevention of "stemness" in normal human fibroblasts by the expression of specific transcription factors (see below).
Human or murine ARF proteins do not contain any recognizable structural motifs and probably need to interact with other proteins to form functional complexes. The first discovered and best-defined function of ARF is the induction of p53 via inhibition of the p53-degrading E3-ubiquitine ligase MDM2 (mouse) or HDM2 (human) (Sherr 2006). In situations of increased cell cycle progression, e.g. when oncogenic signaling stimulates cell cycle entry or loss of pRB function, ARF is transcriptionally induced via E2F1/DP1 and binds to and inhibits MDM2 or HDM2, respectively. This leads to accumulation of p53 and induction of p53-induced response genes, such as p21Cip1 that interferes with cell cycle progression, or the proapoptotic BCL-2 proteins BBC3/PUMA and PMAIP1/Noxa that induce programmed cell death (Villunger et al, 2003). More recently other functions of ARF have been discovered: in response to oncogenic stress ARF enters the nucleolus and retards rRNA transcription thereby inhibiting ribosome biosynthesis (Itahana et al, 2003) and ARF influences the ATM/ATR kinases during the DNA-damage response in a p53-independent manner (Rocha et al, 2005). Moreover, it was shown that independent of p53 ARF antagonizes the activity of two other critical factors for cell cycle entry, namely E2F and Myc (Sherr 2006). The detailed investigation of how p16INK4A and ARF control cell survival and proliferation in distinct cell types will remain a highly interesting field of research in the next years, in particular the physiologic role of these two unrelated twins in non-transformed somatic cells.

4. The role of the INK4A locus for the generation of induced pluripotent stem cells (iPS)

Tissue repair and permanent replacement of damaged or aged cells are essential for the life of complex organisms and usually depend on a distinct, unspecialized stem cell population with almost unlimited proliferative capacity. With age, the capacity of these stem cells to proliferate and generate progenitors declines, which may also contribute for many age-related symptoms. The reprogramming of normal, differentiated cells by the three transcription factors Oct4, Klf4, and Sox2 has opened a completely new field of research and raised the hope to regenerate almost all cell types and tissues within the human body by generating stem cells from somatic cells of a patient. However the process that is initiated by these three transcription factors works at low efficiency and remains poorly understood. In embryonal stem cells and in induced progenitor stem (iPS) cells the INK4A gene locus is completely silenced and neither p16INK4A nor ARF are expressed. The lack of INK4A proteins seems to be a hallmark of different kinds of stem cells. Interestingly, this epigenetic silencing is not due to enhanced DNA-methylation of the INK4A promoters but results from so called "bivalent chromatin" which is present at the INK4A gene locus (Ohm et al, 2007). "Bivalent" means that repressive methylation marks (H3K27me3) and activating methylation marks (H3K4me3) are present on the same histone molecule, leading to a chromatin state that silences gene expression but can be reversed during differentiation of a cell. Such domains are characteristics of embryonal stem cells and are frequently associated with binding sites for Oct4 and Sox2. Although such binding sites are absent in the INK4A gene locus the presence of these bivalent domains suggests that the INK4A gene locus adopts a silent configuration in stem cells, but, in contrast to DNA-methylation-induced silencing, retains the ability to be re-activated during differentiation processes (Li et al, 2009). It is well established that the rate of induced pluripotent stem cells generated from somatic cells significantly drops with the age of the organism they are obtained from. In humans also the cellular levels of p16INK4A increase with age. Back to back several different groups showed in 2009 that the INK4A gene locus critically impairs successful reprogramming to pluripotent stem cells and that it represents a main barrier to iPS cell programming (Utikal et al, 2009; Marion et al, 2009; Banito et al, 2009; Li et al, 2009). Also in these papers the differences of p16INK4A and ARF between murine and human cells become evident: In mouse cells, the ARF-p53 pathway has more impact on preventing the generation of pluripotent stem cells from somatic cells, whereas p16INK4A seems to play a minor role in the mouse. In human fibroblasts, knockdown of ARF does not affect at all the generation of iPS cells whereas knockdown of p16INK4A significantly improved reprogramming efficiency. This suggests that depending on the species, either p16INK4A or ARF represent a barrier to "back-differentiation" of normal somatic cells and prevent the induction of "stemness" in cells that have differentiated into a certain lineage. This makes this gene locus so important for the medical application of induced progenitor cells to e.g. replace damaged tissue of a patient, but also underlines that p16INK4A and/or ARF may be critical for maintaining tissue architecture and function in complex organisms by preventing uncontrolled expansion or "development" of somatic cells with stem cell-like abilities.

5. Regulation of INK4A in hematopoietic stem cells and their progenitors

As discussed before the INK4A gene locus represents a main barrier to the generation of iPS cells. In hematopoietic stem cells and many other stem cell types e.g. neuronal stem cells (Molofsky et al, 2006), the INK4A gene locus is not active. In particular the downregulation and silencing of p16INK4A seems to be essential for the enhanced self-renewal and proliferative capacity of human hematopoietic stem cells (Janzen et al, 2006). At the transcriptional level the INK4A expression is modulated by three main regulators, beta lymphoma Mo-MLV insertion region (BMI1), ETS1 and inhibitor of DNA binding 1 (Id1) whereas age-related induction of p16INK4A and ARF in human cells is mainly related to the balance between ETS1 and Id1 proteins (Ohtani et al, 2001). The reversible silencing of this gene locus in hematopoietic stem cells can be ascribed to the activity of the BMI1 protein. BMI1 belongs to the polycomb group genes, which are transcriptional repressors that control gene expression patterns during differentiation and development (Simon and Kingston 2009). The polycomb group genes fall into two subgroups that are either part of polycomb repression complex 1 (PRC1) or polycomb-repression complex 2 (PRC2). PRC2 is the so called "initiation complex" that functions as a histone-methyltransferase which specifically methylates histone H3 on lysine 27 causing gene silencing. As outlined above methylation of histone H3 on lysine 27 (H3K27me3) and on lysine 4 (H3K4me3) are hallmarks of "bivalent" chromatin that is silenced but retains the ability to be reactivated upon cell differentiation processes. BMI1 is part of PRC1 which is the so called "maintenance complex" that in a second step recognizes trimethylated H3K27. BMI1 directly associates with the INK4A locus and it was demonstrated that repression of the INK4A gene locus depends on the continuous presence of the PRC2 complex (Bracken et al, 2007). Several lines of evidence suggest that BMI1 is critical for maintaining "stemness" at least in human hematopoietic stem cells (Figure 2). In cord blood hematopoietic cells BMI1 expression is highest expressed in the hematopoietic stem cell population and gradually decreases when these cells maturate into more differentiated progenitor cells. Overexpression of BMI1 enhances the self-renewal of hematopoietic stem cells, increases the engraftment potential and results in stem cell maintenance. Knockdown of BMI1 in cord blood CD34+ and in acute myeloid leukemia (AML) CD34+ cells reduces progenitor-forming capacity, stem cell marker expression and long-term culture-initiating cell frequencies significantly suggesting that loss of BMI impairs the maintenance of stem cells and progenitor cells. In parallel, because of the gene-silencing effect of the BMI1 containing PRC1 complex on the INK4A gene locus, loss of BMI1 in C34+ cord blood and AML cells causes the induction of p14ARF and p16INK4A, significantly increased apoptosis and the production of cellular reactive oxygen species (Rizo et al, 2009). Lack of BMI1 in hematopoietic cells from BMI1 knockout mice also resulted in an increased expression of p16INK4A and p19ARF. The fact that the deletion of INK4A/ARF in the BMI1-/- background partly restored the self-renewal capacity of hematopoietic stem cells demonstrates the importance of silencing of the INK4A gene locus by BMI1 for the maintenance of hematopoietic stem cells (Oguro et al, 2006).

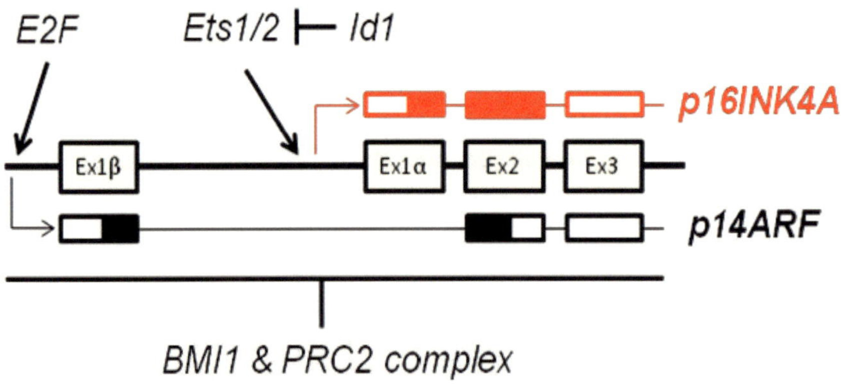

Fig. 2. The INK4A gene locus generates the two unrelated tumor suppressor proteins p16INK4A and ARF by alternative promoter usage and splicing, which are subjected to a complex regulation in hematopoietic stem cells and progenitor cells. Stress and senescence activate p16INK4A via Ets1/2 transcription factors and accelerated cell cycle entry triggers ARF expression. Id1 heterodimerizes and blocks Ets1/2 in young unstressed cells or stem cells. In stem cells BMI1 as part of the polycomb complex PRC2 causes epigenetic gene silencing of the entire locus by bivalent histone methylation (see text).

6. Is p16INK4A critical for the development of hematologic malignancies?

The almost unlimited replicative capacity of stem cells and efficient generation of progenitors may be a double edged sword for a multicellular organism. On one hand this proliferative capacity allows efficient repair, regeneration and plasticity of tissues, on the other hand it increases the risk of acquiring genetic defects in this stem cell population that may result in hyperproliferative diseases, among them malignant transformation and cancer. Considering the fact that the INK4A gene locus codes for two tumor suppressors with completely different functions which either critically control the pRB or the p53 gene network, it becomes clear that genetic abnormalities of this gene locus may have a dramatic impact on progression of a damaged hematopoietic stem cell into precancerous cells that give rise to leukemia. Due to the unusual structure of this gene locus, mutations often affect both, p16INK4A and p14ARF gene products, thereby deleting the gatekeepers of two essential check points. This may explain why mutations of the INK4A gene locus are observed in almost all human cancers. However, the effects of the INK4A gene products are also cell lineage specific, which might explain why some malignancies, for example T-ALL, show very high frequencies of homozygous deletion of the INK4A gene locus. Deletions frequently affect exon 2, thereby destroying both, p16INK4A and p14ARF, but there are also patients with alterations in either exon 1α or exon 1β which only affect one of the tumor suppressors (Cayuela et al, 1996; Cayuela et al, 1997; Hebert et al, 1994; Quelle et al, 1995). In addition methylation of the p16INK4A promoter was reported in T-ALL patients, leading to permanent silencing of the INK4A gene (Gardie et al, 1998; Drexler 1998). From a prognostic point of view inactivation of the INK4A locus seems also highly important for human lymphoblastic leukemia. Loss of INK4A predicts relaps in children with acute lymphoblastic leukemia suggesting a critical role of this locus in disease development and also highlighting the need for additional therapies to treat this subgroup of T-ALL patients (Kees et al, 1997); (Okuda et al, 1995). Several attempts have been undertaken to better understand, why inactivation of the INK4A gene locus is critical in particular for the development of hematopoietic malignancies. One oncogene that is thought to initiate T-cell leukemia is the TAL1/SCL oncogene. TAL1/SCL expressing T-ALL patients have a high incidence (up to 90%) of deletion of exon 2 in the INK4A gene locus. Although TAL1/SCL overexpression induces leukemia in transgenic mice, leukemia by this oncogene is characterized by a long latency suggesting that additional genetic events are required (Condorelli et al, 1996). To elucidate the contribution of the INK4A gene locus to leukemogenesis Shank-Calvo and colleagues (Shank-Calvo et al, 2006) mated TAL1 transgenic mice with single knockout mice for either p16INK4A or p19ARF. Of note, each of these mice developed T-cell leukemia rapidly, indicating that loss of either p16INK4A or p19ARF accelerates TAL1-induced leukemia in mice.

The fact that the INK4A genes are inactivated at high incidence in hematopoietic malignancies might be ascribed to the specific roles of these two proteins in slowing down the proliferation of hematopoietic progenitor cells, as discussed above. INK4A-/- mice possess increased thymus size and cellularity suggesting involvement of p16INK4A in the control of thymocyte proliferation. These animals exhibit increased numbers of CD4 and CD8 T lymphocytes in thymus and spleen (Bianchi et al, 2006) which also reflects increased proliferative potential. By using somatic, tissue specific ablation of p16INK4A in the T- or the B-lymphoid progenitor cells it was recently demonstrated that in the T-cell lineage loss of p16INK4A attenuated age-dependent thymic involution or increased production of naive T-cells. In the B-cell lineage p16INK4A inactivation significantly accelerated lymphoid tumorigenesis. Interestingly, the animals mainly suffered from tumors that manifested in the central nervous system but still expressed CD45 leukocyte-common antigen. These tumor cells were negative for a neuromeningeal marker, proving that they are not brain tumors and expressed B-lymphocyte markers demonstrating their B-cell origin (Liu et al, 2011). In this paper the authors argued therefore that in the T-cell linage p16INK4A merely regulates cell senescence in the mouse, whereas in the B-cell lineage loss of p16INK4A contributes to lymphoid cancer. These results are contradictory to the high prevalence of p16INK4A loss in human T-cell leukemia progenitor cells and may be ascribed to the already above discussed differences of the role of p16INK4A and ARF between mice and men. Senescence, cell cycle arrest and cell death are three possible physiologic fates of a cell that may be triggered by the two tumor suppressors of the INK4A gene locus. In the next chapter we will discuss how p16INK4A affects programmed cell death.

7. p16INK4A regulates programmed cell death and death sensitivity in leukemia cells

When a cell is hit by a genotoxic insult it will either try to repair the genetic damage or, if not possible, undergo programmed cell death. Otherwise the mutation will be inherited to the daughter cells, which may give rise to precancerous cells that slowly proceed into malignancy. Slowing down cell cycle progression upon genotoxic stress may therefore help cells to get time for efficient damage repair and thereby prevent programmed cell death. On the other hand cell cycle arrest in the presence of oncogenic signaling may constitute a death signal per se since apoptosis may be the only way for a precancerous cell to respond to this "conflicting signaling" situation. INK4A gene products are not expressed in hematopoietic stem cells and therefore may not play an essential role for the quiescence state that every stem cell has to enter after division to preserve its replicatory potential. Instead, INK4A proteins accumulate in the progenitor cell population and seem to limit their proliferation.

As a consequence of p16INK4A deficiency rapid movement through the cell cycle may sensitize leukemia cells to genotoxic stress, which has been shown in different types of cancer cells. In p16INK4A-deficient MEFs and U2OS osteosarkoma cells the lack of p16INK4A sensitizes these cells to cell death induction by UV irradiation, whereas p16INK4A-proficient cells are largely resistant. The authors also observed that UV-induced apoptosis in p16INK4A-deficient cells coincided with decreased levels of pro-survival BCL2 and increased levels of pro-apoptotic BAX proteins (Al Mohanna et al, 2004). Moreover, in p16INK4A-deficient mice increased numbers of CD4 and CD8 T-cells are found in thymus and spleen and these increased cell numbers correlated with reduced T-cell apoptosis in the thymus rather than increased proliferation rates (Bianchi et al, 2006). The increased rates of DNA-synthesis in p16INK4A-deficient cells may expose an "archilles heel" to DNA-damage-induced cell death, but there are also data that highlight that p16INK4A reconstitution sensitizes T-ALL cells to certain forms of apoptosis. This suggests that p16INK4A may exert also additional effects beyond cell cycle inhibition, such as the regulation of proteins critical for cell death initiation and cell death decision in mammalian cells. We demonstrated already ten years ago that tetracycline-regulated p16INK4A reconstitution in p16INK4A-deficient CCRF-CEM cells, a human T-ALL cell line, sensitizes these leukemia cells to physiologic levels of cortisol, a glucocorticoid that also plays a significant role during T-cell selection and T-cell maturation in the thymus. In this early study we were able to show that p16INK4A significantly induces the expression of endogenous glucocorticoid receptor thereby markedly lowering the threshold for glucocorticoid-induced apoptosis (Ausserlechner et al, 2001). In this paper we discussed that loss of p16INK4A in precancerous hematopoietic cells may render them resistant to glucocorticoid-induced cell death by physiologic levels of cortisol. Since the strikingly increased sensitivity was difficult to explain by increases in receptor levels alone we sought for additional mechanisms further downstream of the glucocorticoid receptor that may contribute to p16INK4A-regulated death sensitivity. Indeed, also in T-ALL cells activation of p16INK4A affects the balance of death inducers and death protectors at the level of mitochondria, but also activates death ligands. For studying p16INK4A effects in different T-ALL cell lines we applied a tightly controlled tetracycline-regulated expression system, based on different tetracycline-activated transactivators and repressors (Ausserlechner et al, 2006). In Molt4 T-ALL cells, for example, p16INK4A causes increased sensitivity to UV-irradiation, which is associated with induction of the pro-apoptotic BH3-only protein BBC3/Puma (Obexer et al, 2009a).

In principle programmed cell death can be initiated by a number of different signals originating either from outside of the cell (extrinsic pathway) or from intrinsic signals (Strasser 2005). Soluble or cell bound death ligands such as FASLG/FAS ligand or TRAIL bind to their cognate receptors, thereby inducing the formation of the so called death-inducing signaling complex (DISC) which contains the adaptor molecule FADD and procaspase-8. The autocatalytic cleavage and activation of procaspase-8 triggers the downstream caspase cascade. Mitochondria are central decision makers of apoptosis that integrate death signals originating from DNA-damage, growth factor withdrawal, glucocorticoid-treatment and anoikis. These stimuli trigger cell death either by directly regulating cell survival/cell death genes, or by deregulating cellular networks, which leads to apoptosis. Pro- and anti-apoptotic BCL2 proteins, referred to as the "BCL2-rheostat", are involved in this cell death decision either as direct targets or as sensors for cellular stress. BCL2-proteins can be divided into three groups. The prosurvival multi-domain BCL2-proteins BCL2, BCL2L2/Bcl-w, BCL2L1/Bcl-x_L, BCL2A1/A1 and MCL1 share four BCL2-homology (BH) domains, whereas multi-domain proapoptotic proteins BAX and BAK1/Bak are characterized by three BH-domains (Strasser 2005). The third group is the family of BH3-only proteins which contain only the BH3-domain and heterodimerize with prosurvival BCL2-proteins. The two models that have been proposed for apoptosis

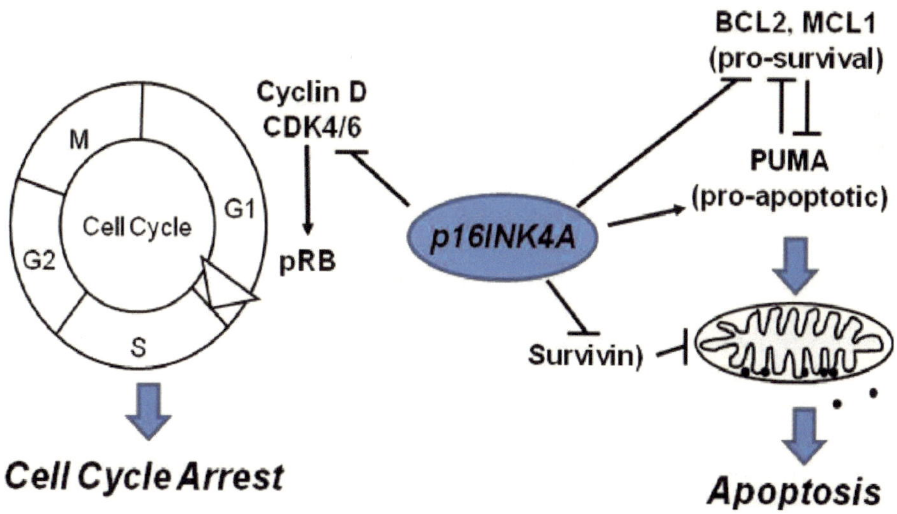

Fig. 3. Expression of p16^{INK4A} induces growth arrest in the G1 phase of the cell cycle and shifts the balance of pro- and anti-apoptotic BCL2 proteins towards the edge of cell death (detailed explanations in the text).

induction by BH3-only proteins suggest that either strong BH3-only proteins such as BCL2L11/Bim, truncated Bid or BBC3/Puma directly activate BAX or BAK1 ("direct activator/de-repressor model") (Kim et al, 2006) or that these BH3-only proteins neutralize the pro-survival function of anti-apoptotic BCL2-proteins ("displacement model") (Labi et al, 2006; Willis et al, 2007). Upon cell death decision BAX or BAK1 oligomerize in the mitochondrial outer membrane which causes cytochrome *c* release from mitochondria and activation of the further downstream apoptosome complex.

Interestingly, the apoptosis-regulatory effect of conditional reconstitution of p16INK4A in T-ALL leukemia cells depends on the therapeutic agent that is applied to the cells: p16INK4A markedly protects against programmed cell death induced by doxorubicin, etoposide and vinblastine (Figure 4), but in parallel sensitizes these cells to FAS- and GC-induced apoptosis (Figure 4 and (Obexer et al, 2009a)). Since p16INK4A induces an almost complete cell cycle arrest in these cells and uncouples growth from cell cycle arrest (Ausserlechner et al, 2005) we believe that this protective effect is merely a consequence of accumulation of cells in the G1 phase of the cell cycle. DNA-damaging agents such as doxorubicin or etoposide and tubulin-destabilzing compounds such as vinblastine exert their effects mainly on proliferating cells in S-phase or mitosis, respectively. Slowly proliferating cells or cells that are arrested in the G1-phase of the cell cycle may be therefore more resistant (Bacher et al, 2006). However, conditional p16INK4A also protects T-ALL cells against bortezomib-induced cell death (Figure 4). Although, the proteasome-inhibitor bortezomib/Velcade™ may perturb the correct degradation of cell cycle regulators such as cyclins, it has been shown that bortezomib is highly effective on slowly proliferating cancer cells such as chronic myeloid leukemia. This suggests that p16INK4A has a direct or indirect affect on cell death regulators at the level of death receptors and/or BCL2-proteins. When analyzing the expression of death receptors and their ligands it became evident that p16INK4A induces FAS-ligand mRNA expression in these cells, but does not change the FAS-receptor expression. Since CCRF-CEM cells are FAS-sensitive, this might cause an autocrine death signal that lowers death resistance in general since also the FAS downstream effectors Caspase-8 and Bid showed accelerated cleavage in p16INK4A expressing cells upon FAS-induced apoptosis. However, by introducing a dominant negative FADD mutant that blocks death receptor signaling we provided evidence that increased death sensitivity in p16INK4A expressing T-ALL cells can be ascribed to distinct changes in the composition of pro- and anti-apoptotic BCL2-proteins at the level of mitochondria (Obexer et al, 2009a). Whereas the potent pro-apoptotic protein BBC3/Puma accumulated in p16INK4A expressing CCRF-CEM and Molt4 cells, the pro-survival proteins BCL2 and MCL1 were downregulated after 24 hours and completely lost after 48 hours of p16INK4A expression. Although p16INK4A-expressing T-ALL cells did not undergo programmed cell death spontaneously within 48 hours, these significant changes in the balance of pro- and antiapoptotic BCL2-proteins reduce the capacity of T-ALL cells to cope with additional apoptotic signals such as binding of death-ligands or glucocorticoid-induced cell death (Figure 3). We demonstrated the relevance of Puma, BCL2 and MCL1 by retroviral overexpression and knock down, but did not further investigate other forms of cell death (Obexer et al, 2009a). Concerning the observation that p16INK4A expression renders T-ALL cells less sensitive to bortezomib, we found that p16INK4A reconstitution induced rapid loss of the BH3-only protein PMAIP1/Noxa in both CCRF-CEM T-ALL and Molt4 T-ALL cells (Obexer et al, 2009a). Noxa is a "weak" BH3-only protein that does not neutralize all pro-survival BCL2-proteins, but preferentially binds to MCL1, BCL2A1/A1 (Willis et al, 2007) and, as recently shown by our group also to BCL2L1/Bcl-x_L. Noxa acts as a sensitizer that critically regulates the sensitivity to e.g. proteasome-inhibition-induced cell death (Hagenbuchner et al, 2010). The rapid loss of Noxa upon p16INK4A reconstitution might therefore explain, why p16INK4A-expressing T-ALL cells show reduced sensitivity to bortezomib-induced apoptosis.

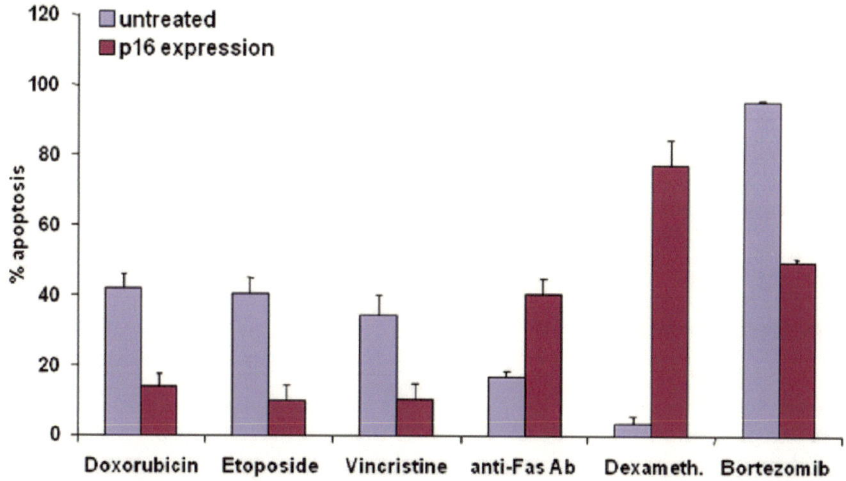

Fig. 4. p16INK4A expression differentially affects the sensitivity of T-ALL cells to various death-inducing agents. T-ALL cells expressing p16INK4A in a tetracycline-regulated manner were cultured for 24 hours in the presence of doxycycline (200 ng/ml) to switch on p16INK4A expression and were then treated with the therapeutic agents doxorubicin (8 µM), etoposide (8 µM), vincristine (8 µM), dexamethasone (10 nM) and bortezomib (10 nM) for additional 24 hours. To activate death receptor signaling an anti-Fas-receptor antibody (clone CH11, 0.1 µg/ml) was applied for 4 hours. Cells were resuspended in hypotonic propidium-iodide containing buffer according Nicoletti et al (Nicoletti et al, 1991) and the percentage of apoptotic cells was assessed in a Beckman-Coulter FC500 flow cytometer. Shown is the mean of three independent experiments.

However, additional levels of apoptosis modulation by p16INK4A in T-ALL cells exist. One protein that is highly expressed in many cancers e.g. in up to 65% of acute lymphoblastic B-cell leukemia is the anti-apoptotic protein BIRC5/Survivin (Troeger et al, 2007). Survivin belongs to the family of Inhibitor of Apoptosis Proteins (IAPs) that are characterized by so called BIR domains that allow them to interact with caspases and other molecules involved in cell death signaling. Survivin has also additional functions since it acts as a chromosomal passenger protein and blocks apoptosis induction at the level of mitochondria (Obexer et al, 2009b). Recently, it was shown that mice overexpressing Survivin in hematopoietic stem cells show a high incidence of hematologic tumors. This pro-oncogenic effect of Survivin was not due to increased proliferative potential but to increased death resistance of hematologic cells (Small et al, 2010).

Interestingly, the loss of p16INK4A during leukemogenesis apparently contributes to high levels of Survivin in T-ALL cells: in leukemia cells engineered to express p16INK4A the Survivin steady state expression levels are completely repressed upon p16INK4A induction (Figure 5A). To directly assess the relevance of Survivin-repression for changes in apoptosis sensitivity we retrovirally transduced human Survivin into T-ALL cells with conditional p16INK4A expression. As shown in Figure 5A this ectopic Survivin compensates for the loss of the endogenous protein during p16INK4A expression. Interestingly, ectopic Survivin prevented FAS-induced death sensitization (Figure 5B), but did not affect the increased sensitivity of p16INK4A-expressing T-ALL cells to glucocorticoid-induced cell death (Figure 5C). These results suggest that in T-ALL cells Survivin interferes with death-receptor-induced apoptosis triggered by FAS-ligand. Therefore, the effects of p16INK4A in leukemia cells by far extend the generally described effect as an inhibitor of cell cycle progression.

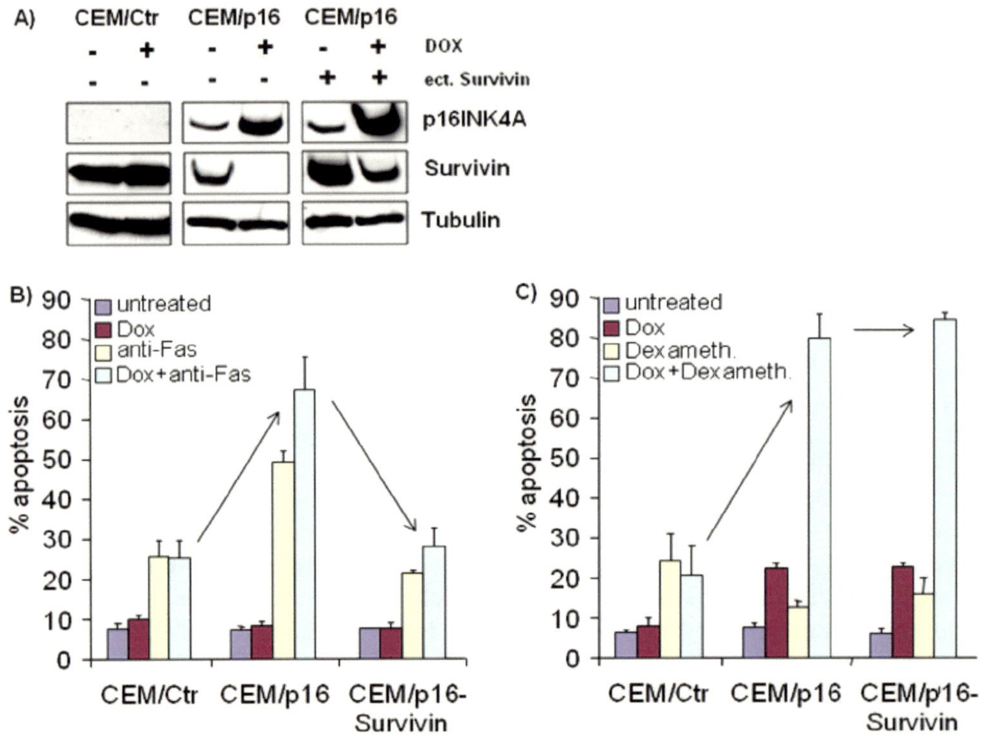

Fig. 5. High levels of p16INK4A in human CCRF-CEM T-ALL cells repress the IAP family member Survivin, which is critical for increased FAS-induced cell death, but not for p16INK4A-induced sensitization to glucocorticoid-induced apoptosis. A) CEM/Ctr cells stably express the reverse tet-transactivator rtTA, CEM/p16 cells are derivatives that contain the rtTA and express human p16INK4A under the control of a tetracycline responsive CMV promoter (Ausserlechner et al, 2001). In presence of 200 ng/ml doxycycline, p16INK4A expression is induced, which causes complete loss of Survivin within 48 hour. Retrovirally transduced Survivin compensates for the loss of the endogenous protein in CEM/p16-Survivin cells. Re-expression of p16INK4A accelerates death-receptor-induced (anti-FAS anibody, 0.1 mg/ml, for four hours) and glucocorticoid-induced apoptosis (10 nM dexamethasone, 24 hours) as shown in B und C (Obexer et al, 2009a). Ectopic expression of Survivin did not change the sensitivity to dexamethasone (C), but prevents increased sensitivity to Fas-induced apoptosis (B). The amount of apoptotic cells was assessed by flow cytometric analysis of propidium-iodide stained nuclei. Each bar represents the mean of three independent experiments.

8. Conclusions

The INK4A genes were discovered in the mid-90s of the last century and intensive studies on their function and regulation have contributed significantly to our current knowledge on cell cycle regulation (and de-regulation) in normal and malignant cells. Despite all this effort and progress, continuously new aspects of p16INK4A and ARF are discovered, which highlight their diverse functions beyond the inhibition of the cell division cycle. In this chapter we reviewed current findings on how these INK4A-encoded genes are regulated in hematopoietic stem cells and that these proteins also represent a barrier to the artificial generation of pluripotent stem cells from normal differentiated tissue. In addition, both proteins also contribute to death sensitivity: ARF by activating p53 via a well defined pathway, p16INK4A by directly or indirectly affecting the expression and activity of critical death regulators such as BCL2 proteins, death ligands or pro-survival proteins such as Survivin. Under normal, physiologic conditions these significant changes in death sensitivity may determine a deadly barrier for cells that try to return to a less differentiated state and also for precancerous cells that lose proliferative control. These novel findings implicate that INK4A proteins are not "only cell cycle brakes" but serve as gatekeepers that keep the doors closed for those cells that want some piece of "stemness".

9. References

Aagaard, L., Lukas J., Bartkova J., Kjerulff A. A., Strauss M. and Bartek J. (1995). Aberrations of P16(Ink4) and Retinoblastoma Tumor-Suppressor Genes Occur in Distinct Sub-Sets of Human Cancer Cell-Lines. *International Journal of Cancer* 61, 115-120.

Al Mohanna, M. A., Manogaran P. S., Al Mukhalafi Z., Al Hussein A. and Aboussekhra A. (2004). The tumor suppressor p16(INK4a) gene is a regulator of apoptosis induced by ultraviolet light and cisplatin. *Oncogene* 23, 201-212.

Ausserlechner, M. J., Obexer P., Deutschmann A., Geiger K. and Kofler R. (2006). A retroviral expression system based on tetracycline-regulated tricistronic transactivator/repressor vectors for functional analyses of anti-proliferative and toxic genes. *Mol. Cancer Ther.* 5, 1927-1934.

Ausserlechner, M. J., Obexer P., Geley S. and Kofler R. (2005). G1 arrest by p16(INK4A) uncouples growth from cell cycle progression in leukemia cells with deregulated cyclin E and c-Myc expression. *Leukemia* 19, 1051-1057.

Ausserlechner, M. J., Obexer P., Wiegers G. J., Hartmann B. L., Geley S. and Kofler R. (2001). The cell cycle inhibitor p16(INK4A) sensitizes lymphoblastic leukemia cells to apoptosis by physiologic glucocorticoid levels. *J. Biol. Chem.* 276, 10984-10989.

Bacher, N., Tiefenthaler M., Sturm S., Stuppner H., Ausserlechner M. J., Kofler R. and Konwalinka G. (2006). Oxindole alkaloids from Uncaria tomentosa induce apoptosis in proliferating, G0/G1-arrested and bcl-2-expressing acute lymphoblastic leukaemia cells. *Br. J. Haematol.* 132, 615-622.

Banito, A., Rashid S. T., Acosta J. C., Li S., Pereira C. F., Geti I., Pinho S., Silva J. C., Azuara V., Walsh M. et al. (2009). Senescence impairs successful reprogramming to pluripotent stem cells. *Genes Dev.* 23, 2134-2139.

Bianchi, T., Rufer N., MacDonald H. R. and Migliaccio M. (2006). The tumor suppressor p16Ink4a regulates T lymphocyte survival. *Oncogene* 25, 4110-4115.

Bracken, A. P., Kleine-Kohlbrecher D., Dietrich N., Pasini D., Gargiulo G., Beekman C., Theilgaard-Monch K., Minucci S., Porse B. T., Marine J. C. et al. (2007). The Polycomb group proteins bind throughout the INK4A-ARF locus and are disassociated in senescent cells. *Genes Dev.* 21, 525-530.

Cayuela, J. M., Gardie B. and Sigaux F. (1997). Disruption of the multiple tumor suppressor gene MTS1/p16(INK4a)/CDKN2 by illegitimate V(D)J recombinase activity in T-cell acute lymphoblastic leukemias. *Blood* 90, 3720-3726.

Cayuela, J. M., Madani A., Sanhes L., Stern M. H. and Sigaux F. (1996). Multiple tumor-suppressor gene 1 inactivation is the most frequent genetic alteration in T-cell acute lymphoblastic leukemia. *Blood* 87, 2180-2186.

Cobrinik, D. (2005). Pocket proteins and cell cycle control. *Oncogene* 24, 2796-2809.

Condorelli, G. L., Facchiano F., Valtieri M., Proietti E., Vitelli L., Lulli V., Huebner K., Peschle C. and Croce C. M. (1996). T-cell-directed TAL-1 expression induces T-cell malignancies in transgenic mice. *Cancer Res.* 56, 5113-5119.

Drexler, H. G. (1998). Review of alterations of the cyclin-dependent kinase inhibitor INK4 family genes p15, p16, p18 and p19 in human leukemia-lymphoma cells. *Leukemia* 12, 845-859.

Ekholm, S. V. and Reed S. I. (2000). Regulation of G(1) cyclin-dependent kinases in the mammalian cell cycle. *Curr. Opin. Cell Biol.* 12, 676-684.

Gardie, B., Cayuela J. M., Martini S. and Sigaux F. (1998). Genomic alterations of the p19ARF encoding exons in T-cell acute lymphoblastic leukemia. *Blood* 91, 1016-1020.

Grana, X., Garriga J. and Mayol X. (1998). Role of the retinoblastoma protein family, pRB, p107 and p130 in the negative control of cell growth. *Oncogene* 17, 3365-3383.

Hagenbuchner, J., Ausserlechner M. J., Porto V., David R., Meister B., Bodner M., Villunger A., Geiger K. and Obexer P. (2010). The Antiapoptotic Protein BCL2L1/BCL-XL is Neutralized by Proapoptotic PMAIP1/Noxa in Neuroblastoma Thereby Determining Bortezomib-Sensitivity Independent of Prosurvival MCL1 Expression. *J. Biol. Chem.* 285, 6904-6912.

Hebert, J., Cayuela J. M., Berkeley J. and Sigaux F. (1994). Candidate tumor-suppressor genes MTS1 (p16INK4A) and MTS2 (p15INK4B) display frequent homozygous deletions in primary cells from T- but not from B-cell lineage acute lymphoblastic leukemias. *Blood* 84, 4038-4044.

Itahana, K., Bhat K. P., Jin A., Itahana Y., Hawke D., Kobayashi R. and Zhang Y. (2003). Tumor suppressor ARF degrades B23, a nucleolar protein involved in ribosome biogenesis and cell proliferation. *Mol. Cell* 12, 1151-1164.

Janzen, V., Forkert R., Fleming H. E., Saito Y., Waring M. T., Dombkowski D. M., Cheng T., DePinho R. A., Sharpless N. E. and Scadden D. T. (2006). Stem-cell ageing modified by the cyclin-dependent kinase inhibitor p16INK4a. *Nature* 443, 421-426.

Kamijo, T., Zindy F., Roussel M. F., Quelle D. E., Downing J. R., Ashmun R. A., Grosveld G. and Sherr C. J. (1997). Tumor suppression at the mouse INK4a locus mediated by the alternative reading frame product p19ARF. *Cell* 91, 649-659.

Kees, U. R., Burton P. R., Lu C. and Baker D. L. (1997). Homozygous deletion of the p16/MTS1 gene in pediatric acute lymphoblastic leukemia is associated with unfavorable clinical outcome. *Blood* 89, 4161-4166.

Kim, H., Rafiuddin-Shah M., Tu H. C., Jeffers J. R., Zambetti G. P., Hsieh J. J. and Cheng E. H. (2006). Hierarchical regulation of mitochondrion-dependent apoptosis by BCL-2 subfamilies. *Nat. Cell Biol.* 8, 1348-1358.

Labi, V., Erlacher M., Kiessling S. and Villunger A. (2006). BH3-only proteins in cell death initiation, malignant disease and anticancer therapy. *Cell Death. Differ.* 13, 1325-1338.

Li, H., Collado M., Villasante A., Strati K., Ortega S., Canamero M., Blasco M. A. and Serrano M. (2009). The Ink4/Arf locus is a barrier for iPS cell reprogramming. *Nature* 460, 1136-1139.

Liu, Y., Johnson S. M., Fedoriw Y., Rogers A. B., Yuan H., Krishnamurthy J. and Sharpless N. E. (2011). Expression of p16(INK4a) prevents cancer and promotes aging in lymphocytes. *Blood* 117, 3257-3267.

Marion, R. M., Strati K., Li H., Murga M., Blanco R., Ortega S., Fernandez-Capetillo O., Serrano M. and Blasco M. A. (2009). A p53-mediated DNA damage response limits reprogramming to ensure iPS cell genomic integrity. *Nature* 460, 1149-1153.

Matsushime, H., Ewen M. E., Strom D. K., Kato J. Y., Hanks S. K., Roussel M. F. and Sherr C. J. (1992). Identification and properties of an atypical catalytic subunit (p34PSK-J3/cdk4) for mammalian D type G1 cyclins. *Cell* 71, 323-334.

Meyerson, M. and Harlow E. (1994). Identification of G1 kinase activity for cdk6, a novel cyclin D partner. *Mol. Cell. Biol.* 14, 2077-2086.

Molofsky, A. V., Slutsky S. G., Joseph N. M., He S., Pardal R., Krishnamurthy J., Sharpless N. E. and Morrison S. J. (2006). Increasing p16INK4a expression decreases forebrain progenitors and neurogenesis during ageing. *Nature* 443, 448-452.

Murray, A. and T. Hunt. 1993. The cell cycle: an introduction. Oxford University Press, Oxford, UK.

Nicoletti, I., Migliorati G., Pagliacci M. C., Grignani F. and Riccardi C. (1991). A rapid and simple method for measuring thymocyte apoptosis by propidium iodide staining and flow cytometry. *J. Immunol. Methods* 139, 271-279.

Obexer, P., Hagenbuchner J., Rupp M., Salvador C., Holzner M., Deutsch M., Porto V., Kofler R., Unterkircher T. and Ausserlechner M. J. (2009a). p16INK4A sensitizes human leukemia cells to FAS- and glucocorticoid-induced apoptosis via induction of BBC3/Puma and repression of MCL1 and BCL2. *J. Biol. Chem.* 284, 30933-30940.

Obexer, P., Hagenbuchner J., Unterkircher T., Sachsenmaier N., Seifarth C., Bock G., Porto V., Geiger K. and Ausserlechner M. (2009b). Repression of BIRC5/survivin by FOXO3/FKHRL1 sensitizes human neuroblastoma cells to DNA damage-induced apoptosis. *Mol. Biol. Cell* 20, 2041-2048.

Oguro, H., Iwama A., Morita Y., Kamijo T., van Lohuizen M. and Nakauchi H. (2006). Differential impact of Ink4a and Arf on hematopoietic stem cells and their bone marrow microenvironment in Bmi1-deficient mice. *J. Exp. Med.* 203, 2247-2253.

Ohm, J. E., McGarvey K. M., Yu X., Cheng L., Schuebel K. E., Cope L., Mohammad H. P., Chen W., Daniel V. C., Yu W. et al. (2007). A stem cell-like chromatin pattern may predispose tumor suppressor genes to DNA hypermethylation and heritable silencing. *Nat. Genet.* 39, 237-242.

Ohtani, N., Zebedee Z., Huot T. J., Stinson J. A., Sugimoto M., Ohashi Y., Sharrocks A. D., Peters G. and Hara E. (2001). Opposing effects of Ets and Id proteins on p16INK4a expression during cellular senescence. *Nature* 409, 1067-1070.

Okuda, T., Shurtleff S. A., Valentine M. B., Raimondi S. C., Head D. R., Behm F., Curcio-Brint A. M., Liu Q., Pui C. H., Sherr C. J. et al. (1995). Frequent deletion of p16INK4a/MTS1 and p15INK4b/MTS2 in pediatric acute lymphoblastic leukemia. *Blood* 85, 2321-2330.

Parry, D., Bates S., Mann D. J. and Peters G. (1995). Lack of cyclin D-Cdk complexes in Rb-negative cells correlates with high levels of p16INK4/MTS1 tumour suppressor gene product. *EMBO J.* 14, 503-511.

Quelle, D. E., Ashmun R. A., Shurtleff S. A., Kato J. Y., Bar S. D., Roussel M. F. and Sherr C. J. (1993). Overexpression of mouse D-type cyclins accelerates G1 phase in rodent fibroblasts. *Genes Dev.* 7, 1559-1571.

Quelle, D. E., Zindy F., Ashmun R. A. and Sherr C. J. (1995). Alternative reading frames of the INK4a tumor suppressor gene encode two unrelated proteins capable of inducing cell cycle arrest. *Cell* 83, 993-1000.

Rizo, A., Olthof S., Han L., Vellenga E., de Haan G. and Schuringa J. J. (2009). Repression of BMI1 in normal and leukemic human CD34(+) cells impairs self-renewal and induces apoptosis. *Blood* 114, 1498-1505.

Rocha, S., Garrett M. D., Campbell K. J., Schumm K. and Perkins N. D. (2005). Regulation of NF-kappaB and p53 through activation of ATR and Chk1 by the ARF tumour suppressor. *EMBO J.* 24, 1157-1169.

Shank-Calvo, J. A., Draheim K., Bhasin M. and Kelliher M. A. (2006). p16Ink4a or p19Arf loss contributes to Tal1-induced leukemogenesis in mice. *Oncogene* 25, 3023-3031.

Sharpless, N. E., Bardeesy N., Lee K. H., Carrasco D., Castrillon D. H., Aguirre A. J., Wu E. A., Horner J. W. and DePinho R. A. (2001). Loss of p16Ink4a with retention of p19Arf predisposes mice to tumorigenesis. *Nature* 413, 86-91.

Sharpless, N. E., Ramsey M. R., Balasubramanian P., Castrillon D. H. and DePinho R. A. (2004). The differential impact of p16(INK4a) or p19(ARF) deficiency on cell growth and tumorigenesis. *Oncogene* 23, 379-385.

Sherr, C. J. (2006). Divorcing ARF and p53: an unsettled case. *Nat. Rev. Cancer* 6, 663-673.

Sherr, C. J. and Roberts J. M. (1999). CDK inhibitors: positive and negative regulators of G1-phase progression. *Genes Dev.* 13, 1501-1512.

Sherr, C. J. and Roberts J. M. (2004). Living with or without cyclins and cyclin-dependent kinases. *Genes Dev* 18, 2699-2711.

Simon, J. A. and Kingston R. E. (2009). Mechanisms of polycomb gene silencing: knowns and unknowns. *Nat. Rev. Mol. Cell Biol.* 10, 697-708.

Small, S., Keerthivasan G., Huang Z., Gurbuxani S. and Crispino J. D. (2010). Overexpression of survivin initiates hematologic malignancies in vivo. *Leukemia* 24, 1920-1926.

Strasser, A. (2005). The role of BH3-only proteins in the immune system. *Nat. Rev. Immunol.* 5, 189-200.

Troeger, A., Siepermann M., Escherich G., Meisel R., Willers R., Gudowius S., Moritz T., Laws H. J., Hanenberg H., Goebel U. et al. (2007). Survivin and its prognostic significance in pediatric acute B-cell precursor lymphoblastic leukemia. *Haematologica* 92, 1043-1050.

Utikal, J., Polo J. M., Stadtfeld M., Maherali N., Kulalert W., Walsh R. M., Khalil A., Rheinwald J. G. and Hochedlinger K. (2009). Immortalization eliminates a roadblock during cellular reprogramming into iPS cells. *Nature* 460, 1145-1148.

Villunger, A., Michalak E. M., Coultas L., Mullauer F., Bock G., Ausserlechner M. J., Adams J. M. and Strasser A. (2003). p53- and drug-induced apoptotic responses mediated by BH3-only proteins puma and noxa. *Science* 302, 1036-1038.

Willis, S. N., Fletcher J. I., Kaufmann T., van Delft M. F., Chen L., Czabotar P. E., Ierino H., Lee E. F., Fairlie W. D., Bouillet P. et al. (2007). Apoptosis initiated when BH3 ligands engage multiple Bcl-2 homologs, not Bax or Bak. *Science* 315, 856-859.

8

Accumulation of Specific Epigenetic Abnormalities During Development and Progression of T Cell Leukemia/Lymphoma

Takashi Oka[1], Hiaki Sato[1], Mamoru Ouchida[1], Atae Utsunomiya[2], Daisuke Ennishi[1], Mitsune Tanimoto[1] and Tadashi Yoshino[1]

[1]Okayama University, Okayama,
[2]Imamura Bun-in Hospital, Kagoshima
Japan

1. Introduction

The genetic abnormalities found in various types of leukemia and lymphoma do not provide a complete picture of the molecular mechanism(s) responsible for hematopoietic malignancies. Aberrant changes in epigenetics, including systems controlling DNA methylation, histone modifications, chromatin remodeling and miRNAs, are additional mechanisms that contribute to the malignant phenotype. DNA methylation is one of the basic mechanisms that controls the development and differentiation, and maintains the normal physiological status, in mammalian cells. DNA methylation is also involved in the regulation of imprinted gene expression and X-chromosome inactivation, and in the fine-tuning of tissue specific differentiation and development from stem cells. However, aberrant promoter hypermethylation of CpG islands leads to epigenetic silencing of multiple genes, including tumor suppressor genes, and has been recognized as an important mechanism involved in carcinogenesis. Furthermore, multiple genes have been shown to be methylated simultaneously (a condition termed the CpG island methylator phenotype: CIMP) in various types of human malignancies. This mechanism is a fundamental process involved in the development of many tumors. A comprehensive knowledge of the methylation profile of a given tumor may provide important information for risk assessment, diagnosis, monitoring, and treatments.

Adult T cell leukemia/lymphoma (ATLL) is an aggressive malignant disease of CD4-positive T lymphocytes caused by infection with human T-lymphotropic virus type I (HTLV-1). HTLV-1 causes ATLL in 3-5% of infected individuals after a long latent period of 40-60 years. Such a long latent period suggests that a multi-step leukemogenic/lymphomagenic mechanism is involved in the development of ATLL, although the critical event(s) involved in the progression have not been characterized in details. The pathogenesis of HTLV-1 has been investigated intensively in terms of the viral regulatory proteins HTLV-1 Tax and Rex, which are supposed to play key roles in the HTLV-1 leukemogenesis/lymphomagenesis, as well as the HTLV-1 basic leucine zipper factor (HBZ). The mechanism(s) underlying the progression of ATLL have been reported from various genetic aspects, including specific chromosome abnormalities and changes in

the characteristic HTLV-1 Tax and Rex protein expression pattern, although the detailed mechanism(s) triggering the onset and progression of ATLL remains to be elucidated.
In this chapter, the current state of knowledge about the epigenetic abnormalities that occur during the development and progression of T cell leukemia/lymphoma, especially during adult T- cell leukemia/lymphoma (ATLL), will be reviewed, as will the basic mechanism of epigenetic regulation of gene expression and various clinical aspects of T cell leukemia/lymphoma. In addition, the relevance of this knowledge to leukemia/lymphoma risk assessment, prevention and early detection will be discussed.

2. Epigenetic regulation on gene expression

The term "epigenetics" was coined by Conrad H. Waddinton in the 1940s, fusing the word "genetics" with "epigenesis". The classical definition proposed by Waddinton involves the heritability of a phenotype, passed on through either mitosis or meiosis. Recently, epigenetics has been proposed as "a stably heritable phenotype resulting from changes in a chromosome without alterations in the DNA sequence" (Berger et al., 2009). The pigenetic regulation of gene expression falls mainly into two categories, DNA methylation and histone modification (Figure 1).

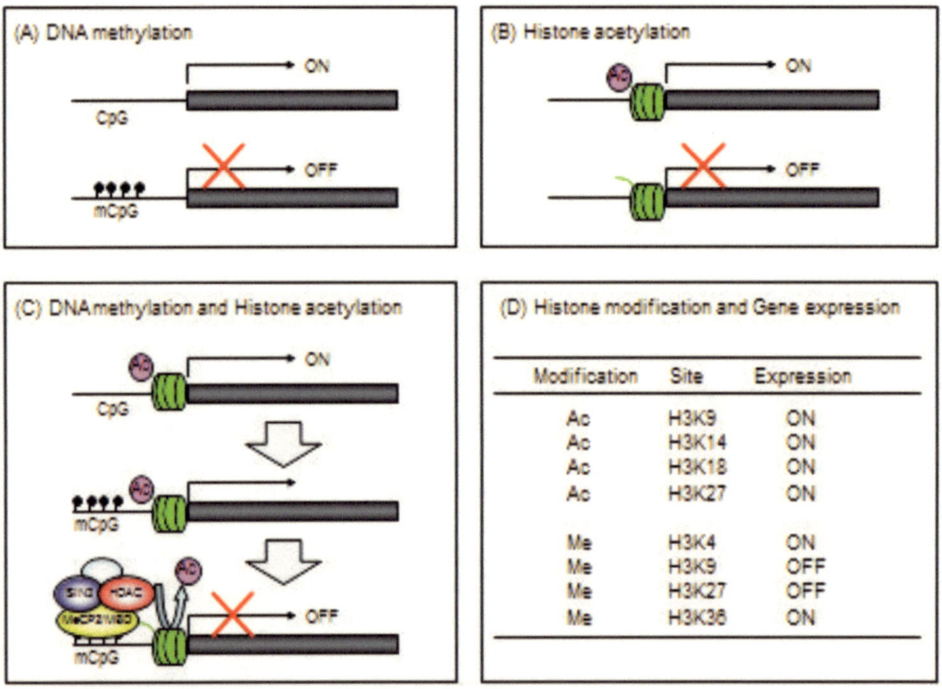

Fig. 1. (A) DNAmethylation of CpG islands in the 5′ transcriptional regulatory region occurs gene silencing. (B) Histone acetylation and deacetylation regulate gene expression. (C) DNA methylation recruits methyl-CpG binding proteins such as MeCP2, MBD1, MBD2 and MBD4, followed by association with co-repressors such as HDAC complexes, resulting in gene silencing. (D) Histone modification and gene expression state. Ac, acetylation; Me, methylation; H3, histone 3; K, lysine.

2.1 DNA methylation

In the case of eukaryotes, especially in vertebrates, 5-methylcytosine is the predominant modified base in DNA. The 5'-methylation of cytosine residues is a physical modification, and does not inhibit its pairing with guanine nucleotide. In mammals, cytosine methylation is essentially confined to the sequence 5'-CpG-3' (Razin & Riggs, 1980). In certain areas of the genome of mammals, especially in regulatory regions of genes like promoters and enhancers, a high concentration of these CpG dinucleotides is found, and these are referred to as "CpG islands" (CGIs). The methyl-residue is exposed to the major groove of double stranded DNA, and the modification of cytosine in regulatory regions results in the alteration (inhibition or activation) of the interactions between DNA and DNA binding proteins. The methylation of cytosine is catalyzed by DNA methyltransferase enzymes, which can transfer the methyl residue supplied by S-adenosylmethionine (SAM) to cytosine on DNA. In mammals, three DNA methyltransferases, DNMT1, DNMT3A, and DNMT3B, are known to carry out methylation and maintenance.

DNA methyltransferase I (DNMT1) is known as a "maintenance methyltransferase". This enzyme has been shown to have a 10-fold preference for hemi-methylated sites as a substrate. This enzyme can transfer a methyl residue specifically to a newly synthesized strand after semi-conservative replication of methylated DNA, and copies the methylation status of the parental DNA during the division of somatic cells. UHRF1 (also known as NP95) preferentially binds to hemi-methylated sites, and it has been suggested that DNMT1 might be recruited to DNA replication foci by UHRF1 (Sharif et al., 2007; Bostick et al., 2007). Mammalian cells use DNMT1 primarily to maintain the DNA methylation profile in a stable fashion throughout cell division.

De novo methylation of unmodified DNA is required to form methylation patterns in response to embryogenesis, cell differentiation and extracellular signals. DNMT3A and DNMT3B are known as "*de novo* methyltransferases" which are used to methylate previously unmethylated DNA during development and differentiation. These DNMTs function to discontinuously change the methylation profile for specific compartments of the genome in a tissue-specific manner in vertebrates. In mammals, during the early stage of embryonic development and the early development of primordial germ cells, DNA methylation is erased, followed by introduction of DNA methylation by *de novo* methyltransferases at different sites (Reik, 2007). The *de novo* methylation is carried by DNMT3A and DNMT3B during the early stage of embryonic development, and DNMT3A and its cofactor, DNMT3-like (DBMT3L), are active during germ cell development. Recently, a new model was proposed, in which DNMT3A and DNMT3B, compartmentalized to CpG islands, complete the methylation process and correct errors left by DNMT1 (Jones & Liang, 2009).

In general, the DNA methylation profile is associated with gene repression, and CpG island methylation is involved in the regulation of imprinted gene expression and X-chromosome inactivation, in addition to the fine-tuning of the specific differentiation of cells and their development from stem cells (Csankovszki et al., 2001; Jones & Takai, 2001; Kaneda et al., 2004; Meissner et al., 2008). Aberrant methylation of DNA is also known to be associated with many diseases including malignant tumors, imprinting disorders, and neuronal diseases. Aberrant promoter hypermethylation of tumor suppressor genes is a prevalent phenomenon in human cancers, as well as malignant leukemia/lymphoma, and inhibits the expression of these genes, leading to tumorigenesis in these cells. Recently, it has been reported that aberrant promoter hypermethylation, referred to as the CpG island methylator phenotype (CIMP), is associated with specific clinical conditions in colorectal cancer, brain tumors, and malignant leukemia/lymphoma, as we will describe later in detail. On the other hand, it is also known that genome-wide hypomethylation is commonly observed in human tumors, and global loss of DNA methylation leads to widespread tumorigenesis as a result of chromosomal instability (Holm et al., 2005).

2.2 Histone modification

Large eukaryotic genomes in the nucleus are tightly packed, forming the fundamental repeating units referred to as nucleosomes. The nucleosome core particle consists of approximately 147 base pairs of DNA wrapped in left-handed superhelical turns around a histone octamer consisting of 2 copies each of the core histones H2A, H2B, H3, and H4. The N-terminal tail domains of histones comprise 25~30% of the mass of individual histones, and pass through a channel formed by the minor grooves of two DNA strands, and protrude from the surface of the chromatin. The tails of histones are subject to many posttranslational modifications, including methylation of arginines, methylation, acetylation, ubiquitination, ADP-ribosylation, and sumolation of lysines, and phosphorylation of serine and threonine residues. These modifications on the tail domains are considered to be a histone language that is read by other proteins. This language is referred to as the "histone code" (Strahl & Allis, 2000), and also as the "epigenetic code" with regard to histone modification and DNA methylation.

2.2.1 Histone acetylation

Histone acetylation that occurs at multiple lysine residues of histone 3 (H3) and histone 4 (H4) is associated with active transcription, commonly observed in euchromatin, and is usually carried out by a variety of histone acetyltransferase complexes (HATs) such as p300, CBP and MOZ, which are known as fusion genes in acute myeloid leukemia. Histone acetylation results in a change in the net charge of nucleosomes, which can lead to the decrease of inter- or intranucleosomal DNA-histone interactions. On the other hand, deacetylation of histones occurs as a result of interactions with histone deacetylase complexes (HDACs), and is associated with transcriptional repression. Histone deacetylase complexes, HDAC1 and HDAC2, contain the SIN3 complex and MiNuRD (nucleosome remodeling and deacetylase) complex, and these complexes interact with methylated DNA on gene promoters through methylated DNA binding proteins, MeCP2 and MBD2/MBD3, respectively. SIRT1 is an NAD(+)-dependent histone deacetylase, and is a stress-response and chromatin-silencing factor, which is involved in various nuclear events such as transcription, DNA replication, and DNA repair (Abdelmohsen et al., 2007). The PML-RARA fusion protein induces a block on hematopoietic differentiation and acute promyelocytic leukemia by inactivating target genes via its ability to recruit HDAC3, MBD1 and DNA methyltransferases (Villa et al., 2006). The AML protein, a partner of fusion proteins detected in acute myeloid leukemia, interacts with p300, CBP, MOZ, PML, SIN3A and HDAC.

2.2.2 Histone methylation

Promoter regions in actively transcribed genes are marked by the presence of a trimethyl mark on histone 3 lysine 4 (H3K4me3), in addition to hypomethylated promoter CpG islands and histone hyperacetylation. The transcribed body of an active gene is characterized by trimethylation of histone 3 at lysine 36 (H3K36me3), while transcriptionally repressed genes exhibit the trimethylation of histone 3 at lysine 27 (H3K27me3). Permanently silenced genes are characterized by trimethylation at lysine 9 (H3K9me3), with histone hypoacetylation and hypermethylation of CpG islands on their promoters. For these histone methylations, polycomb group (PcG) and Trithorax group (Trx) proteins work on alternative systems of epigenetic memory to regulate gene expression and chromatin structure via modification of histone tails in a heritable manner (Bantignies & Cavalli, 2006; Cernilogar & Orlando, 2005; Cunliffe, 2003).

The multiprotein polycomb complexes are important mediators of transcriptional repression. The PRC2 (Polycomb repressive complex) is responsible for adding methyl groups to H3K27 (Kirmizis et al., 2004). The catalytic component of the PRC2 complex is EZH2, a histone methyltransferase. The cofactors SUZ12 and EED induce EZH2 activity and interact with nucleosomes. The H3K27-methylated histones recruit the PRC1 complex, and PC2, a component of the PRC1 complex, binds to H3K27-methylated histones and blocks gene activation by interfering with the movement of nucleosomes. H3K27-methylated histones also recruit the PRC2 complex to nucleosomes of the nascent DNA strand during DNA replication to continue gene silencing (Hansen et al., 2008). The mutation and over-expression of EZH2 has been reported in malignant cells, especially in diffuse large B-cell lymphomas (Morin et al., 2010). Histone demethylation is mediated by the Jumonji domain (JMJD) enzymes, which remove tri-, di- or monomethyl modifications. H3K27me3 is similarly removed by the JMJD3 and UTX proteins. Alterations of UTX have been found in a variety of tumors (van Haaften et al., 2009). However, the mechanism by which loss of the H3K27 methylation system leads to cancer remains poorly characterized.

Trithorax (Trx) group molecules, such as the MLL/ALL family of genes are methyltransferases for H3K4, and positively regulate the expression of target genes, including multiple HOX genes. MLL is a frequent target for recurrent translocations in acute leukemias that may be characterized as acute myeloid leukemia (AML), acute lymphoblastic leukemia (ALL), or mixed lineage leukemia (MLL). More than 50 different MLL fusion partners have been identified so far. Leukemogenic MLL translocations encode MLL fusion proteins that have lost H3K4 methyltransferase activity, and loss of H3K4 methyltransferase activity is strongly associated with disorders of hematopoietic progenitor cells. LSD1 (lysine-specific demethylase-1) removes di- and monomethyl modifications from H3K4 (Kouzarides, 2007).

2.3 Transcriptional regulation of genes

In addition to epigenetic regulation by DNA methylation and histone modifications, the other major regulation system is concerned with transcriptional regulation as a result of remodeling of the chromatin structure. Chromatin is actively remodeled by the SWI/SNF family protein complexes, referred to as chromatin remodeling complexes, which have DNA helicase activity (DNA-dependent ATPase activity) to alter the histone-DNA contacts. Chromatin remodeling complexes carry out transient unwrapping of the DNA end from histone octamers, forming a DNA loop, and moving nucleosomes to different translational positions (sliding). These chromatin remodeling complexes are mainly thought to exert activities that precede transcriptional activation of genes. Among the ATPase subunit group (SMARCA1-6) of chromatin remodeling complexes, SMARCA2/BRM and

SMARCA4/BRG1 interact with chromatin-modifying enzymes, such as HDAC1, HDAC2, SIN3, and poly (ADP-ribose) polymerase (PARP) 1, and methyl-CpG binding protein MeCP2 (Calvin et al., 2010; Harikrishnan et al., 2005; Sif et al., 2001). In many tumor cells, alterations of the SMARCA2, 4, and 6 genes have been reported (Gunduz et al., 2005; Wong et al., 2000; Yano et al., 2004).

Chromatin remodeling and epigenetic regulation are involved in the intricate control of gene expression. The methyl-CpG binding protein, MeCP2, is involved in histone methyltransferase activity (Fuks et al., 2003) and in regulating DNA methyltransferase DNMT1 (Kimura & Shiota, 2003). Methylated CpG islands in the 5′ transcriptional regulatory region recruit methyl-CpG binding proteins such as MeCP2, MBD1, MBD2 and MBD4, followed by association with co-repressors such as HDAC complexes, histone methyltransferases, and chromatin remodeling complexes, thus resulting in the formation of a repressive chromatin structure that leads to gene silencing. This may provide "epigenetic memory" by helping progeny cells to "remember" their cellular identity (Bird, 2002). The epigenetic landscape of the whole genome is different in malignant cells compared to that in normal cells. Epigenetic processes have been implicated in the development of various malignancies, including leukemia/lymphoma, in which the repression or silencing of tumor suppressor genes is remarkably common (Costello et al., 2000; Esteller, 2005; Esteller et al., 2001; Herman & Baylin, 2003; Miremadi et al., 2007).

3. Clinical characteristics of T-cell lymphoma

T-cell lymphoma is distinct clinicopathological entity classified by the WHO. T-cell lymphoma is a neoplasm with geographical variations in frequency, and the pathogenesis and clinical behavior, including the prognosis, are different from other lymphomas, such as B-cell lymphoma and Hodgkin's lymphoma. In this section, we mainly discuss the clinical features and management of T-cell lymphoma.

3.1 Clinical features of T-cell lymphoma

3.1.1 Epidemiology

The incidence of T-cell lymphoma demonstrates interesting geographical variations; in North America and Europe, about 5-10% of lymphomas are T-cell lymphomas (Anderson et al., 2002). However, in Asia, T-cell and natural killer (NK)-cell lymphomas account for 15-25% of all lymphomas (Au et al., 2005). The higher prevalence of T-cell lymphoma in Asia is reported to be influenced by endemic virus infections, such as human T-cell lymphotropic virus type-I (HTLV-1) and Epstein-Barr virus (EBV). The establishment of management recommendations by Asian oncologists in collaboration with international experts is urgently needed.

3.1.2 Clinical behavior of T-cell lymphoma

The WHO's classification includes 15 different T-cell lymphomas. Peripheral T-cell lymphoma not otherwise specified (PTCL-NOS), angioimmunoblastic T-cell lymphoma (AITL), and anaplastic large cell lymphoma (ALCL) account for 70-80% of T-cell lymphomas (Armitage et al., 1998). The other subtypes of T-cell lymphoma are rare entities.

PTCL-NOS is a heterogeneous subtype that cannot be defined as another specific T-cell lymphoma. Both nodal and extranodal sites can be involved in this lymphoma. The nodal type can be well characterized histologically, but the extranodal type often does not show a definite histopathological pattern. In particular, cutaneous PTCL has specific histological features, and this lymphoma is defined as a distinct subtype; cutaneous T-cell lymphoma, in the WHO classification. Therefore, PTCL-NOS is often diagnosed by demonstration of a T-cell lineage. The relatively high proportion of patients with PTCL-NOS described in some series of T-cell lymphomas might thus reflect inadequate classification into other T-cell lymphoma subtypes. The clinical behavior of PTCL-NOS is not specific, but it generally has an aggressive clinical course similar to aggressive B-cell lymphoma, but the outcome of PTCL-NOS is poorer than that of aggressive B-cell lymphomas, such as diffuse large B-cell lymphoma (Tomita et al., 2007).

The clinicopathological features of ALCL depend on the presence of anaplastic large cell lymphoma kinase (ALK). ALK-positive ALCL typicallys arise in 20-30-year-old patients, and mainly in males (Suzuki et al., 2000). The presentation can be both nodal and extranodal, involving the skin, bones, soft tissues, lungs, and liver. On the other hand, ALK-negative ALCL occurs primarily in elderly patients, and its presentation is usually nodal. The prognosis of ALCL is clearly divided into two groups by ALK expression, with the ALK-positive ALCL patients having a better prognosis than the ALK-negative patients (Suzuki et al., 2000).

AITL occurs in elderly patients, who are often initially described as having an atypical reactive process with generalized lymphoadenopathy, skin rash, hepatosplenomegaly, fever and hypergammaglobulinemia. The prognosis of AITL is poor and comparable to that of PTCL-NOS, and many patients will die of infectious complications that may be the result of underlying immunodeficiency (Armitage et al., 1998).

Other uncommon T-cell lymphomas include enteropathy-associated T-cell lymphoma (EATL), adult T-cell leukemia/lymphoma (ATLL), hepatosplenic T-cell lymphoma (10), and subcutaneous panniculitis-like T-cell lymphoma. EATL is associated with gluten-sensitive enteropathy and has a fatal clinical course. ATLL is caused by infection with HTLV-1, and this entity is also described in other sections in this issue.

3.2 Management of T-cell lymphomas

3.2.1 Initial assessment and staging of T-cell lymphomas

In the process of diagnosing T-cell lymphoma, the assessment of viral infection should be done as early as possible. The histological features and immunophenotype of ATLL are not specific among other T-cell lymphomas, and the detection of HTLV-1 is the only clue to the diagnosis of ATLL. The detection of EBV infection in the serum and lymphoma tissue is also important in T-cell lymphoma patients. In NK-cell lymphoma, the detection of EBV in tissues is an important diagnostic tool. When EBV is detectable in lymphoma or non-lymphoma cells, quantification of EBV DNA by quantitative PCR is a useful surrogate marker of the disease burden.

Radiological procedures including CT and MRI are critical methods used in the staging of T-cell lymphomas. In addition, [18F]-fluorodeoxyglucose (FDG) has recently been reported to be avid in T-cell lymphoma patients, and PET/CT might be a useful procedure for the initial assessment of T-cell lymphoma patients (Kako et al., 2007).

3.3 Treatment

3.3.1 Initial chemotherapy

In the past several decades, conventional anthracycline-based chemotherapy has been the mainstay for the treatment of lymphoma, including T-cell lymphoma. The large international group trial established that cyclophosphamide, doxorubicin, vincristine, and predonisone (CHOP) was equally effective and less toxic than intensive second and third generation chemotherapy for aggressive lymphoma (Fisher et al., 1993). CHOP or CHOP-type chemotherapy is now considered to be the standard treatment for peripheral T-cell lymphomas, including PTCL-NOS, AITL and ALCL. However, the results of treatment with a CHOP-like regimen for T-cell lymphoma is poor, with 5-year overall survival (OS) of 10-45% (Armitage et al., 1998; López-Guillermo et al., 1998). Due to the low incidence of T-cell lymphoma, the optimum treatment regimen for T-cell lymphoma has not been studied prospectively in randomized controlled trials, and no effective regimen other than CHOP has been established. Although ALK-positive ALCL patients have a good prognosis even when treated using the CHOP regimen (Suzuki et al., 2000), other PTCL patients will need more efficacious regimens.

Recently, modern dose-intense regimens have been investigated for aggressive lymphoma. A cyclophosphamide, doxorubicin, vincristine, dexamethasone (hyper CVAD) regimen was reported to be effective against Burkitt's lymphoma or mantle cell lymphoma, and a study of the hyper CVAD regimen for T-cell lymphoma patients showed a 3-year OS that was similar to that obtained using CHOP (49% and 43%)(Escalón et al., 2005). A French group showed that the cyclophosphamide, doxorubicin, vincristine, bleomycin, and prednisone (ACVBP) regimen was associated with a significant better 5-year OS than CHOP (46% vs 38%) in a randomized trial of patients with various types of aggressive lymphomas (Tilly et al., 2003). However, T-cell lymphoma patients accounted for only 15% of the cases evaluated in this study. Randomized trials will be necessary for more accurate assessment of the efficacy of this regimen for T-cell lymphoma.

3.3.2 Hematopoietic stem cell transplantation

Because of the generally poor outcome obtained with initial conventional chemotherapy, high-dose chemotherapy with autologous stem cell transplantation (ASCT) has been considered as a part of initial treatment for T-cell lymphoma. Numerous studies have shown favorable outcomes with low treatment-related mortality (TRM) (median OS was 50-70 months), particularly in advanced stage patients (Rodriguezet al., 2003 & 2007; Feyler et al., 2007). One study excluding ALK-positive ALCL patients, who are known to have a good prognosis with chemotherapy alone, showed that the median OS was 54 months, which was similar to the results of chemotherapy alone (Mounier et al., 2004). The trial conducted by the EBMT including 146 AILT patients reported that the median OS was 59 months, with low TRM (7%), indicating that ASCT should be considered as a useful treatment strategy for AITL patients (Kyriakou et al., 2008). Although most studies were retrospective and included ALK-positive ALCL patients, the favorable results and low toxicity indicated that ASCT is a promising strategy for PTCL patients. To clarify the patients who would benefit most from ASCT, further investigations in a prospective randomized setting are warranted.

Allogeneic HSCT is considered as a salvage treatment for relapsed or refractory patients. Corradini et al conducted a Phase 2 study of 17 relapsed or refractory patients, and showed that there was a good outcome, with 64% and 80% 1-year disease-free survival (DFS) and OS respectively. Of interest, several patients responded to donor lymphocyte infusion, suggesting that there was a graft-versus lymphoma effect (Corradini et al., 2004). Another author reported their retrospective experience with seventy-seven PTCL patients who received an allogeneic HSCT. This study showed that the 5-year OS and event-free survival

(EFS) rates were 57% and 53%, respectively, in almost non-complete response (CR) patients (Le Gouill et al., 2008). However the 1-year TRM was 32% in patients treated using a myeloablative conditioning regimen, indicating that further prospective trials, including reduced induction stem cell transplantation, will be necessary.

3.3.3 Novel therapeutic agents

Several new agents, including molecular targeting drugs, have been studied. Gemcitabine has been investigated in several combination chemotherapy regimens. When gemcitabine was combined with etoposide and CHOP for the treatment of 26 patients with T-cell lymphoma, favorable results were demonstrated, including an overall response rate of 77%, with 62% achieving a CR. However, 54% of patients experienced severe neutropenia, and the EFS was only 7 months (O'Connor, 2010).

Alemtuzumab is a humanized monoclonal antibody against CD52, which is expressed on both T cells and B cells. In 24 patients with T-cell lymphomas, alemtuzumab plus CHOP treatment resulted in a CR in 71% of patients, and a 1-year OS of 70%, and 2-year OS of 53%. However, severe infective complications, such as invasive aspergillosis and cytomegalovirus disease, were often observed (Gallamini et al., 2007).

Romidepin was the first histone deacetylase inhibitor (HDACi) to show efficacy in patients with PTCL or cutaneous T-cell lymphoma (CTCL). In a report of four patients treated in a phase 1 study, one patient with PTCL-NOS had a CR, and prompted a subsequent phase 2 study to assess its efficacy in patients with CTCL (Sandor et al., 2002). These two trials resulted in the FDA approval of the agent for patients with CTCL. Romideptin was also studied in patients with PTCL in a multicenter study; leading to an overall response rate of 33%, with a CR rate of 11% (Piekarz et al., 2009). On the basis of these results, a confirmatory international study of romideptin in PTCL patients is ongoing.

In conclusion, T-cell lymphoma is a distinct subtype of lymphoma, based on its unique epidemiology and clinical behavior. However, the optimal treatment strategy is undefined, and a prognostic model remains unclear due to the rarity of this entity. PTCL, the most common T-cell lymphoma, has a poor prognosis when patients are treated with conventional chemotherapy, and a large scale study is needed to establish more effective chemotherapy regimens, including HSCT. Novel targeted agents have been and are currently being examined for efficacy against the disease and to decrease the toxicity for the patients, and an improved understanding of the biology of PTCLs may give rise to new treatment options.

4. Leukemogenesis/lymphomagenesis and the progression of adult T-cell leukemia-lymphoma -The clinical aspects-

4.1 Epidemiology, etiology, and leukemogenesis

Adult T-cell leukemia-lymphoma (ATLL) is a mature T-cell malignancy, caused by human T-cell leukemia virus type-I (HTLV-1)(Poiesz *et al.*, 1980), and is characterized by lymphadenopathy, hepatosplenomegaly, skin lesions, the appearance of abnormal lymphocytes with convoluted or lobulated nuclei in the peripheral blood (PB) and specific geographic distributions (Uchiyama *et al.*, 1977). ATLL cells are often resistant to conventional chemotherapeutic agents associated with the expression of P-glycoprotein (Kuwazuru *et al.*, 1990) or functional lung resistance-related protein (Ohno *et al.*, 2001), and

ATLL patients often present with opportunistic infections (Shimoyama *et al.*, 1991). At present, the therapeutic outcomes of patients with acute or lymphoma type ATLL are still very poor.

It is estimated that over one million peoples infected by HTLV-1 live in Japan (Yamaguchi *et al.*, 2002) and that 15-20 million peoples are infected worldwide (Proietti *et al.*, 2005). Only a small percentage of HTLV-1 carriers develop ATLL at a median age of 67 in Japan, whose median age is older than those in other countries. The cumulative risk of ATLL development in HTLV-1 carriers from 30 to 79 years of age was estimated to be 2.1% for females and 6.6% for males (Arisawa *et al.*, 2000). Recently, the Joint Study on Predisposing Factors on ATLL Development (JSPFAD) Group performed a large scale cohort study between 2002 and 2008 for HTLV-1 carriers in order to clarify the risk factors for the development of ATLL. During this period, 14 cases out of 1,218 HTLV-1 carriers developed ATLL. This study revealed 4 major risk factors for the development of ATLL in HTLV-1 carriers using a multivariate analysis, i.e., high HTLV-1 proviral loads (in other words, an increase in HTLV-1 infected cells) in the PB, advanced age (over 40 years of age), the existence of a family history of ATLL, and detecting HTLV-1 antibody positivity during treatment for other diseases (Iwanaga *et al.*, 2010). Familial ATLL cases were reported by several researchers (Miyamoto *et al.*, 1985; Ratner *et al.*, 1990; Wilks *et al.*, 1993). Surprisingly, we experienced a family with accumulated familial ATLL, in which six of seven siblings (excluding one who died during World War II) developed acute type ATLL between 1978 and 1989 (Nomura *et al.*, 2006).

In HTLV-1 leukemogenesis, the HTLV-1 viral protein Tax activates nuclear factor-κB (NF-κB), represses p53, and is associated with various other protein-protein interactions (Yoshida, 2001). In particular, Tax plays an important role in the early phase of HTLV-1 leukemogenesis by immortalization of HTLV-1 infected T cells. On the other hand, cells expressing Tax are eradicated by the normal immune surveillance system by Tax- specific cytotoxic T lymphocytes (CTL). The accumulation of gene impairment finally results in leukemogenesis/lymphomagenesis of ATLL in HTLV-1 infected cells that escape from the CTL. However, ATLL cells frequently lack Tax expression or carry deletions in the Tax gene. Therefore, the Tax gene has been suggested to be non-essential for the proliferation of ATLL cells. On the other hand, HTLV-1 basic leucine zipper factor gene (HBZ) is expressed on the ATLL cells in all ATLL patients, and supports the proliferation of ATLL cells (Satou *et al.*, 2006). HBZ is now considered to be vital for the leukemogenesis and progression of ATLL.

Interestingly, there is a distinct mechanism of flower cell formation in ATLL cells which is a characteristic feature of the acute type ATLL demonstrated by Fukuda *et al* (2005). The multilobulated nuclear formation in ATLL cells is induced by overactivation of phosphatidylinositol 3-kinase signaling cascades resulting from disruption of phosphatidylinositol-3,4,5-triphosphate inositol phosphatases such as the phosphatase and tensin homolog deleted on chromosome 10 (PTEN) and Src homology 2 domain containing inositol polyphosphate phosphatase (SHIP). Moreover this aberrantly activated signaling pathway is suggested to have an essential role in the development of ATLL in patients.

Recently, it has been reported that ATLL cells are derived from regulatory T (Treg) cells or helper T cell type 2 (Th2) cells both of which express CD4 and CD25 on their cell surface. Because ATLL cells express CC chemokine receptor 4 (CCR4) which is expressed on both Treg and Th2 cells, and forkhead/winged helix transcription factor (FoxP3) which is expressed on Treg cells in most ATLL patients, ATLL cells are now thought to be mainly of Treg cell origin (Karube *et al.*, 2004).

4.2 Clinical features

The signs or symptoms frequently seen at the onset of ATLL include lymph node swelling, hepatosplenomegaly and skin lesions. ATLL patients also often suffer from abdominal symptoms such as abdominal pain or refractory diarrhea due to infiltration of ATLL cells into the gastrointestinal (GI) tract (Utsunomiya *et al.*, 1988), and headache or disturbance of consciousness due to infiltration of ATLL cells into the central nervous systems (CNS). In addition, cough or dyspnea due to pleural effusion or lung infiltration of ATLL cells, abdominal distension due to lymph node swelling in the abdominal cavity, hepatosplenomegaly and/or ascites often distress ATLL patients. General fatigue, muscle weakness, constipation, and disturbance of consciousness are also seen, and are caused by the hypercalcemia associated with ATLL.

Opportunistic infections are common in ATLL patients due to impairment of cellular immunity. In particular, fungal (cutaneous, pulmonary, oral, esophageal and meningeal) and protozoal (*Pneumocystis carinii, Strongyloides stercoralis*) infections are often seen at diagnosis, mainly in the acute or chronic, rather than the lymphoma type, of ATLL (Shimoyama *et al.*, 1991).

4.3 Hematological and laboratory features

Leukocytes often increase from moderate to marked levels in leukemic type ATLL, while anemia and thrombocytopenia are rarely seen or mild, if they occur at all. Increases in the serum level of lactate dehydrogenase (LDH), serum calcium and soluble interleukin-2 receptor (sIL-2R) are frequently observed. Neutrophilia and/or eosinophilia are also observed due to the increased level of cytokines produced by the ATLL cells. Eosinophilia is a poor prognostic factor in ATLL patients (Utsunomiya *et al.*, 2007). Hypercalcemia occurs more frequently in patients with aggressive ATLL, not only at the onset but also at relapse or upon transformation from an indolent to aggressive form. The mechanism underlying hypercalcemia is thought to be associated with the expression of parathyroid hormone-related peptides (PTHrP) (Watanabe *et al.*, 1990) or tumor necrosis factor-β (TNF-β) (Ishibashi *et al.*, 1991). In addition, over expression of receptor activator of nuclear factor-κB ligand (RANKL) on ATLL cells was found to correlate with hypercalcemia in ATLL patients (Nosaka *et al.*, 2002). The tumor suppressor lung cancer 1 (TSLC1) gene was initially identified as a novel cell surface marker for ATLL. Afterward the expression of TSLC1 was found to be associated with tumor growth and organ infiltration of ATLL cells (Dewan *et al.*, 2008).

4.4 Diagnosis and classification

ATLL is diagnosed as peripheral T-cell leukemia or lymphoma by cytology and the surface phenotype of tumor cells, and/or pathology combined with immunohistochemical findings. Positivity for anti-HTLV-1 antibodies in the sera is mandatory for a diagnosis of ATLL. Most ATLL cells have a CD4+CD8- surface phenotype, and other unusual phenotypes such as CD4+CD8+, CD4-CD8+, CD4-CD8- are seen in about 20% of ATLL patients. The patients with these unusual phenotypes have a poorer prognosis than the patients with the typical phenotype (Kamihira, *et al.*, 1992). ATLL cells also express CD25, CCR4 and FoxP3. Histologically, the lymph nodes are occupied by diffuse proliferation of lymphoma cells with resultant destruction of the lymph node structure. Extranodal lesions such as those in the GI tract, skin or lungs should be diagnosed by histological examination. In addition to the presence of HTLV-1 antibodies in the sera, the detection of monoclonal integration of HTLV-1 proviral DNA in leukemia cells or tumor cells is necessary for a definite diagnosis of ATLL.

After the diagnosis of ATLL, subclassification of ATLL should be performed to determine the optimal therapeutic regimen. ATLL is divided into four clinical subtypes; the acute, lymphoma, chronic and smoldering types, according to the percentage of ATLL cells in the PB, the involvement of the CNS, bone, peritoneum, pleura and GI tract, and whether there are increases in the serum LDH and calcium (Table 1) (Shimoyama *et al*, 1991). An increase in the serum LDH and blood urea nitrogen, and a decrease in the serum albumin level are poor prognostic factors in patients with chronic type ATLL, so patients who have at least one of these poor prognostic factors have been considered to belong to the unfavorable subgroup (Shimoyama, 1994). The acute, lymphoma and chronic types with at least one of poor prognostic factors are considered to be aggressive ATLL, while chronic type, without any poor prognostic factors, and the smoldering types are called indolent ATLL.

	Smoldering	Chronic	Lymphoma	Acute
Anti-HTLV-1 antibody	+	+	+	+
Lymphocyte (×10⁹/l)	<4	≧4*3	<4	*
Abnormal T-lymphocytes	≧5%	+*4	≦1%	+*4
Flower cells of T cell marker	Occasionally	Occasionally	-	+
LDH	≦1.5N	≦2N	*	*
Corrected Ca (mEq/l)	<5.5	<5.5	*	*
Histology-proven lymphadenopathy	-	*	+	*
Tumor lesion				
Skin	*2	*	*	*
Lung	*2	*	*	*
Lymph node	-	*	+	*
Liver	-	*	*	*
Spleen	-	*	*	*
CNS	-	-	*	*
Bone	-	-	*	*
Ascites	-	-	*	*
Pleural effusion	-	-	*	*
GI tract	-	-	*	*

Table 1. Diagnostic criteria for clinical subtype of ATLL

N: normal upper limit, CNS: central nervous system, GI tract: gastrointestinal tract.

* : No essential qualification except terms required for other subtype(s).

*2: No essential qualification if other terms are fulfilled, but histology-proven malignant lesion(s) is required in case abnormal T-lymphocytes are less than 5% in peripheral blood.

*3: Accompanied by T-lymphocytosis (3.5×10^9/l or more).

*4: In case abnormal T-lymphocytes are less than 5% in peripheral blood, histology-proven tumor lesion is required.

A specific subtype of ATLL whose main lesions are limited to the skin, and does not have marked leukemic cells (<5%), a serum LDH level without exceeding 1.5-fold the normal upper limit, and a serum calcium level in the normal range was proposed as cutaneous type ATLL. The percentage of abnormal T-lymphocytes in the PB of such patients is less than 5% (Amano *et al.*, 2008).

4.5 Progression/acute transformation

Indolent ATLL often progresses into acute type ATLL during the long period of the natural course of the disease. The rapid growth of lymph nodes, hepatosplenomegaly, and/or marked skin manifestations suddenly occur in previously indolent ATLL, often accompanied by marked leukocytosis, an increase in the serum LDH, sIL-2R and/or hypercalcemia. In particular, the sIL-2R level has been considered to be an indicator of disease progression and prognosis (Kamihira *et al.*, 1994). Multi-step aberrant CpG island hyper-methylation was detected in ATLL patients, which was associated with the progression and transformation (crisis) of ATLL (Sato *et al.*, 2010). Clonal evolution of ATLL cells often occurs at the time of acute transformation in ATLL patients.

4.6 Spontaneous regression

Few ATLL patients show spontaneous regression of tumors (Shimamoto *et al.*, 1993). We experienced two chronic type ATLL patients, both of whom had a poor prognostic factor (increased serum LDH), who obtained a complete remission (CR) without any therapeutic intervention. In one patient, the systemic lymphadenopathy and ATLL cells in the PB disappeared, and the serum LDH level was normalized after surgical excision of an inguinal lymph node. However, he suffered from bone pain due to multiple bone lesions infiltrated by ATLL cells about 10 months after the CR. In another patient, the leukocytes and abnormal lymphocytes in the PB, and the serum LDH level gradually decreased to normal range. The ATLL cells in her PB had disappeared completely about 6 years after the diagnosis of ATLL without any therapy. She is now in an HTLV-1 carrier state, and has been free from ATLL for about 7 years after the complete disappearance of the ATLL cells in her PB. Although the mechanisms of spontaneous regression of ATLL have not been elucidated, it is suggested that the cytotoxic activity of peripheral mononuclear cells or the apoptosis of ATLL cells are associated with this phenomenon (Jinnohara *et al.*, 1997; Matsushita *et al.*, 1999). Clarification of this interesting phenomenon might be useful for the development of new immunological therapy for ATLL patients.

4.7 Therapy

Treatment for patients with ATLL differs according to the clinical subtypes. It therefore is very important to make an accurate diagnosis of the clinical subtype of ATLL in order to ensure that the appropriate therapy is selected. In patients with indolent ATLL including those with the smoldering type or the chronic type without any unfavorable prognostic factors, watchful waiting is the standard of care in Japan except when the patients are suffering from symptomatic skin lesions.

Generally, intensive combination chemotherapy for aggressive ATLL has been performed immediately after the diagnosis because the prognoses of aggressive ATLL are poorer than those of other non-Hodgkin's lymphomas (NHL) free from HTLV-1 infection (Shimoyama *et al.*, 1988). The results of chemotherapy in studies performed by the Japan Clinical Oncology Group-Lymphoma Study Group (JCOG-LSG) from the 1980's to early 1990's were unsatisfactory for ATLL. The CR rate was 17-42%, and the median OS time was 5-13 months, and the OS rate at 3 years was only 13-24% (Uozumi, 2010). Recently, Tsukasaki *et al* (2007) reported the results of a randomized phase III trial for aggressive ATLL. They revealed that the CR rate was higher in the patients treated with sequential combination chemotherapy consisting of VCAP (vincristine, cyclophosphamide, doxorubicin, and prednisone), AMP (doxorubicin, ranimustine, and prednisone), and VECP (vindesine, etpoposide, carboplatin, and prednisone) (mLSG15) than in those treated with biweekly CHOP (vincristine, cyclophosphamide, doxorubicin, and prednisone: bi-CHOP) (40% vs

25%, respectively). Furthermore, the OS rate at 3 years was higher in the mLSG15 arm than in the bi-CHOP arm (24% vs 13%, respectively) (Tsukasaki *et al.*, 2007).
On the other hand, Bazarbachi *et al* (2010) reported that excellent results were obtained using combination therapy with zidovudine (AZT) and interferon-α (IFN) for ATLL patients. The OS rate at 5 years was 46% for their 75 patients who received first-line antiviral therapy. In particular, the OS rate at 5 years for patients with the chronic and smoldering types of ATLL was 100%. However, the results for aggressive type ATLL obtained using AZT/IFN therapy were inferior to those obtained during the JCOG-LSG study (JCOG9303, JCOG9801)(Yamada *et al.*, 2001; Tsukasaki *et al.*, 2007). Nevertheless, as the results of chemotherapy for aggressive ATLL are unsatisfactory, new strategies using approaches other than conventional chemotherapy are needed for ATLL to improve the survival of the patients.
We previously reported that allogeneic hematopoietic stem cell transplantation (allo-HSCT) was useful for aggressive ATLL (Utsunomiya *et al.*, 2001). Following our report, many other researchers reported the possibility of long-term survival in ATLL patients who received allo-HSCT using conventional or reduced intensity conditioning (Fukushima *et al.*, 2005; Okamura *et al.*, 2005; Shiratori *et al.*, 2008; Hishizawa *et al.*, 2010). A graft-versus-Tax (Gv-Tax) response in ATLL patients after allo-HSCT was demonstrated by Harashima *et al* (2004). The Gv-Tax response, which has been suggested to induce a graft versus-ATLL (Gv-ATLL) effect may bring about the eradication of not only ATLL cells but also of HTLV-1 infected cells in general (Okamura *et al.*, 2005; Yonekura *et al.*, 2008).
New agents, especially an anti-CCR4 antibody (KW-0761) are promising for ATLL therapy. Recently, promising results for relapsed ATLL patients who had been treated by intravenous administration of KW-0761 indicated that the overall response rate was 31% in a phase I study (Yamamoto *et al.*, 2010) and 50% in a phase II study (Ishida *et al.*, 2010). Other novel agents, such as lenalidomide (a thalidomide analogue) and bortezomib, which inhibits proteasome and thereby inhibits activation of NF-κB, are now being evaluated in clinical trials for relapsed ATLL in Japan. In addition, immunotherapy using dendric cells stimulated by Tax peptides is now being prepared for ATLL patients who had previously obtained remission by chemotherapy.
In conclusion, ATLL presents diverse features, and the mechanisms of leukemogenesis induced by HTLV-1 development and the progression of ATLL have not been well elucidated. Clarification of these mechanisms will therefore give ATLL patients a chance to obtain a cure. Furthermore, our final goals are not only to cure ATLL patients, but also to completely eradicate HTLV-1 by preventing HTLV-1 infection or by eradicating infections once they are established.

5. Epigenetics of leukemia and lymphoma

5.1 Modulation of the expression profile in the immune system through epigenetic mechanism

Epigenetic mechanisms control the development and differentiation, and maintain the normal physiological status in mammalian cells, and epigenetic events link a subjects' genotype to their phenotype. Epigenetic regulatory mechanisms are a central system to control the differentiation and function of the immune system and to ensure an appropriate gene expression profile in immune cells (Natoli G, 2010). This mechanism changes the gene expression profile, permitting cells to adapt to multiple environmental pressures. Pathogenic factors may be considered such an environmental pressure (Arens & Schoenberger; 2010). Consequently, cellular differentiation and adaptation might be considered as an epigenetic phenomenon. Many of the recent epigenetic investigations have focused on DNA methylation, histone modifications and chromatin remodeling. Non-coding RNAs, such miRNAs, also play important roles in epigenetic pathways (Thai et al. 2010).

5.2 Epigenetic abnormalities in leukemia and lymphoma

Lymphoma and leukemia, as well as other cancers, have been thought to be predominantly induced by acquired genetic changes such as mutations, deletions, and amplifications of genes and chromosome translocations. However, it is now becoming clear that microenvironment-mediated epigenetic alterations also play important roles. Although many genetic changes have been reported, it is difficult to discriminate cause from consequence. It is also unclear whether genetic or epigenetic changes occur first. Recent data suggest that cancer has a fundamentally common basis that is grounded in a polyclonal epigenetic disruption of stem/progenitor cells, mediated by 'tumor-progenitor genes'. Furthermore, tumor cell heterogeneity is due, in part, to epigenetic variation in progenitor cells, and epigenetic plasticity, together with genetic lesions, drives tumor progression (Feinburg et al, 2006). The epigenetic disruption of key genes is supposed to occur at the earliest stage of cancer development. Some of the most convincing evidence for epigenetic disruption of progenitor cells derives from the ubiquitous nature of genome-wide hypomethylation, which is present in almost of all malignant tumors. In addition, gene-silencing induced by hypermethylation of genes involved in DNA repair (MGMT, hMLH1), cell cycle progression (p16INK4a, p15INK4b, p14ARF), signal transducing molecules (SHP1), apoptosis (DAPK) and cell adhesion (CHD1, HCAD) (Flanagan, 2007) is also common. Therefore, non-neoplastic, but epigenetically disrupted, stem/progenitor cells might be a crucial target for cancer risk assessment and chemoprevention.

5.3 Frequent gene silencing of hematopoietic cell-specific protein tyrosine phosphatase (SHP1) in hemetopoietic cell malignancies

Genome-wide studies of gene expression on a genomic scale using cDNA microarrays make it easy to measure the transcription levels of almost every gene at once. Various types of leukemia/lymphoma have been analyzed using cDNA microarrays to investigate the molecular basis of leukemogenesis/ lymphomagenesis. From the cDNA microarray analyses of gene expression pattern of the human NK/T cell line (NK-YS), followed by comprehensive and systematic tissue microarrays, RT-PCR and Western blotting analysis, it has been demonstrated that strongly decreased expression of hematopoietic cell specific protein-tyrosine-phosphatase *SHP1* mRNA was present in malignant cells (Oka et al., 2001). A further analysis using standard immunohistochemistry and tissue microarrays, which utilized 207 paraffin-embedded specimens of various kinds of malignant lymphomas, showed that 100% of NK/T lymphomas and more than 95% of malignant leukemia/lymphoma patient specimens of DLBCL, follicular lymphoma (FL), Hodgkin's lymphoma (HL) (Hodgkin's disease (HD)), mantle cell lymphoma (MCL), peripheral T-cell lymphoma (PTCL), ATLL and plasmacytoma were negative for SHP1 protein expression.
The promoter region of the *SHP1* gene has been revealed to be highly methylated in patient samples of adult T cell leukemia (methylation frequency: 90%), natural killer (NK)/T cell

lymphoma (91%), diffuse large B-cell lymphoma (93%), MALT lymphoma (82%), mantle cell lymphoma (75%), plasmacytoma (100%) and follicular lymphoma (96%). The methylation frequency was significantly higher in high grade-MALT lymphoma cases (100%) than in low grade-MALT lymphoma cases (70%), correlating well with the frequency of the lack of SHP1 protein in high grade- (80%) and low grade-MALT lymphoma (54%) (Oka et al., 2002; Koyama et al., 2003). This suggests that the *SHP1* gene silencing with aberrant CpG methylation is related to the progression of lymphoma, in addition to the malignant transformation. Furthermore, the promoter methylation of the *SHP1* gene was clearly correlated with the clinical stage, such as complete remission or relapse. Loss of heterozygosity with microsatellite markers near the *SHP1* gene was shown in 79% of informative ALL cases. These findings indicate that the *SHP1* gene is a relevant novel biomarker of a wide range of hematopoietic malignancies. Additionally, these results suggest that loss of *SHP1* gene expression plays an important role in multistep lymphomagenesis/leukemogenesis.

SHP1 negatively regulates the Janus kinase/signal transducer and activator of transcription (Jak/STAT) signaling pathway (Chim et al., 2004a; Chim et al., 2004b). SHP1 in myeloma showed hypermethylation, with constitutive STAT3 phosphorylation. Demethylating reagent-treated myeloma samples showed restored SHP1 expression in accordance with down-regulation of phosphorylated STAT3 (Chim et al., 2004a). SHP1 methylation thus leading to the induction of epigenetic activation of the Jak/STAT pathway might play a key role in the pathogenesis of myeloma. Similarly, frequent methylation of SHP1 was observed in mantle cell and follicular lymphomas (Oka et al., 2001 & 2002; Chim et al., 2004c) and also in acute myeloid leukemia (Oka et al., 2001; Chim et al., 2004b). The hypermethylation of SHP1 led to the activation of the Jak/STAT signaling pathway, along with the upregulation of cyclin D1 and *BCL2,* and could be the basis for the lymomagenesis of follicular lymphoma (Koyama et al., 2003; Chim et al., 2004c).

6. Epigenetic alterations induced by infectious agents

6.1 Oncogenic infectious agents

Infectious agents, including viruses, bacteria and parasites, have been reported to be associated with various human malignancies (Oka et al., 2011). These include Epstein-Barr virus (EBV), human T lymphotropic virus type-I (HTLV-1), human T lymphotropic virus type-II (HTLV-2), hepatitis viruses (hepatitis B virus (HBV) and hepatitis C virus (HCV)), human papilloma virus (HPV), polyoma viruses (JC virus, BK virus, SV40) and Kaposi's sarcoma-associated herpesvirus/human herpesvirus-8 (KSHV/HHV-8). EBV is associated with Burkitt's lymphoma and diffuse large B-cell lymphoma (DLBCL), NK/T lymphoma, nasopharyngeal carcinoma and Hodgkin's disease (Lindstrom et al., 2002; Kwong et al., 2002; Bravender, 2010). HTLV-1 is associated with adult T-cell leukemia/lymphoma (ATLL) (Poiesz et al. 1980; Hinuma et al., 1981; Yoshida et al., 1982), HTLV-2 with hairy cell leukemia (Feuer et al., 2005; Kaplan, 1993; Hielle, 1991), HHV-8 with Kaposi's sarcoma and primary effusion lymphomas (Zhang et al., 2010; Du, 2007), HBV and HCV with hepatocellular carcinoma (HCC) (Miroux et al., 2010; Alavian et al., 2010), HPV with cervical carcinoma (Tota et al., 2010; Grce et al., 2010) and JCV with brain and colon cancer (Parkin, 2006; Selgrad et al.,2009). The bacterium *Helicobacter pylori,* a major contributor to gastric cancer and MALT lymphoma, and parasitic infections such as particular *Schistosoma hematobium,* a major cause of bladder cancer in Egypt, and liver flukes (Zur Hausen, 2009) are also associated with human cancers. The molecular mechanisms by which these infectious agents contribute to the carcinogenesis and lymphomagenesis are not always clear. However, some of the evidence discussed below suggests an important role for epigenetic changes and aberrant DNA methylation in the onset and progression of malignancies associated with infectious agents.

6.2 Epigenetic changes induced by virus infection

More than 20% of cancers have been causally linked to human pathogens (Zur Hausen, 2009). Why virus infection is sometimes controlled, and on the other occasions leads to the progression to malignant tumors is still mystery. However, recent evidence suggests that epigenetic changes induced by infection play a causative role. Oncogenic viruses have been revealed to increase DNA methylation activity and decrease histone acetylation activity (Flanagan, 2007). The latent membrane protein 1 (LMP-1), one of the virus proteins of EBV, has been shown to be an oncoprotein with transforming activity. LMP-1 activates DNMT1, DNMT3a and DNMT3b to initiate epigenetic alterations, followed by hypermethylation and gene silencing of the *E-cadherin* gene (Tsai et al., 2002). Human epithelial cells expressing LMP-1 have been shown to have higher invasive activity, in accordance with reduced expression of the *E-cadherin* gene (Kim et al., 2000). Integration-defective HIV-I was shown to increase DNMT1 expression, followed by increased methylation of CpG islands in the promoter region of the *p16^{INK4A}* and *IFN-gamma* genes to induce gene silencing (Fang et al., 2001; Mikovits et al., 1998). Overall increases in DNA methyltransferase activity in malignant cells compared with normal tissues is also common in non-virus-related cancers (Esteller, 2006)

The ability to alter histone modifications and chromatin structure is also common to many oncogenic viruses, including EBV, HPV, adenoviruses and HTLV-1. EBV nuclear antigens EBNA2 and EBNA 3c alter histone acetylation by interacting with p300/CBP, PCAF histone acetyltransferase (HAT) complexes or with histone deacetylase (HDAC), respectively (Wang et al., 2000; Knight et al., 2003). The HPV E6 oncoprotein binds and inhibits the histone acetyltransferase activity of the p300/CBP complex (Patel et al., 1999). The HTLV-1 Tax protein also interacts with the p300/CBP complex to mediate transcriptional repression (Kwok et al., 1996). Disruption or alteration of p300/CBP histone acetyltransferase activity is common to many oncogenic viruses, suggesting that it may be one of the critical early events in virus-induced tumorigenesis. Further evidence of the early involvement of p300/CBP in various non-viral cancers has also been observed, suggesting that abrogation or perturbation of the histone acetyltransferase activity of p300/CBP may be one of the critical early events in all malignant tumors (Flanagan, 2007).

6.3 Accumulation of epigenetic abnormalities during the development and progression of ATLL

ATLL is an aggressive malignant disease of CD4-positive T lymphocytes caused by infection with HTLV-1 (Poiesz et al., 1980; Hinuma et al., 1981). HTLV-1 causes ATLL in 3-5% of infected individuals after a long latent period of 40–60 years (Tajima et al., 1990). Such a long latent period suggests that a multi-step leukemogenic/lymphomagenic mechanism is involved in the development of ATLL, although the critical events in its progression have not been well characterized. The pathogenesis of HTLV-1 has been intensively investigated in terms of the viral regulatory proteins HTLV-1 Tax and Rex, which are supposed to play key roles in the HTLV-1 leukemogenesis/lymphomagenesis, as well as the HTLV-1 basic leucine zipper factor

(HBZ) (Matsuoka et al., 2003, 2007; Gaudray et al.2002). The mechanism responsible for the progression of ATLL have been investigated from various genetic aspects, including specific chromosome abnormalities (Okamoto et al., 1989; Oka et al.1992, 2006; Ariyama et al.1999; Fujimoto et al., 1999), changes in the characteristic HTLV-1 Tax, Rex and HBZ protein expression patterns (Oka et al., 1992; Selgrad et al., 2009) and aberrant expression of the *SHP1* (Oka et al., 2002, 2006), *P53* (Yamato et al., 1993; Tawara et al., 2006), *DRS* (Shimakage et al. 2007), and *ASY/Nogo* (Shimakage et al. 2006) genes, although the detailed mechanisms triggering the onset and progression of ATLL remains to be elucidated. Frequent epigenetic aberration of DNA hypermethylation associated with *SHP1* gene silencing has been identified in a wide range of hematopoietic malignancies (Oka et al., 2001, 2002; Koyama et al., 2003). Recently, the number of genes methylated CpG islands, including the *SHP1, P15, P16, P73, HCAD, DAPK,* and *MGMT* genes, has been reported to increase with disease progression, and aberrant hypermethylation in specific genes has been detected even in HTLV-1 carriers, and correlated with eventual progression to ATLL (Sato et al., 2010). CIMP was observed most frequently in the lymphoma type ATLL, and was also closely associated with the progression and crisis of ATLL. The high number of methylated genes, and the increased incidence of CIMP were shown to be unfavorable prognostic factors for ATLL (Sato et al., 2010) and correlated with a shorter overall survival as calculated by a Kaplan-Meyer analysis. These findings strongly suggest that the multi-step accumulation of aberrant CpG methylation in specific target genes and the presence of CIMP are deeply involved in the crisis, progression and prognosis of ATLL, and that CpG methylation and CIMP may provide new diagnostic and prognostic biomarkers for patients with this disease (Figure 2).

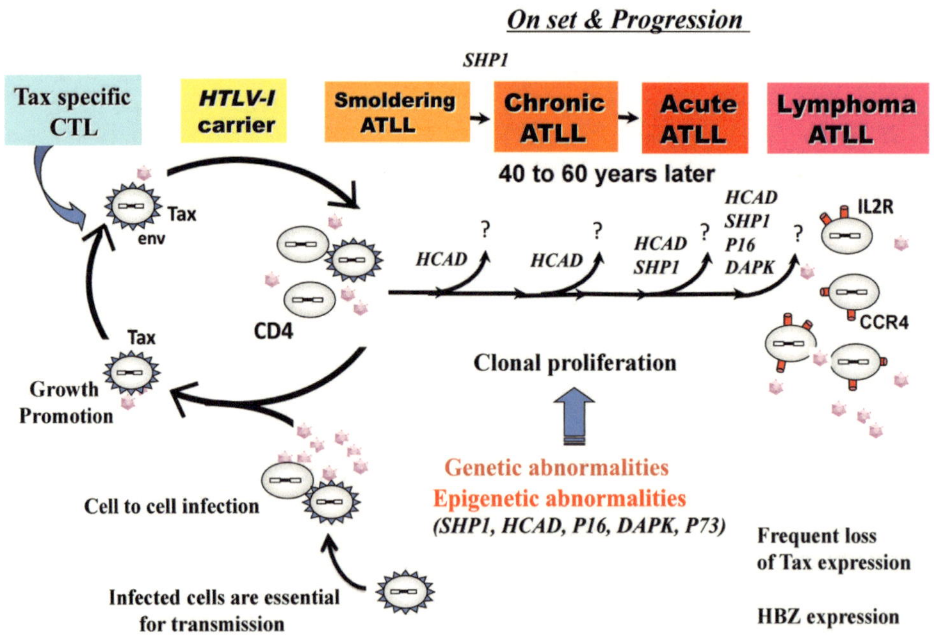

Fig. 2. Natural course from infection of human T lymphotropic virus type-I (HTLV-1) to onset and progression of adult T-cell leukemia/lymphoma (ATLL). Accumulation of genetic and epigenetic changes in host and virus genome during long latent period induce onset of ATLL.

It will be of interest to determine whether there is a direct link between HTLV-1 induction of DNMTs causing CIMP and hypermethylation of specific target genes, and how or what kind of viruses induce deregulation of the epigenetic machinery. Such discoveries may provide new insights into the understanding of the molecular mechanisms responsible for virus-induced lymphomagenesis and leukemogenesis.

The HTLV-1 Tax protein has been demonstrated to activate the nuclear factor-κB (NF-κB) and Akt pathways as major cellular pro-survival pathways (Yoshida, 2001). However, Tax transcripts are detected in only about 40% of transformed ATLL cells and are sometimes mutated. On the other hand, it has been demonstrated that the Hbz transcript is ubiquitously expressed in all ATLL cells, and possesses a pro-proliferative function in cells (Satou et al., 2006). It has therefore been proposed that Tax initiates transformation, while HBZ is required to maintain the transformed phenotype late in ATLL when Tax expression is extinguished (Matsuoka & Jeang, 2011). During malignant progression, tumor cells need to acquire novel characteristics that lead to uncontrolled growth and reduced immunogenicity. The loss of Tax expression *in vivo* could facilitate the escape of HTLV-1 infected cells from CTL-surveillance to induce disease progression. In the Bovine Leukemia Virus (BLV)-induced ovine (sheep) leukemia model, silencing of viral gene expression has been proposed as a mechanism leading to immune evasion (Merimi et at., 2007). They showed that there was a correlation between the complete suppression of provirus expression and tumor onset, providing experimental evidence that virus and Tax silencing are critical, if not mandatory, for the progression to overt malignancy. This suggests that epigenetic and/or genetic changes in the host genome induced by HTLV-1 infection are crucial for the onset and progression, independent of virus genome expression.

This raises questions about whether it might be possible to maintain the leukemic phenotype, on for cells to progress to ATLL without Tax expression. One possibility is that the genetic changes are associated with multipolar mitosis and aneuploidy. Aberrant centrosome replication is linked to oncogenesis, disregulating the intact spindle assembly checkpoint, accurate centrosome cycle and proper cytokinesis (Chi & Jeang, 2007). A second possibility is that there is aberrant expression of miRNAs (microRNAs) in ATLL leukemic cells, which occur independent of Tax expression. Yeung et al. reported that the tumor suppressor protein, TP53INP1, in HTLV-1 infected/transformed cells was targeted for repression by upregulated expression of miR-93 and miR-130b (Yeung et al., 2008). Pichler et al also reported that TP53INP1 was targeted in HTLV-1 infected/transformed cells by miR-21, -24, 146a and -155 (Pichler et al., 2008). Bellon et al described that ATLL cells show increased expression of miR155 (Bellon et al., 2009). These aberrant expression levels of onco-miR may disregulate downstream gene expression. A third possibility is that aberrant gene expression induced by epigenetic abnormalities, including aberrant DNA methylation, abnormal changes in histone modifications and dysregulation of chromatin remodeling, are maintained by daughter cells though epigenetic machinery.

6.4 Possible link to host-pathogen interaction

Experimental interspecies-transmission of BLV to sheep shows the shorter latency period preceding disease onset: leukemia occurs usually 1-4 years after infection in contrast to 4-10 years in cows. In addition, the incidence of virus-induced leukemia is much higher: almost all infected sheep will succumb within normal life time compared to only about 5% in cattle, suggesting that it is related to the lack of natural transmission of BLV to sheep (Florins et al.,

2008). In nature it is often observed that interspecies transmission of viruses results in a high incidence of disease in the new host. Genetic analyses of several human and simian T-cell leukemia virus type-I (HTLV-1/STLV-1) strains of African and Asian origin suggest recent interspecies transfer between species within primate genera, including humans. The phylogenetic analyses suggest that at least three independent human-simian exchanges have occurred during the evolution of these retroviruses (Dekaban et al., 1996). The incidence of ATLL within normal lifetime is about 5%, suggesting that HTLV-1 is in the process to establish a new relationship to human as a natural host. Elucidation of symbiotic evolution mechanisms may provides new insights to find out the strategy to reduce the virulence of HTLV-1 and suppress the onset of diseases.

7. Epigenetic therapy for leukemia/ lymphoma

Abnormalities of the epigenetic machinery have been associated with a broad range of diseases, including hematologic disorders and malignant leukemia/lymphoma. The malignancies have specific epigenetic profiles related to their histological type, and show many common phenotypes such as self-sufficiency of growth signals, resistance to anti-proliferative or pro-apoptotic signals, and so on. As previously reported, epigenetic markers can be used for various clinical applications, including for determing the risk of the onset and progression, for early detection, prediction of prognosis, and for predicting treatment outcomes and evaluating the response to treatment.

Moreover, there are already several systems with high sensitivity for detecting epigenetic profiles, such as the methylation-specific polymerase chain reaction (MSP) assay, which have been developed using leukemia/lymphoma samples (Oka et al., 2002; Sato et al., 2010). The epigenetic modifications are characterized by reversible reactions. On the basis of this point, inhibitors to reverse these modifications as therapeutic interventions have been developed and exploited, and good results have been reported for various malignant leukemias/lymphomas.

It is important to determine why T cell leukemia/lymphoma shows a worse prognosis than other disease, and to use this information to design a effective treatment. It is noteworthy that epigenetic therapy is now regarded as an innovative approach to the treatment of T cell leukemia/lymphoma (Piekarz et al., 2009a). In fact, treatment of tumor cells with epigenetic drugs can induce a range of antitumor effects, including apoptosis, cell cycle arrest, differentiation and senescence, modulation of immune responses, and angiogenesis (Bolden et al., 2006). The current drugs targeted for epigenetic mechanisms are categorized as either histone deacetylase (HDAC) inhibitors (HDACi) such as vorinostat, romidepsin and DNA methyltransferase (DNMT) inhibitors, such as 5-aza-2'-deoxycytidine (DAC) or 5-azacytidine (5-AC).

HDACi have diverse structures, and include sodium butyrate, vorinostat, MS-275, TSA, and FK228 (Prince et al., 2009). However, regardless of their structures, similarities have been observed with regard to their efficacy, and their timing- and dose-dependence, although some profiles on gene expression induced by HDACi seem to be agent-specific (Gray et al., 2004; Peart et al., 2005). Several HDACi have also been reported to predominantly improve the patient prognosis (Prince et al., 2009). However, the mechanism responsible for the marked efficacy of HDACi in T cell lymphoma is not yet understood, nor is there an understanding of the differences among the various HDACi. Piekarz et al. speculated that the responsive subset of T cell lymphomas has its origin in an as-yet unknown chromosomal rearrangement that recruits the class I HDACs to the promoter of a gene, and T cell lymphoma is therefore distinctly susceptible to different therapeutic interventions that affect HDACs (Piekarz et al., 2009b). In particular, Vorinostat (suberoylanilide hydroxamic acid, SAHA), which is a hydroxamic acid derivative that inhibits both class I and II HDACs, showed a good response for the treatment of relapsed and refractory cutaneous T-cell lymphoma (CTCL) (O'Connor et al., 2006; Mann et al., 2007; Duvic et al., 2007; Olsen et al., 2007; Garcia-Manero et al., 2008). Romidepsin (depsipeptide, FR901228, FK228, NSC 630176) is generally classified as a broad-spectrum inhibitor, as it inhibits class II enzymes. Romidepin was the first HDACi reported to show efficacy as monotherapy (complete or partial response) in patients with PTCL and CTCL (Piekarz et al., 2001). Favorable responses have been confirmed in CLL (Byrd et al., 2005; Dai et al., 2008; Inoue et al., 2009), CTCL (Piekarz et al., 2009b; Bates et al., 2010; Whittaker et al., 2010), and in additional PTCL patients (Bates et al., 2010; Piekarz et al., 2011). Panobinostat (LBH589) induces clinical responses in patients with refractory CTCL (Ellis et al., 2008). Peart et al. described that the specific attributes of each individual HDACi could be clarified, and that "matching" an individual HDACi to particular tumors or genetic profiles might help improve the clinical responses (Peart et al., 2003).

The two main analogs of DNMT inhibitors, such as DAC and 5-AC, are incorporated into DNA to trap and target DNMTs for degradation. The subsequent absence of these enzymes during DNA synthesis causes hypomethylation, and finally, reactivation of silenced gene expression in the daughter cells. The activated gene expression has effects on multiple pathways, contributing to a clinical response (Yoo et al., 2006). However, caution should be exercised, because the hypomethylation resulting from treatment these drugs can also likely activate oncogenes that are generally known to be silenced (e.g., *COX2, EGFR*, etc) (Toyota et al., 2005). Recent data show that hypomethylation by treatment with a single DAC is insufficient for the induction of gene expression (Si et al., 2010). Therefore, combination therapies using DNA demethylating agents with HDACi are well established. Indeed, HDACi enhance the activation of aberrantly methylated tumor suppressor gene promoters in tumor cells by DNA demethylating agents (Cameron et al., 1999; Steiner et al., 2005). These results suggest that potentiation of DAC-mediated gene induction by HDACi may be more complex than mere additive activities. However, the previous trials have mostly involved patients with AML and MDS (Silverman et al., 2009), not including those with T cell leukemia/lymphoma.

Approximately 30–40% cases of PTCL-NOS express CCR4+, and CCR4 expression is an unfavorable prognostic factor (Ohshima et al., 2004; Ishida et al., 2004). Additionally, PTCL originating from a CCR4+ Treg cell often shows a tendency to be "PTCL-NOS with genomic alterations" (Ishida et al., 2011). Tumor cells from most ATLL patients are characterized by the Treg phenotype (CD4+CD25+CCR4+FOXP3+) (Yoshie et al., 2002; Karube et al., 2008). Consequently, anti-CCR4 mAbs (KW-0761) have been developed, and have shown notable anti-tumor effects (Yamamoto et al., 2010; Ishii et al., 2010).

Interestingly, a recent investigation showed that the CCR4 expression on human $CD4^+$ T cells is regulated by histone H3 acetylation and methylation (Singh et al., 2010). In ATLL, it was noted that the indolent type is associated with a worse survival (mean survival time: 4.1 years) (Takasaki et al., 2010), and the proliferation of HTLV-1 infected cells seems to determine the viral burden during the carrier state (Matsuoka et al., 2011). These reports

suggest that early detection and treatment are essential for preventing transformation, or for decreasing the tumor burden in patients with the disease. Tax expression is regulated by the SUV39H1 histone methyltransferase (Kamoi et al., 2006) and HDAC1 (Ego et al., 2002), which negatively regulate the viral gene expression. These findings indicate that the presence of epigenetic abnormalities, including those that occur as a result of Tax regulation, play crucial roles in the pathogenesis of ATLL. A previous report showed that a histone deacetylase inhibitor, valproate, reduced the HTLV-1 proviral load in HAM/TSP through induction of tax gene expression and subsequent activation of CTLs (Lezin et al., 2007). However, it is important to note that the downstream effectors affected by these epigenetic agents have not been elucidated, although their primary enzymatic targets are known. In addition, it is necessary to confirm the optimal dosing schedule, potency, pharmacology, and longterm toxicity for each cell type.
Recent reports have evaluated additional combinations of HDACi with other agents, such as anthracyclines, in patients with AML and MDS (Zxu et al., 2010) and AMG 655 (anti-TRAIL receptor 2 antibody) in patients with various B cell lymphomas (National Cancer Institute (NCI), USA; http://www.cancer.gov). It appears that combination therapy using epigenetic agents with another therapy, such as immunotherapy, will make it possible to create an effective treatment strategy for intractable T cell leukemia/lymphoma. Additional larger studies of epigenetic therapy in subjects with intractable T cell leukemia/lymphoma are warranted.

8. Conclusions and perspective

Increased activity of DNA methyltransferases and decreases in p300/CBP-mediated histone acetylation are common in both virus-induced and non-viral malignancies, which suggests that epigenetic therapy would be effective for a wide range of malignancies. Aberrant DNA methylation has been shown to be the most consistent molecular changes present in many neoplasms. Hypermethylation of specific target genes, which can be detected at various stages and in different types of lymphomas and leukemias, can be detected with high sensitivity and accuracy. In the near future, we hope to be able to identify the specific signature of the methylation profile and biomarkers of hypermethylated genes for each specific type and stage of malignancy. Moreover, some epigenetic markers might be present prior to the development of lymphoma and leukemia. Thus, epigenetic markers may crucial for identifying the risk of leukemia/lymphoma development and also indicate the possibility of cancer prevention for such high-risk patients. Epigenetic changes, in contrast to genetic changes, can be easily reversed by the use of therapeutic interventions at various stages. The hypermethylated genes found in various cancers, in addition to leukemia/lymphoma, seem to be particularly sensitive to reactivation by demethylating reagents and HDACi. Therefore, restoration of multiple gene functions at the same time may be possible by therapeutic targeting of DNA methylation and histone acetylation. This could have profound implications for the diagnosis and treatment of malignancies.
The newer technologies that enable the global analyses of the epigenome are developing with remarkable speed, and include methods such as ChIP-on-chip (Chromatin ImmunoPrecipitation with microarray) and ChIP-sequencing, with deep sequencing by next generation sequencers for mapping global methylation and chromatin modifications, which will provide information about the landscape of infection-induced alterations, and about the

dynamic nature of microbe-host interactions and the human epigenome itself with regard to the various diseases. Such findings will greatly assist in improving human health.

9. Acknowledgements

The authors would like to acknowledge to John Wiley & Sons Ltd for kindly giving us a permission to reproduce Table I, which has been originally published in *Br J Haematol* (1991) 79, 428-437.

10. References

Abdelmohsen, K., Pullmann, R.Jr., Lal, A., Kim, H.H., Galban, S., Yang, X., Blethrow, J.D., Walker, M., Shubert, J., Gillespie, D.A., Furneaux, H. and Gorospe, M. (2007). Phosphorylation of HuR by Chk2 regulates SIRT1 expression. *Mol Cell* 25(4), 543-557.

Alavian, S.M., Behnava, B., Tabatabaei, S.V. (2010). Comparative efficacy and overall safety of different doses of consensus interferon for treatment of chronic HCV infection: a systematic review and meta-analysis. *Eur J Clin Pharmacol 66*, 1071-1079.

Amano, M., Kurokawa, M., Ogata, K., Itoh, H., Kataoka, H., and Setoyama, M. (2008). New entity, definition and diagnostic criteria of cutaneous adult T-cell leukemia/lymphoma: human T-lymphotropic virus type 1 proviral DNA load can distinguish between cutaneous and smoldering types. *J Dermatol* 35, 270-275.

Anderson, J. R., Armitage, J.O., and Weisenburger, D.D. (2002). Epidemiology of the non-Hodgkin's lymphomas: distributions of the major subtypes differ by geographic locations. *Non-Hodgkin's Lymphoma Classification Project* 9, 717-720.

Arens, R., and Schoenberger, S. P. (2010). Plasticity in programming of effector and memory CD8 T-cell formation. *Immunol Rev* 235(1),190-205.

Arisawa, K., Soda, M., Endo, S., Kurokawa, K., Katamine, S., Shimokawa, I., Koba, T., Takahashi, T., Saito, H., Doi, H., Shirahama, S. (2000). Evaluation of adult T-cell leukemia/lymphoma incidence and its impact on non-Hodgkin lymphoma incidence in southwestern Japan. *Int J Cancer* 85, 319-324.

Armitage, J.O., Greer, J.P., Levine, A.M., Weisenburger, D.D., Formenti, S.C., Bast, M., Conley, S., Pierson, J., Linder, J. and Cousar J.B. (1998). Peripheral T-cell lymphoma. *Cancer* 63, 158-163.

Ariyama, Y., Mori, T., Shinomiya, T., Sakabe, T., Fukuda, Y., Kanamaru, A., Yamada, Y., Isobe, M., Seto, M., Nakamura, Y., and Inazawa, J. (1999). Chromosomal imbalances in adult T-cell leukemia revealed by comparative genomic hybridization: gains at 14q32 and 2p16–22 in cell lines. *J Hum Genet 44*, 357–363.

Au, W.Y., Ma, S.Y., Chim, C.S., Choy, C., Loong, F., Lie, A. K., Lam, C.C., Leung, A.Y., Tse, E., Yau, C.C., Liang, R., and Kwong, Y.L. (2005). Clinicopathologic features and treatment outcome of mature T-cell and natural killer-cell lymphomas diagnosed according to the World Health Organization classification scheme: a single center experience of 10 years. *Ann of Oncol* 16, 206-214.

Bantignies, F., and Cavalli, G. (2006). Cellular memory and dynamic regulation of polycomb group proteins. *Curr Opin Cell Biol* 18, 275-283.

Bates, S.E., Zhan, Z., Steadman, K., Obrzut, T., Luchenko, V., Frye, R., Robey, RW., Turner, M., Gardner, E.R., Figg, W.D., Steinberg, S.M., Ling, A., Fojo, T., To, K.W. and

Piekarz, R.L. (2010). Laboratory correlates for a phase II trial of romidepsin in cutaneous and peripheral T-cell lymphoma. *Br J Haematol* 148(2), 256-267.

Bazarbachi, A., Plumelle, Y., Ramos, J. C., Tortevoye, P., Otrock, Z., Taylor, G., Gessain, A., Harrington, W., Panelatti, G., and Hermine, O. (2010). Meta-analysis on the use of zidovudine and interferon-alfa in adult T-cell leukemia/lymphoma showing improved survival in the leukemic subtypes. *J Clin Oncol* 28, 4177-4183.

Berger, S.L., Kouzarides, T., Shiekhattar, R., and Shilatifard, A. (2009). An operational definition of epigenetics. *Genes Dev* 23(7), 781-783.

Bird, A. (2007). DNA methylation patterns and epigenetic memory. *Genes Dev* 16, 6-21.

Bolden, J.E., Peart, M.J., and Johnstone, R.W. (*2006*). Anticancer activities of histone deacetylase inhibitors. *Nat Rev Drug Discov 5, 769*–784.

Bostick, M., Kim, J.K., Estève, P.O., Clark, A., Pradhan, S., and Jacobsen, S.E. (2007). UHRF1 plays a role in maintaining DNA methylation in mammalian cells. *Science* 317(5845), 1760-1764.

Bravender, T. (2010). Epstein-Barr virus, cytomegalovirus, and infectious mononucleosis. *Adolesc Med State Art Rev 21*, 251-264.

Byrd, J.C., Marcucci, G., Parthun, M.R., Xiao, J.J., Klisovic, R.B., Moran, M., Lin, T.S., Liu, S., Sklenar, AR., Davis, M.E., Lucas, D.M., Fischer, B., Shank, R., Tejaswi, S.L., Binkley, P., Wright, J., Chan, K.K., and Grever, M.R. (2005). A phase1and pharmacodynamic study of depsipeptide (FK228) in chronic lymphocytic leukemia and acutemyeloid leukemia. *Blood* 105, 959-967.

Cameron, E.E., Bachman, K.E., Myohanen, S., Herman, J.G., and Baylin, S.B. (1999). Synergy of demethylation and histone deacetylase inhibition in the re-expression of genes silenced in cancer. *Nat Gene,* 21, 103-107.

Cancer. gov [homepage on the Internet]. Bethesda (MD): National Cancer Institute, U.S. National Institutes of Health. Available from: http://www.cancer.gov.

Cernilogar, F.M., and Orlando, V. (2005). Epigenome programming by polycomb and trithorax proteins. *Biochem Cell Biol* 83, 322-331.

Chim, C. S., Fung, T. K., Cheung, W. C., Liang, R., and Kwong, Y. L. (2004a). SOCS1 and SHP1 hypermethylation in multiple myeloma: implications for epigenetic activation of the Jak/STAT pathway. *Blood* 103(12), 4630-4635.

Chim, C. S., Wong, A. S., and Kwong, Y. L. (2004b). Epigenetic dysregulation of the Jak/STAT pathway by frequent aberrant methylation of SHP1 but not SOCS1 in acute leukaemias. *Ann Hematol* 83(8), 527-532.

Chim, C. S., Wong, K. Y., Loong, F., Srivastava, G. (2004c). SOCS1 and SHP1 hypermethylation in mantle cell lymphoma and follicular lymphoma: implications for epigenetic activation of the Jak/STAT pathway. *Leukemia* 18(2), 356-358.

Corradini, P., Dodero, A., Zallio, F., Caracciolo, D., Casini, M., Bregni, M., Narni, F., Patriarca, F., Boccadoro, M., Benedetti, F., Rambaldi, A., Gianni, A. M., and Tarella, C. (2004). Graft-versus-lymphoma effect in relapsed peripheral T-cell non-Hodgkin's lymphomas after reduced-intensity conditioning followed by allogeneic transplantation of hematopoietic cells. *J Clin Oncol* 22, 2172-2176.

Costello, J.F., Fruhwald, M.C., Smiraglia, D.J., Rush, L.J., Robertson, G.P., Gao, X., Wright, F.A., Feramisco, J.D., Peltomaki, P., Lang, J.C., Schuller, D.E., Yu, L., Bloomfield, C.D., Caligiuri, M.A., Yates, A., Nishikawa, R., Su Huang, H., Petrelli, N.J., Zhang, X.,

O'Dorisio, M.S., Held, W.A., Cavenee, W.K., and Plass, C. (2000). Aberrant CpG-island methylation has non-random and tumour-typespecific patterns. *Nat Genet* 24, 132–138.

Csankovszki, G., Nagy, A., and Jaenisch, R. (2001). Synergism of Xist RNA, DNA methylation, and histone hypoacetylation in maintaining X chromosome inactivation. *J Cell Biol* 153, 773-784.

Cunliffe, V.T. (2003). Memmory by modification: the influence of chromatin structure on gene expression during vertebrate development. *Gene* 305, 141-150.

Dai, Y., Chen, S., Kramer, L.B., Funk, V.L., Dent, P., and Grant, S. (2008). Interactions between bortezomib and romidepsin and belinostat in chronic lymphocytic leukemia cells. *Clin Cancer Res* 14 (2), 549-558.

Dekaban, G., Coulthart, M., Franchini, G. (1996). Natural history of HTLVs/STLVs, In: *Human T-cell lymphotropic virus type I,* Edited by Hollsberg, P., and Hafler, D.A. pp11-32, John Wiley & Sons Ltd, UK. ISBN 0-471-96676-2.

Dewan, M. Z., Takamatsu, N., Hidaka, T., Hatakeyama, K., Nakahata, S., Fujisawa, J., Katano, H., Yamamoto, N., and Morishita, K. (2008). Critical role for TSLC1 expression in the growth and organ infiltration of adult T-cell leukemia cells in vivo. *J Virol* 82, 11958-11963.

Du, M.Q.; Bacon, C.M.; Isaacson. P.G. Kaposi sarcoma-associated herpesvirus/human herpesvirus 8 and lymphoproliferative disorders. *J. Clin. Pathol.* 2007, *60*, 1350-1357.

Duvic, M., Talpur, R., Ni, X., Zhang, C., Hazarika, P., Kelly, C., Chiao, J.H., Reilly, J.F., Ricker, J.L., Richon, V.M., and Frankel, S.R. (2007). Phase 2 trial of oral vorinostat (suberoylanilide hydroxamic acid, SAHA) for refractory cutaneous T-cell lymphoma (CTCL). *Blood* 109, 31- 39.

Ego, T., Ariumi, Y., and Shimotohno, K. (2002). The interaction of HTLV-1 Tax with HDAC1 negatively regulates the viral gene expression. *Oncogene* 21, 7241-7246.

Ellis, L., Pan, Y., Smyth, G.K., George, D.J, McCormack, C., Williams-Truax, R., Mita, M., Beck, J., Burris, H., Ryan. G., Atadja, P., Butterfoss, D., Dugan, M., Culver, K., Johnstone, R.W., and Prince, H.M. (2008). Histone deacetylase inhibitor panobinostat induces clinical responses with associated alterations in gene expression profiles in cutaneous T-cell lymphoma. *Clin Cancer Res* 14, 500 -510.

Escalón, M.P., Liu, N.S., Yang, Y., Hess, M., Walker, P.L., Smith, T.L., and Dang, N.H. (2005). Prognostic factors and treatment of patients with T-cell non-Hodgkin lymphoma: the M. D. Anderson Cancer Center experience. *Cance,* 103, 2091-2098.

Esteller, M. (2003). Relevance of DNA methylation in the management of cancer. *Lancet Oncol 4*, 351–358.

Esteller, M. (2005). Dormant hypermethylated tumour suppressor genes: questions and answers. *J Pathol* 205, 172–180.

Esteller, M. (2006). Epigenetics provides a new generation of oncogenes and tumour-suppressor genes. Br J Cancer 3094(2), 179-183.

Esteller, M., Corn, P.G., Baylin, S.B., and Herman, J.G. (2001). A gene hypermethylation profile of human cancer. *Cancer Res* 61, 3225–3229.

Fang, J.Y., Mikovits, J.A., Bagni, R., Petrow-Sadowski, C.L., and Ruscetti, F.W. (2001). Infection of Lymphoid Cells by Integration-Defective Human Immunodeficiency Virus Type 1 Increases De Novo Methylation. *J Virol 75*, 9753-9761.

Florins, A., Boxus, M., Vandermeers, F., Verlaeten, O., Bouzar, A. B., Defoiche, J., Hubaux, R., Burny, A., Kettmann, R., and Willems, L. (2008). Emphasis on cell turnover in two hosts infected by bovine leukemia virus: a rationale for host susceptibility to disease. *Vet Immunol Immunopathol* 125(1-2), 1-7.

Feinberg, A. P., Ohlsson, R., Henikoff, S. (2006). The epigenetic progenitor origin of human cancer. *Nat Rev Genet* 7(1), 21-33.

Feuer, G., and Green, P.L. (2005). Comparative biology of human T-cell lymphotropic virus type 1 (HTLV-1) and HTLV-2. *Oncogene 24*, 5996-6004.

Feyler, S., Prince, H.M., Pearce, R., Towlson, K., Nivison-Smith, I., Schey, S., Gibson, J., Patton, N., Bradstock, K., Marks, D.I., and Cook, G. (2007). The role of high-dose therapy and stem cell rescue in the management of T-cell malignant lymphomas: a BSBMT and ABMTRR study. *Bone Marrow Transplant* 40, 443-450.

Fisher, R.I., Gaynor, E.R., Dahlberg, S., Oken, M.M., Grogan, T.M., Mize, E.M., Glick, J.H., Coltman, C.A., and Jr, Miller, T.P. (1993). Comparison of a standard regimen (CHOP) with three intensive chemotherapy regimens for advanced non-Hodgkin's lymphoma. *N Engl J Med* 328, 1002-1006.

Flanagan, J. M. (2007). Host epigenetic modificationas by oncogenic viruses. *Br J Cancer* 96(2), 183-188.

Fujimoto, T., Hata, T., Itoyama, T., Nakamura, H., Tsukasaki, K., Yamada, Y., Ikeda, S., Sadamori, N., and Tomonaga, M. (1999). High rate of chromosomal abnormalities in HTLV-1-infected T-cell colonies derived from prodromal phase of adult T-cell leukemia: a study of IL-2-stimulated colony formation in methylcellulose. *Cancer Genet. Cytogenet 109*, 1–13.

Fuks, F., Hurd, P.J., Wolf, D., Nan, X., Bird, A.P., and Kouzarides, T. (2003). The methyl-CpG-binding protein MeCP2 links DNA methylation to histone methylation. *J Biol Chem* 278(6), 4035-4040.

Fukuda, R., Hayashi, A., Utsunomiya, A., Nukada, Y., Fukui, R., Itoh, K., Tezuka, K., Ohashi, K., Mizuno, K., Sakamoto, M., Hamanoue, M., and Tsuji, T. (2005). Alteration of phosphatidylinositol 3-kinase cascade in the multilobulated nuclear formation of adult T cell leukemia/lymphoma (ATLL). *Proc Natl Acad Sci USA* 102, 15213-15218.

Fukushima, T., Miyazaki, Y., Honda, S., Kawano, F., Moriuchi, Y., Masuda, M., Tanosaki, R., Utsunomiya, A., Uike, N., Yoshida, S., Okamura, J., and Tomonaga, M. (2005). Allogeneic hematopoietic stem cell transplantation provides sustained long-term survival for patients with adult T-cell leukemia/lymphoma. *Leukemia* 19, 829-834.

Gallamini, A., Zaja, F., Patti, C., Billio, A., Specchia, M. R., Tucci, A., Levis, A., Manna, A., Secondo, V., Rigacci, L., Pinto, A., Iannitto, E., Zoli, V., Torchio, P., Pileri, S., and Tarella, C. (2007). Alemtuzumab (Campath-1H) and CHOP chemotherapy as first-line treatment of peripheral T-cell lymphoma: results of a GITIL (Gruppo Italiano Terapie Innovative nei Linfomi) prospective multicenter trial. *Blood* 110, 2316-2123.

Garcia-Manero, G., Yang, H., Bueso-Ramos, C., Ferrajoli, A., Cortes, J., Wierda, W. G., Faderl, S., Koller, C., Morris, G., Rosner, G., Loboda, A., Fantin, V.R., Randolph, S.S., Hardwick, J.S., Reilly, J.F., Chen, C., Ricker, J. L., Secrist, J. P., Richon, V. M., Frankel, S. R., and Kantarjian, H. M. (2008). Phase 1 study of the histone deacetylase inhibitor vorinostat (suberoylanilide hydroxamic acid [SAHA]) in patients with advanced leukemias and myelodysplastic syndromes. *Blood* 111, 1060 -1066.

Gaudray, G., Gachon, F., Basbous, J., Biard-Piechaczyk, M., Devaux, C., and Mesnard, J.M. (2002). The complementary strand of the human T-cell leukemia virus type 1 RNA genome encodes a bZIP transcription factor that down-regulates viral transcription. *J Virol 76*, 12813-12822.

Gray, S.G., Qian, C.N., Furge, K., Guo, X., and Tehm B.T. (2004). Microarray profiling of the effects of histone deacetylase inhibitors on gene expression in cancer cell lines. *Int J Oncol* 24, 773-795.

Grce, M., Matovina, M., Milutin-Gasperov, N., and Sabol, I. (2010). Advances in cervical cancer control and future perspectives. *Coll Antropol 34*, 731-736.

Gunduz, E., Gunduz, M., Ouchida, M., Nagatsuka, H., Beder, L., Tsujigiwa, H., Fukushima, K., Nishizaki, K., Shimizu, K., and Nagai, N. (2005). Genetic and epigenetic alterations of BRG1 promote oral cancer development. *Int J Oncol* 26(1), 201-210.

Hang, C.T., Yang, J., Han, P., Cheng, H. L., Shang, C., Ashley, E., Zhou, B., and Chang, C.P. (2010). Chromatin regulation by Brg1 underlies heart muscle development and disease. *Nature* 466(7302), 62–67.

Hansen, K.H., Bracken, A.P., Pasini, D., Dietrich, N., Gehani, S.S., Monrad, A., Rappsilber, J., Lerdrup, M., and Helin, K. (2008). A model for transmission of the H3K27me3 epigenetic mark. *Nat Cell Biol* 10(11), 1291-1300.

Harashima, N., Kurihara, K., Utsunomiya, A., Tanosaki, R., Hanabuchi, S., Masuda, M., Ohashi, T., Fukui, F., Hasegawa, A., Masuda, T., Takaue, Y., Okamura, J., and Kannagi, M. (2004). Graft-*versus*-Tax response in adult T-cell leukemia patients after hematopoietic stem cell transplantation. *Cancer Res* 64, 391-399.

Harikrishnan, K.N., Chow, M.Z., Baker, E.K., Pal, S., Bassal, S., Brasacchio, D., Wang, L., Craig, J.M., Jones, P.L., Sif, S., and El-Osta, A. (2005). Brahma links the SWI/SNF chromatin-remodeling complex with MeCP2-dependent transcriptional silencing. *Nat Genet* 37(3), 254-264.

Hatta, Y., Yamada, Y., Tomonaga, M., Miyoshi, I., Said, J.W., and Koeffler, H.P. Detailed deletion mapping of the long arm of chromosome 6 in adult T-cell leukemia. *Blood 93*, 613–616.

Herman, J.G., and Baylin, S.B. (2003). Gene silencing in cancer in association with promoter hypermethylation. *N Engl J Med* 349, 2042–2054.

Hinuma, Y., Nagata, K., Hanaoka, M., Nakai, M., Matsumoto, T., Kinoshita, K., Shirakawa, S., and Miyoshi, I. Adult T-cell leukemia: antigen in an ATL cell line and detection of antibodies to the antigen in human sera. *Proc Natl Acad Sci USA 78*, 6476-6480.

Hishizawa, M., Kanda, J., Utsunomiya, A., Taniguchi, S., Eto, T., Moriuchi, Y., Tanosaki, R., Kawano, F., Miyazaki, Y., Nagafuji, K., Hara, M., Takanashi, M., Kai, S., Atsuta, Y., Suzuki, R., Kawase, T., Matsuo, K., Nagamura-Inoue, T., Kato, S., Sakamaki, H., Morishima, Y., Okamura, J., Ichinohe, T., and Uchiyama, T. (2010). Transplantation of allogeneic hematopoietic stem cells for adult T-cell leukemia: a nationwide retrospective study. *Blood* 116, 1369-1376.

Hjelle, B. (1991). Human T-cell leukemia/lymphoma viruses. Life cycle, pathogenicity, epidemiology, and diagnosis. *Arch Pathol Lab Med 115*, 440-450.

Holm, T.M., Jackson-Grusby, L., Brambrink, T., Yamada, Y., Rideout, W. M. 3rd., and Jaenisch, R. (2005). Global loss of imprinting leads to widespread tumorigenesis in adult mice. *Cancer Cell* 8(4), 275-285.

Inoue, S., Harper, N., Walewska, R., Dyer, M.J., a Cohen, G. (2009). M.Enhanced Fas-associated death domain recruitment by histone deacetylase inhibitors is critical for the sensitization of chronic lymphocytic leukemia cells to TRAIL-induced apoptosis. *Mol Cancer Ther* 8(11), 3088-3097.

Ishibashi, K., Ishitsuka, K., Chuman, Y., Otsuka, M., Kuwazuru, Y., Iwahashi, M., Utsunomiya, A., Hanada, S., Sakurami, T., and Arima, T. (1991). Tumor necrosis Factor-® in the serum of adult T-cell leukemia with hypercalcemia. *Blood* 77, 2451-2455.

Ishida, T., Inagaki, H., Utsunomiya, A., Takatsuka, Y., Komatsu, H., Iida, S., Takeuchi, G., Eimoto, T., Nakamura, S., and Ueda, R. (2004). CXCR3 and CCR4 expression in Tcell and NK-cell lymphomas with special reference to clinicopathological significance for peripheral T-cell lymphoma, unspecified. *Clin Cancer Res* 10, 5494–5500.

Ishida, T., Joh, T., Uike, N., Yamamoto, K., Utsunomiya, A., Yoshida, S., Saburi, Y., Miyamoto, T., Takemoto, S., Suzushima, H., Tsukasaki, K., Nosaka, K., Fujiwara, H., Ishitsuka, K., Inagaki, H., Ogura, M., Akinaga, S., Tomonaga, M., Tobinai, K., and Ueda, R. (2010). Multicenter phase II study of KW-0761, a defucosylated anti-CCR4 antibody, in relapsed patients with adult T-cell leukemia-lymphoma (ATL). American Society of Hematology Annual Meeting and Exposition, #285, December 6, Orlando, FL,

Ishida, T., and Ueda, R. (2011). Immunopathogenesis of lymphoma: focus on CCR4. *Cancer Sci* 102(1), 44-50.

Ishida, T., Utsunomiya, A., Iida, S., Inagaki, H., Takatsuka, Y., Kusumoto, S., Takeuchi, G., Shimizu, S., Ito, M., Komatsu, H., Wakita, A., Eimoto, T., Matsushima, K., and Ueda, R. (2003). Clinical significance of CCR4 expression in adult T-cell leukemia/lymphoma: its close association with skin involvement and unfavorable outcome. *Clin Cancer Res* 9, 3625-3634.

Ishii, T., Ishida, T., Utsunomiya, A., Inagaki, A., Yano, H., Komatsu, H., Iida, S., Imada, K., Uchiyama, T., Akinaga, S., Shitara, K., and Ueda. R. (2010). Defucosylated humanized anti-CCR4 monoclonal antibody KW-0761 as a novel immunotherapeutic agent for adult T-cell leukemia/lymphoma. *Clin Cancer Res* 16, 1520–1531.

Iwanaga, M., Watanabe, T., Utsunomiya, A., Okayama, A., Uchimaru, K., Koh, K., Ogata, M., Kikuchi, H., Sagara, Y., Uozumi, K., Mochizuki, M., Tsukasaki, K., Saburi, Y., Yamamura, M., Tanaka, J., Moriuchi, Y., Hino, S., Kamihira, S., Yamaguchi, K., for the Joint Study on Predisposing Factors of ATL Development investigators. (2010). Human T-cell leukemia virus type I (HTLV-1) proviral load and disease progression in asymptomatic HTLV-1 carriers: a nationwide prospective study in Japan. *Blood* 116, 1211-1219.

Jinnohara, T., Tsujisaki, M., Sasaki, S., Hinoda, Y., and Imai, K. (1997). Cytotoxic activity in a case of adult T-cell leukemia/ lymphoma with spontaneous regression. *Int J Hematol* 65, 293-298.

Jones, P.A., and Liang, G. (2009). Rethinking how DNA methylation patterns are maintained. *Nat Rev Genet* 10(11), 805-811.

Jones, P.A., and Takai, D. (2001). The role of DNA methylation in mammalian epigenetics. *Science* 293, 1068-1070.

Kako, S., Izutsu, K., Ota, Y., Minatani, Y., Sugaya, M., Momose, T., Ohtomo, K., Kanda, Y., Chiba, S., Motokura, T., and Kurokawa, M. (2007). FDG-PET in T-cell and NK-cell neoplasms. *Ann Oncol* 18, 1685-1690.

Kalebic, T. (2003). Epigenetic changes: potential therapeutic targets. *Ann NY Acad Sci 983,* 278–285.

Kamihira, S., Sohda, H., Atogami, S., Toriya, K., Yamada, Y., Tsukazaki, K., Momita, S., Ikeda, S., Kusano, M., Amagasaki, T., Kinoshita, K., and Tomonaga, M. (1992). Phenotypic diversity and prognosis of adult T-cell leukemia. *Leukemia Res* 16, 435-441.

Kamihira, S., Atogami, S., Sohda, H., Momita, S., Yamada, Y., and Tomonaga, M. (1994). Significance of soluble interleukin-2 receptor levels for evaluation of the progression of adult T-cell leukemia. *Cancer* 73, 2753-2758.

Kamoi, K., Yamamoto, K., Misawa, A., Miyake, A., Ishida, T., Tanaka, Y., Mochizuki, M., and Watanabe, T. (2006). SUV39H1 interacts with HTLV-1 Tax and abrogates Tax transactivation of HTLV-1 LTR. *Retrovirology* 13, 3-5.

Kaneda, M., Okano, M., Hata, K., Sado, T., Tsujimoto, N., Li, E., and Sasaki, H. (2004). Essential role for de novo DNA methylatransferase Dnmt3a in paternal and maternal imprinting. *Nature* 429, 900-903.

Kaplan, M. H. (1993). Human retroviruses and neoplastic disease. *Clin Infect Dis 2,* S400-S406.

Karube, K., Aoki, R., Sugita, Y., Yoshida, S., Nomura, Y., Shimizu, K., Kimura, Y., Hashikawa, K., Takeshita, M., Suzumiya, J., Utsunomiya, A., Kikuchi, M., and Ohshima, K. (2008). The relationship of FOXP3 expression and clinicopathological characteristics in adult T-cell leukemia/lymphoma. *Mod Pathol* 21(5), 617-625.

Karube, K., Ohshima, K., Tsuchia, T., Yamaguchi, T., Kawano, R., Suzumiya, J., Utsunomiya, A., Harada, M., Kikuchi, M. (2004). Expression of FoxP3, a key molecule in CD4+CD25+ regulatory T cells, in adult T-cell leukemia/lymphoma cells. *Br J Haematol* 126, 81-84.

Kim, K. R., Yoshizaki, T., Miyamori, H., Hasegawa, K., Horikawa, T., Furukawa, M., Harada, S., Seiki, M., and Sato, H. (2000). Transformation of Madin-Darby canine kidney (MDCK) epithelial cells by Epstein-Barr virus latent membrane protein 1 (LMP1) induces expression of Ets1 and invasive growth. *Oncogene 19,* 1764-1771.

Kimura, H., and Shiota, K. (2003). Methyl-CpG-binding protein, MeCP2, is a target molecule for maintenance DNA methyltransferase, Dnmt1. *J Biol Chem* 278(7), 4806-4812.

Kirmizis, A., Bartley, S. M., Kuzmichev, A., Margueron, R., Reinberg, D., Green, R., and Farnham, P. J. (2004). Silencing of human polycomb target genes is associated with methylation of histone H3 Lys 27. *Genes Dev* 18(13), 1592-1605.

Knight, J. S., Lan, K., Subramanian, C., and Robertson, E. S. (2003). Epstein-Barr virus nuclear antigen 3C recruits histone deacetylase activity and associates with the corepressors mSin3A and NCoR in human B-cell lines. *J Virol* 77(7), 4261-4272.

Kondo, T., Oka, T., Sato, H., Shinnou, Y., Washio, K., Takano, M., Morito, T., Takata, K., Ohara, N., Ouchida, M., Shimizu, K., Yoshino, T. (2009). Accumulation of aberrant CpG hypermethylation by *Helicobacter pylori* infection promotes development and progression of gastric MALT lymphoma. *Int J Oncol 35,* 547-557. 5

Kouzarides, T. (2007). Chromatin modifications and their function. *Cell* 128(4), 693-705.

Kuwazuru, Y., Hanada, S., Furukawa, T., Yoshimura, A., Sumizawa, T., Utsunomiya, A., Ishibashi, K., Saito, T., Uozumi, K., Maruyama, M., Ishizawa, M., Arima, T., and Akiyama, S. (1990). Expression of P-glycoprotein in adult T-cell leukemia cells. *Blood* 76, 2065-2071.

Kwok, R. P., Laurance, M. E., Lundblad, J. R., Goldman, P. S., Shih, H., Connor, L. M., Marriott, S. J., and Goodman, R. H. (1996). Control of cAMP-regulated enhancers by the viral transactivator Tax through CREB and the co-activator CBP. *Nature* 380(6575), 642-646.

Kwong, J., Lo, K.W., To, K.F., Teo, P.M., Johnson, P.J., and Huang, D.P. (2002). Promoter hypermethylation of multiple genes in nasopharyngeal carcinoma. *Clin Cancer Res 8*, 131-137.

Kyriakou, C., Canals, C., Goldstone, A., Caballero, D., Metzner, B., Kobbe, G., Kolb, H.J., Kienast, J., Reimer, P., Finke, J., Oberg, G., Hunter, A., Theorin, N., Sureda, A., and Schmitz, N., Outcome-Lymphoma Working Party of the European Group for Blood and Marrow Transplantation. (2008). High-dose therapy and autologous stem-cell transplantation in angioimmunoblastic lymphoma: complete remission at transplantation is the major determinant of Outcome-Lymphoma Working Party of the European Group for Blood and Marrow Transplantation. *J Clin Oncol* 26, 218-224.

Le Gouill, S., Milpied, N., Buzyn, A., De Latour, R.P., Vernant, J.P., Mohty, M., Moles, M.P., Bouabdallah, K., Bulabois, C.E., Dupuis, J., Rio, B., Gratecos, N., Yakoub-Agha, I., Attal, M., Tournilhac, O., Decaudin, D., Bourhis, J.H., Blaise, D., Volteau, C., and Michallet, M., Société Française de Greffe de Moëlle et de Thérapie Cellulaire.(2008). Graft-versus-lymphoma effect for aggressive T-cell lymphomas in adults: a study by the Société Francaise de Greffe de Moëlle et de Thérapie Cellulaire. *J Clin Oncol* 26, 2264-2271.

Lezin, A., Gillet, N., Olindo, S., Signate, A., Grandvaux, N., Verlaeten, O., Belrose, G., de Carvalho Bittencourt, M., Hiscott, J., Asquith, B., Burny, A., Smadja, D., Césaire, R., and Willems, L. (2007). Histone deacetylase mediated transcriptional activation reduces proviral loads in HTLV-1 associated myelopathy/tropical spastic paraparesis patients. *Blood* 110(10), 3722-3728.

Lindstrom, M. S., Wiman, K. G. (2002). Role of genetic and epigenetic changes in Burkitt lymphoma. *Semin Cancer Biol 12*, 381-387.

López-Guillermo, A., Cid, J., Salar, A., López, A., Montalbán, C., Castrillo, J. M., González, M., Ribera, J.M., Brunet, S., García-Conde, J., Fernández de Sevilla, A., Bosch, F., and Montserrat, E. (1998). Peripheral T-cell lymphomas : initial features, natural history, and prognostic factors in a series of 174 patients diagnosed according to the R.E.A.L. Classification. *Ann Oncol* 9, 849-855.

Maekita, T., Nakazawa, K., Mihara, M., Nakajima, T., Yanaoka, K., Iguchi, M., Arii, K., Kaneda, A., Tsukamoto, T., Tatematsu, M., Tamura, G., Saito, D., Sugimura, T., Ichinose, M., and Ushijima, T. (2006). High levels of aberrant DNA methylation in Helicobacter pylori-infected gastric mucosae and its possible association with gastric cancer risk, *Clin Cancer Res 12*, 989-995.

Mann, B. S., Johnson, J. R., He, K., Sridhara, R., Abraham, S., Booth, B. P., Verbois, L., Morse, D. E., Jee, J. M., Pope, S., Harapanhalli, R. S., Dagher, R., Farrell, A., Justice, R., and Pazdur, R. (2007).Vorinostat for treatment of cutaneous manifestations of advanced primary cutaneous T-cell lymphoma. *Clin Cancer Res* 13, 2318-2322.

Matsuoka, M. (2003). Human T-cell leukemia virus type I and adult T-cell leukemia. *Oncogene 22*, 5131-5140.

Matsuoka, M., and Jeang, K. T. (2007). Human T-cell leukemia virus type 1 (HTLV-1) infectivity and cellular transformation. *Nat Rev Cancer 7*, 270-280.

Matsuoka, M., and Jeang, K. T (2011). Human T-cell leukemia virus type 1 (HTLV-1) and leukemic transformation: viral infectivity, Tax, HBZ and therapy. *Oncogene* 30, 12, 1379-1389.

Matsushita, K., Arima, N., Fujiwara, H., Hidaka, S., Ohtsubo, H., Arimura, K., Kukita, T., Okamura, M., and Tei, C. (1999). Spontaneous regression associated with apoptosis in a patient with acute-type adult T-cell leukemia. *Am J Hematol* 61, 144-148.

Meissner, A., Mikkelsen, T. S., Gu, H., Wernig, M., Hanna, J., Sivachenko, A., Zhang, X., Bernstein, B. E., Nusbaum, C., Jaffe, D. B., Gnirke, A., Jaenisch, R., and Lander, E. S. (2008). Genome-scale DNA methylation maps of pluripotent and differentiated cells. *Nature* 454, 766-771.

Mikovits, J.A., Young, H. A., Vertino, P., Issa, J. P., Pitha, P. M., Turcoski-Corrales, S., Taub, D. D., Petrow, C. L., Baylin, S. B., and Ruscetti, F. W. (1998). Infection with human immunodeficiency virus type 1 upregulates DNA methyltransferase, resulting in de novo methylation of the gamma interferon (IFN-gamma) promoter and subsequent downregulation of IFN-gamma production. *Mol Cell Biol 18*, 5166-5177.

Miremadi, A., Oestergaard, M.Z., Pharoah, P.D., and Caldas, C. (2007). Cancer genetics of epigenetic genes. *Hum Mol Genet* 15, 28–49.

Miroux, C., Vausselin, T., and Delhem N. (2010). Regulatory T cells in HBV and HCV liver diseases: implication of regulatory T lymphocytes in the control of immune response. *Expect Opin Biol Ther 10*, 1563-1572.

Miyamoto, Y., Yamaguchi, K., Nishimura, H., Takatsuki, K., Motoori, T., Morimatsu, M., Yasaka, T., Ohya, I., Koga, T. (1985). Familial adult T-cell leukemia. *Cancer* 55, 181-185.

Morin, R. D., Johnson, N. A., Severson, T. M., Mungall, A. J., An, J., Goya, R., Paul, J. E., Boyle, M., Woolcock, B. W., Kuchenbauer, F., Yap, D., Humphries, R. K., Griffith, O. L., Shah, S., Zhu, H., Kimbara, M., Shashkin, P., Charlot, J. F., Tcherpakov, M., Corbett, R., Tam, A., Varhol, R., Smailus, D., Moksa, M., Zhao, Y., Delaney, A., Qian, H., Birol, I., Schein, J., Moore, R., Holt, R., Horsman, D. E., Connors, J. M., Jones, S., Aparicio, S., Hirst, M., Gascoyne, R. D., and Marra, M. A. (2010). Somatic mutations altering EZH2 (Tyr641) in follicular and diffuse large B-cell lymphomas of germinal-center origin. *Nat Gene.* 42(2), 181-185.

Mounier, N., Gisselbrecht, C., Brière, J., Haioun, C., Feugier, P., Offner, F., Recher, C., Stamatoullas, A., Morschhauser, F., Macro, M., Thieblemont, C., Sonet, A., Fabiani, B., Reyes, F., Groupe d'Etude des Lymphomes de l'Adulte. (2004). Prognostic factors in patients with aggressive non-Hodgkin's lymphoma treated by front-line autotransplantation after complete remission: a cohort study by the Groupe d'Etude des Lymphomes de l'Adulte. *J Clin Oncol* 22, 2826-2834.

Nakajima, T., Maekita, T., Oda, I., Gotoda, T., Yamamoto, S., Umemura, S., Ichinose, M., Sugimura, T., Ushijima, T., and Saito, D. (2006). Higher methylation levels in gastric mucosa significantly correlate with higher risk of gastric cancers. *Cancer Epidemiol Biomark Prev 15*, 2317-2321.

Natoli G. (2010). Maintaining cell identity through global control of genomic organization. *Immunity* 33(1), 12-24.

Nomura, K., Utsunomiya, A., Furushou, H., Tara, M., Hazeki, M., Tokunaga, M., Uozumi, K., Hanada, S., Yashiki, S., Tajima, K., Sonoda, S. (2006). A family predisposing to adult T-cell leukemia. *J Clin Exp Hematopathol* 46, 67-71.

Nosaka, K., Miyamoto, T., Sakai, T., Mitsuya, H., Suda, T., Matsuoka, M.. (2002). Mechanism of hypercalcemia in adult T-cell leukemia: overexpression of receptor activator of nuclear factor κB ligand on adult T-cell leukemia cells. *Blood* 99, 634-640.

O'Connor, O. A. (2010). Novel agents in development for peripheral T-cell lymphoma. *Semin Hematol* 47 Suppl 1, S11-14.

O'Connor, O. A., Heaney, M. L., Schwartz, L., Richardson, S., Willim, R., MacGregor-Cortelli, B., Curly, T., Moskowitz C., Portlock, C., Horwitz, S., Zelenetz, A.D., Frankel, S., Richon, V., Marks, P., and Kelly, W. K. (2006). Clinical experience with intravenous and oral formulations of the novel histone deacetylase inhibitor suberoylanilide hydroxamic acid in patients with advanced hematologic malignancies. *J Clin Oncol* 24, 166 -173.

Ohno, N., Tani, A., Uozumi, K., Hanada, S., Furukawa, T., Akiba, S., Sumizawa, T., Utsunomiya, A., Arima, T., and Akiyama, S. (2001). Expression of functional lung resistance-related protein predicts poor outcome in adult T-cell leukemia. *Blood* 98, 1160-1165.

Ohshima, K., Karube, K., Kawano, R., Tsuchiya, T., Suefuji, H., Yamaguchi, T., Suzumiya, J., and Kikuchii, M. (2004). Classification of distinct subtypes of peripheral T-cell lymphoma unspecified identified by chemokine and chemokine receptor expression: analysis of prognosis. *Int J Oncol* 25, 605–613.

Oka, T., Ouchida, M., Koyama, M., Ogama, Y., Takada, S., Nakatani, Y., Tanaka, T., Yoshino, T., Hayashi, K., Ohara, N., Kondo, E., Takahashi, K., Tsuchiyama, J., Tanimoto, M., Shimizu, K., and Akagi, T. (2002). Gene silencing of the tyrosine phosphatase SHP1 gene by aberrant methylation in leukemias/lymphomas. *Cancer Res 62*, 6390–6394.

Oka, T., Ouchida, M., Tanimoto, M., Shimizu, K., and Yoshino, T. (2006). High frequent gene silencing of hematopoietic cell specific protein tyrosine phosphatase SHP1 in hematopoietic cell malignancies. *Gene Silencing: New Research*; Redberry, G.W., Ed.; Nova Science: New York, NY, USA, pp. 1–34.

Oka, T., Sato, H., Ouchida, M., Utsunomiya A and Yoshino T. (2011). Cumulative Epigenetic Abnormalities in Host Genes with Viral and Microbial Infection during Initiation and Progression of Malignant Lymphoma/Leukemia. *Cancers* 3, 568-581

Oka, T., Sonobe, H., Iwata, J., Kubonishi, I., Satoh, H., Takata, M., Tanaka, Y., Tateno, M., Tozawa, H., Mori, S., Yoshiki, T., and Ohtsuki, Y. (1992). Phenotypical progression of a rat lymphoid cell line immortalized by HTLV-1 to induce lymphoma/leukemia-like disease in rats. *J Virol 66*, 6686–6694.

Oka, T., Yoshino, T., Hayashi, K., Ohara, N., Nakanishi, T., Yamaai, Y., Hiraki, A., Aoki-Sogawa, C., Kondo, E., Teramoto, N., Takahashi, K., Tsuchiyama, J., and Akagi, T. (2001). Reduction of hematopoietic cell-specific tyrosine phosphatase SHP-1 gene expression in natural killer cell lymphoma and various types of lymphomas/leukemias: combination analysis with cDNA expression array and tissue microarray. *Am J Pathol 159*, 1495–1505.

Okamoto, T., Ohno, Y., and Tsugane, S. Multi-step carcinogenesis model for adult T-cell leukemia. *Jpn J Cancer Res 80*, 191-195.

Okamura, J., Utsunomiya, A., Tanosaki, R., Uike, N., Sonoda, S., Kannagi, M., Tomonaga, M., Harada, M., Kimura, N., Masuda, M., Kawano, F., Yufu, Y., Hattori, H., Kikuchi, H., and Saburi, Y. (2005). Allogeneic stem-cell transplantation with reduced conditioning intensity as a novel immunotherapy and antiviral therapy for adult T-cell leukemia/lymphoma. *Blood* 105, 4143-4145.

Olsen, E. A., Kim, Y. H., Kuzel, T. M., Pacheco, T. R., Foss, F. M., Parker, S., Frankel, S. R., Chen, C., Ricker, J. L., Arduino, J. M., and Duvic, M. (2007). Phase IIb multicenter trial of vorinostat in patients with persistent, progressive, or treatment refractory cutaneousT-cell lymphoma. *J Clin Oncol* 25, 3109-3115.

Parkin, D. M. (2006). The global health burden of infection-associated cancers in the year 2002. *Int J Cancer 118*, 3030-3044.

Patel, D., Huang, S. M., Baglia, L. A., and McCance, D. J. (1999). The E6 protein of human papillomavirus type 16 binds to and inhibits co-activation by CBP and p300. *EMBO J* 18(18), 5061-5072.

Peart, M. J., Smyth, G. K., van Laar, R. K., Bowtell, D. D., Richon, V. M., Marks, P. A., Holloway, A. J., and Johnstone, R.W. (2005). Identification and functional significance of genes regulated by structurally different histone deacetylase inhibitors. *Proc Natl Acad Sci U S A* 102, 3697 -3702.

Peart, M. J., Tainton, K. M., Ruefli, A. A., Dear, A. E., Sedelies, K. A., O'Reilly, L. A., Waterhouse, N. J., Trapani, J. A., and Johnstone, R. W. (2003). Novel mechanisms of apoptosis induced by histone deacetylase inhibitors. *Cancer Res* 63, 4460-4471.

Peng, H., Du, M., Diss, T. C., Isaacson, P. G., and Pan, L. (1997). Genetic evidence for a clonal link between low and high-grade components in gastric MALT B-cell lymphoma. *Histopathol 30*, 425-429.

Piekarz, R.L., and Bates, S. E. (2009a). Epigenetic Modifiers: Basic Understanding and Clinical Development. *Clin Cancer Res* 15, 3918-3926.

Piekarz, R. L., Frye, R., Prince, H. M., Kirschbaum, M. H., Zain, J., Allen, S. L., Jaffe, E. S., Ling, A., Turner, M., Peer, C. J., Figg, W. D., Steinberg, S. M., Smith, S., Joske, D., Lewis, I., Hutchins, L., Craig, M., Fojo, A.T., Wright, J. J., and Bates, S. E. (2011). Phase II trial of romidepsin in patients with peripheral T-cell lymphoma. *Blood* 117(22), 5827-5834.

Piekarz, R. L., Frye, R., Turner, M., Wright, J. J., Allen, S. L., Kirschbaum, M. H., Zain, J., Prince, H. M., Leonard, J. P., Geskin, L. J., Reeder, C., Joske, D., Figg, W. D., Gardner, E. R., Steinberg, S. M., Jaffe, E. S., Stetler-Stevenson, M., Lade, S., Fojo, A. T., and Bates, S. E. (2009b). Phase II multi-institutional trial of the histone deacetylase inhibitor romidepsin as monotherapy for patients with cutaneous T-cell lymphoma. *J Clin Oncol* 27(32), 5410-5417.

Piekarz, R.L., Robey, R., Sandor, V., Bakke, S., Wilson, W.H., Dahmoush, L., Kingma, D. M., Turner M. L., Altemus, R., and Bates, S. E. (2001). Inhibitor of histone deacetylation, depsipeptide (FR901228), in the treatment of peripheral and cutaneous T-cell lymphoma: a case report, *Blood* 98, 2865–2868

Prince, H. M., Bishton, M. J., and Harrison, S. J. (2009). Clinical studies of histone deacetylase inhibitors. *Clin Cancer Res* 15(12), 3958-3969.

Poiesz, B. J., Ruscetti, F. W., Gazdar, A. F., Bunn, P. A., Minna, J. D., and Gallo, R. C. (1980). Detection and isolation of type C retrovirus particles from fresh and cultured lymphocytes of a patient with cutaneous T-cell lymphoma. *Proc Natl Acad Sci USA* 77, 7415-7419.

Proietti, F. A., Carneiro-Proietti, A. B., Catalan-Soares, B., and Murphy, E. L. (2005). Global epidemiology of HTLV-I infection and associated diseases. *Oncogene* 24, 6058-6068.

Ratner, L., Heyden, V., Paine, E., Frei-Lahr, D., Brown, R., Petruska, P., Reddy, S., and Lairmore, M. D. (1990). Familial adult T-cell leukemia/lymphoma. *Am J Hematol* 34, 215-222.

Razin, A., and Riggs, A. D. (1980). DNA methylation and gene function. *Science* 210, 604-610.

Reik, W. (2007). Stability and flexibility of epigenetic gene regulation in mammalian development. *Nature* 447, 425-432.

Remstein, E. D., James, C. D., and Kurtin, P. J. (2000). Incidence and subtype specificity of API2-MALT1 fusion translocations in extranordal, nordal, and splenic marginal zone lymphomas. *Am J Pathol 156*, 1183-1188.

Rodriguez, J., Caballero, M. D., Gutierrez, A., Gandarillas, M., Sierra, J., Lopez-Guillermo, A., Sureda, A., Zuazu, J., Marin, J., Arranz, R., Carreras, E., Leon, A., De Sevilla, A. F., San Miguel, J. F., Conde, E., GEL/TAMO Spanish Group. (2003), High dose chemotherapy and autologous stem cell transplantation in patients with peripheral T-cell lymphoma not achieving complete response after induction chemotherapy. The GEL-TAMO experience. *Haematologica* 88, 1372-1377.

Rodríguez, J., Conde, E., Gutiérrez, A., Arranz, R., León, A., Marín, J., Bendandi, M., Albo, C., and Caballero, M. D. (2007). The results of consolidation with autologous stem-cell transplantation in patients with peripheral T-cell lymphoma (PTCL) in first complete remission: the Spanish Lymphoma and Autologous Transplantation Group experience. *Ann Oncol* 18. 652-657.

Sandor, V., Bakke, S., Robey, R. W., Kang, M. H., Blagosklonny, M. V., Bender, J., Brooks, R., Piekarz, R. L., Tucker, E., Figg, W. D., Chan, K. K., Goldspiel, B., Fojo, A. T., Balcerzak, S. P., and Bates, S. E.(2002). Phase I trial of the histone deacetylase inhibitor, depsipeptide (FR901228, NSC 630176), in patients with refractory neoplasms. *Clin Cancer Res* 8, 718-728.

Sato, H., Oka, T., Shinnou, Y., Kondo, T., Washio, K., Takano, M., Takata, K., Morito, T., Huang, X., Tamura, M., Kitamura, Y., Ohara, N., Ouchida, M., Oshima, K., Shimizu, K., Tanimoto, M., Takahashi, K., Matsuoka, M., Utsunomiya, A., and Yoshino, T. (2010). Multi-step aberrant CpG island hyper-methylation is associated with the progression of adult T-cell leukemia/lymphoma. *Am J Pathol* 176, 402-415.

Satou, Y., Yasunaga, J., Yoshida, M., and Matsuoka, M. (2006). HTLV-I basic leucine zipper factor gene mRNA supports proliferation of adult T cell leukemia cells. *Proc Natl Acad Sci USA* 103, 720-725.

Selgrad, M., De Giorgio, R., Fini, L., Cogliandro, R. F., Williams, S., Stanghellini, V., Barbara, G., Tonini, M., Corinaldesi, R., Genta, R. M., Domiati-Saad, R., Meyer, R., Goel, A., Boland, C. R., and Ricciardiello, L. (2009). JC virus infects the enteric glia of patients with chronic idiopathic intestinal pseudo-obstruction. *Gut 58*, 25-32.

Sharif, J., Muto, M., Takebayashi, S., Suetake, I., Iwamatsu, A., Endo, T. A., Shinga, J., Mizutani-Koseki, Y., Toyoda, T., Okamura, K., Tajima, S., Mitsuya, K., Okano, M., and Koseki, H. (2007). The SRA protein Np95 mediates epigenetic inheritance by recruiting Dnmt1 to methylated DNA. *Nature* 450(7171), 908-912.

Shimakage, M., Inoue, N., Ohshima, K., Kawahara, K., Yamamoto, N., Oka, T., Tambe, Y., Yasui, K., Matsumoto, K., Yutsudo, M., and Inoue, H. (2007). Downregu-lation of drs mRNA expression is associated with the progression of adult T-cell leukemia/lymphoma. *Int J Oncol 30*, 1343–1348.

Shimakage, M., Inoue, N., Ohshima, K., Kawahara, K., Yamamoto, N., Oka, T., Yasui, K., Matsumoto, K., Inoue, H., Watari, A., Higashiyama, S., Yutsudo, M. (2006). Down-regulation of ASY/Nogo transcription associated with progression of adult T-cell leukemia/lymphoma. *Int J Cancer 119,* 1648–1653.

Shimamoto, Y., Kikuchi, M., Funai, N., Suga, K., Matsuzaki, M., and Yamaguchi, M. (1993). Spontaneous regression in adult T-cell leukemia/lymphoma. *Cancer* 72, 735-740.

Shimoyama, M., Ota, K., Kikuchi, M., Yunoki, K., Konda, S., Takatsuki, K., Ichimaru, M., Ogawa, M., Kimura, I., Tominaga, S., Tsugane, S., Taguchi, H., Minato, K., Takenaka, T., Tobinai, K., Kurita, S., Oyama, A., Hisano, S., Kozuru, M., Matsumoto, M., Nomura, K., Takiguchi, T., Sugai, S., Yamaguchi, K., Hattori, T., Kinoshita, K., Tajima, K., and Suemasu, K. (1988). Chemotherapeutic results and prognostic factors of patients with advanced non-Hodgkin's lymphoma treated with VEPA or VEPA-M. *J Clin Oncol* 6, 128-141.

Shimoyama, M., and members of The Lymphoma Study Group (1984-87). (1991). Diagnostic criteria and classification of clinical subtypes of adult T-cell leukaemia-lymphoma. A report from the Lymphoma Study Group (1984-87). *Br J Haematol* 79, 428-437.

Shimoyama, M. (1994). Chemotherapy of ATL. In: Takatsuki K, ed. Adult T-cell leukemia. New York, Oxford University Press , pp221-237.

Shiratori, S., Yasumoto, A., Tanaka, J., Shigematsu, A., Yamamoto, S., Nishio, M., Hashino, S., Morita, R., Takahata, M., Onozawa, M., Kahata, K., Kondo, T., Ota, S., Wakasa, K., Sugita, J., Koike, T., Asaka, M., Kasai, M., and Imamura, M. (2008). A retrospective analysis of allogeneic hematopoietic stem cell transplantation for adult T cell leukemia/lymphoma (ATL): clinical impact of graft-versus-leukemia/lymphoma effect. *Biol Blood Marrow transplant* 14, 817-823.

Si, J., Boumber, Y. A., Shu, J., Qin, T., Ahmed, S., He, R., Jelinek, J., and Issa, J. P. (2010). Chromatin remodeling is required for gene reactivation after decitabine-mediated DNA hypomethylation. *Cancer Res* 70(17), 6968-6977.

Sif, S., Saurin, A. J., Imbalzano, A. N., and Kingston, R. E. (2001). Purification and characterization of mSin3A-containing Brg1 and hBrm chromatin remodeling complexes. *Genes Dev* 15(5), 603-618.

Silverman, L. R. (2009). Hypomethylating agents in myelodysplastic syndromes changing the inevitable: the value of azacitidine as maintenance therapy, effects on transfusion and combination with other agents. *Leuk Res* 33, Suppl 2, S18-21.

Singh, S.P., de Camargo, M. M., Zhang, H. H., Foley, J. F.; Hedrick, M. N., and Farber, J. M. (2010). Changes in histone acetylation and methylation that are important for persistent but not transient expression of CCR4 in human CD4+ T cells. *Eur J Immunol* 40(11), 3183-3197.

Steiner, F.A., Hong, J.A., Fischette, M.R., Guo, Z. S., Chen, G. A., Weiser, T. S., Kassis, E. S., Nguyen, D. M., Lee, S., Trepel, J. B., and Schrump, D. S. (2005). Sequential 5-Aza 2'-deoxycytidine/depsipeptide FK228 treatment induces tissue factor pathway inhibitor 2 (TFPI-2) expression in cancer cells. *Oncogene* 24, 2386 -2397.

Strahl, B. D., and Allis, C. D. (2000). The language of covalent histone modifications. *Nature* 403(6765), 41-45.

Suzuki, R., Kagami, Y., Takeuchi, K., Kami, M., Okamoto, M., Ichinohasama, R., Mori, N., Kojima, M., Yoshino, T., Yamabe, H., Shiota, M., Mori, S., Ogura, M., Hamajima, N., Seto, M., Suchi, T., Morishima, Y., and Nakamura, S. (2000). Prognostic significance of CD56 expression for ALK-positive and ALK-negative anaplastic large-cell lymphoma of T/null cell phenotype. *Blood* 96, 2993-3000.

Tajima, K. (1990). The T- and B-cell Malignancy Study Group: the 4th nationwide study of adult T-cell leukemia/lymphoma (ATL) in Japan: estimates of risk of ATL and its geographical and clinical features. *Int J Cancer 45*, 237-243.

Takasaki, Y., Iwanaga, M., Imaizumi, Y., Tawara, M., Joh, T., Kohno, T., Yamada, Y., Kamihira, S., Ikeda, S., Miyazaki, Y., Tomonaga, M., and Tsukasaki, K. (2010). Long-term study of indolent adult T-cell leukemia-lymphoma. *Blood* 115, 4337-4343.

Tawara, M., Hogerzeil, S. J., Yamada, Y., Takasaki, Y., Soda, H., Hasegawa, H., Murata, K., Ikeda, S., Imaizumi, Y., Sugahara, K., Tsuruda, K., Tsukasaki, K., Tomonaga, M., Hirakata, Y., and Kamihira, S. (2006). Impact of p53 aberration on the progression of adult T-cell leukemia/lymphoma. *Cancer Lett 234*, 249-255.

Thai, T. H., Christiansen, P. A., Tsokos, G. C. (2010). Is there a link between dysregulated miRNA expression and disease? *Discov Med* 10(52), 184-194.

Tilly, H., Lepage, E., Coiffier, B., Blanc, M., Herbrecht, R., Bosly, A., Attal, M., Fillet, G., Guettier, C., Molina, T. J., Gisselbrecht, C., Reyes, F., Groupe d'Etude des Lymphomes de l'Adulte. (2003). Intensive conventional chemotherapy (ACVBP regimen) compared with standard CHOP for poor-prognosis aggressive non-Hodgkin lymphoma. *Blood* 102, 4284-4289.

Tomita, N., Motomura, S., Hyo, R., Takasaki, H., Takemura, S., Taguchi, J., Fujisawa, S., Ogawa, K., Ishigatsubo, Y., and Takeuchi, K. (2007). Comparison of peripheral T-cell lymphomas and diffuse large B-cell lymphoma. *Cancer* 109, 1146-1151.

Tota, J., Mahmud, S. M., Ferenczy, A., Coutlée, F., and Franco, E. L. Promising strategies for cervical cancer screening in the post-human papillomavirus vaccination era. *Sex Health 7*, 376-382.

Toyota, M., and Issa, J. P. *(2005)*. Epigenetic changes in solid and hematopoietic tumors. *Semin Oncol 32, 521*-530.

Tsai, C. N., Tsai, C. L., Tse, K. P., Chang, H. Y., and Chang, Y. S. (2002). The Epstein-Barr virus oncogene product, latent membrane protein 1, induces the downregulation of E-cadherin gene expression via activation of DNA methyltransferases. *Proc Natl Acad Sci USA* 99(15), 10084-10089.

Tsukasaki, K., Utsunomiya, A., Fukuda, H., Shibata, T., Fukushima, T., Takatsuka, Y., Ikeda, S., Masuda, M., Nagoshi, H., Ueda, R., Tamura, K., Sano, M., Momita, S., Yamaguchi, K., Kawano, F., Hanada, S., Tobinai, K., Shimoyama, M., Hotta, T., and Tomonaga, M. (2007). VCAP-AMP-VECP compared with biweekly CHOP for adult T-cell leukemia-lymphoma: Japan Clinical Oncology Group Study JCOG9801. *J Clin Oncol* 25, 5458- 5464.

Uchiyama, T., Yodoi, J., Sagawa, K., Takatsuki, K., and Uchino, H. (1977). Adult T-cell leukemia: clinical and hematological features of 16 cases. *Blood* 50, 481-492.

Uozumi, K. (2010). Treatment of adult T-cell leukemia. *J Clin Exp Hematopathol* 50, 9-25.

Utsunomiya, A., Hanada, S., Terada, A., Kodama, M., Uematsu, T., Tsukasa, S., Hashimoto, S., Tokunaga, M. (1988). Adult T-cell leukemia with leukemia cell infiltration into the gastrointestinal tract. *Cancer* 61, 824-828.

Utsunomiya, A., Ishida, T., Inagaki, A., Yano, H., Komatsu, H., Iida, S., Yonekura, K., Takeuchi, S., Takatsuka, Y., Ueda, R. (2007). Clinical significance of a blood eosinophilia in adult T-cell leukemia/lymphoma: a blood eosinophilia is a significant unfavorable prognostic factor. *Leuk Res* 31, 91-95.

Utsunomiya, A., Miyazaki, Y., Takatsuka, Y., Hanada, S., Uozumi, K., Yashiki, S., Tara, M., Kawano, F., Saburi, Y., Kikuchi, H., Hara, M., Sao, H., Morishima, Y., Kodera, Y., Sonoda, S., and Tomonaga, M. (2001). Improved outcome of adult T cell leukemia/lymphoma with allogeneic hematopoietic stem cell transplantation. *Bone Marrow Transplant* 27, 15-20.

van Haaften, G., Dalgliesh, G. L., Davies, H., Chen, L., Bignell, G., Greenman, C., Edkins, S., Hardy, C.,O'Meara, S.,Teague, J., Butler, A., Hinton, J., Latimer, C., Andrews, J., Barthorpe, S., Beare, D., Buck, G., Campbell, P. J., Cole, J., Forbes, S., Jia, M., Jones, D., Kok, C.Y., Leroy, C., Lin, M. L., McBride, D. J., Maddison, M., Maquire, S., McLay, K., Menzies, A., Mironenko, T., Mulderrig, L., Mudie, L., Pleasance, E., Shepherd, R., Smith, R., Stebbings, L., Stephens, P., Tang, G., Tarpey, P. S., Turner, R., Turrell, K., Varian, J., West, S., Widaa, S., Wray, P., Collins, V. P., Ichimura, K., Law, S., Wong, J., Yuen, S. T., Leung, S. Y., Tonon, G., DePinho, R. A., Tai, Y. T., Anderson, K. C., Kahnoski, R. J., Massie ,A., Khoo, S.K., The, B. T., Stratton, M. R., and Futreal, P. A. (2009). Somatic mutations of the histone H3K27 demethylase gene UTX in human cancer. *Nat Genet* 41(5), 521-523.

Villa, R., Morey, L., Raker, V. A., Buschbeck, M., Gutierrez, A., De Santis, F., Corsaro, M., Varas, F., Bossi, D., Minucci, S., Pelicci, P.G., and Di Croce, L. (2006). The methyl-CpG binding protein MBD1 is required for PML-RARalpha function. *Proc Natl Acad Sci USA*. 103(5), 1400-1405.

Wang, D., Liebowitz, D., and Kieff, E. (1985). An EBV membrane protein expressed in immortalized lymphocytes transforms established rodent cells. *Cell 43*, 831-840.

Wang, L., Grossman, S. R., and Kieff, E. (2000). Epstein-Barr virus nuclear protein 2 interacts with p300, CBP, and PCAF histone acetyltransferases in activation of the LMP1 promoter. *Proc Natl Acad Sci USA* 97(1):430-435.

Watanabe, T., Yamaguchi, K., Takatsuki, K., Osame, M., Yoshida, M. (1990). Constitutive expression of parathyroid hormone-related protein gene in human T cell leukemia virus type 1 (HTLV-1) carriers and adult T cell leukemia patients that can be trans-activated by HTLV-1 tax gene. *J Exp Med* 172, 759-765.

Whittaker, S. J., Demierre, M. F., Kim, E. J., Rook, A. H., Lerner, A., Duvic, M., Scarisbrick, J., Reddy, S., Robak, T., Becker, J. C., Samtsov, A., McCulloch, W., and Kim, Y. H. (2010). Final results from a multicenter, international, pivotal study of romidepsin in refractory cutaneous T-cell lymphoma. *J Clin Oncol* 28(29), 4485-4491.

Wilks, R. J., LaGrenade, L., Hanchard, B., Campbell, M., Murphy, J., Cranston, B., Blattner, W. A., and Manns, A. (1993). Sibling adult T-cell leukemia/lymphoma and clustering of human T-cell lymphotropic virus type I infection in a Jamaican family. *Cancer* 72, 2700-2704.

Wong, A. K., Shanahan, F., Chen, Y., Lian, L., Ha, P., Hendricks, K., Ghaffari, S., Iliev, D., Penn, B., Woodland, A. M., Smith, R., Salada, G., Carillo, A., Laity, K., Gupte, J., Swedlund, B., Tavtigian, S. V., Teng, D. H., and Lees, E. (2000). BRG1, a component of the SWI-SNF complex, is mutated in multiple human tumor cell lines. *Cancer Res* 60(21), 6171-6177.

Yamada, Y., Tomonaga, M., Fukuda, H., Hanada, S., Utsunomiya, A., Tara, M., Sano, M., Ikeda, S., Takatsuki, K., Kozuru, M., Araki, K., Kawano, F., Niimi, M., Tobinai, K.,

Hotta, T., and Shimoyama, M. (2001). A new G-CSF-supported combination chemotherapy, LSG15, for adult T-cell leukemia-lymphoma: Japan Clinical Oncology Group Study 9303. *Br J Haematol* 113, 375-382.

Yamaguchi, K., and Watanabe, T. (2002). Human T lymphotropic type-I and adult T-cell leukemia in Japan. *Int J Hematol* 76 (Suppl 2), 240-250.

Yamamoto, K., Utsunomiya, A., Tobinai, K., Tsukasaki, K., Uike, N., Uozumi, K., Yamaguchi, K., Yamada, Y., Hanada, S., Tamura, K., Nakamura, S., Inagaki, H., Ohshima, K., Kiyoi, H., Ishida, T., Matsushima, K., Akinaga, S., Ogura, M., Tomonaga, M., and Ueda, R. (2010). Phase I study of KW-0761, a defucosylated humanized anti-CCR4 antibody, in relapsed patients with adult T-cell leukemia-lymphoma and peripheral T-cell lymphoma. *J Clin Oncol* 28, 1591-1598.

Yamato, K., Oka, T., Hiroi, M., Iwahara, Y., Sugito, S., Tsuchida, N., and Miyoshi, I. (1993). Aberrant expression of the p53 tumor suppresser gene in adult T-cell leukemia and HTLV-1-infected cells. *Jpn J Cancer Res 84*, 4–8.

Yano, M., Ouchida, M., Shigematsu, H., Tanaka, N., Ichimura, K., Kobayashi, K., Inaki, Y., Toyooka, S., Tsukuda, K., Shimizu, N., and Shimizu, K. (2004). Tumor-specific exon creation of the HELLS/SMARCA6 gene in non-small cell lung cancer. *Int J Cancer* 112(1), 8-13.

Yonekura, K., Utsunomiya, A., Takatsuka, Y., Takeuchi, S., Tashiro, Y., Kanzaki, T., Kanekura, T. (2008). Graft-versus-adult T-cell leukemia/lymphoma effect following allogeneic hematopoietic stem cell transplantation. *Bone Marrow Transplant* 41, 1029-1035.

Yoo, C. B., and Jones, P. A. *(2006)*. Epigenetic therapy of cancer: past, present and future. *Nat Rev Drug Discov 5, 37*–50.

Yoshida M. (2001). Multiple viral strategies of HTLV-1 dysregulation of cell growth control. *Annu Rev Immunol* 19, 475-496.

Yoshida, M., Miyoshi, I., and Hinuma, Y. (1982). Isolation and characterization of retrovirus from cell lines of human adult T-cell leukemia and its implication in the disease. *Proc. Natl. Acad. Sci. USA 79*, 2031-2035.

Yoshie, O., Fujisawa, R., Nakayama, T., Harasawa, H., Tago, H., Izawa, D., Hieshima, K., Tatsumi, Y., Matsushima, K., Hasegawa, H., Kanamaru, A., Kamihira, S., and Yamada, Y. (2002). Frequent expression of CCR4 in Adult T-cell leukemia and human T-cell leukemia virus type 1-transformed T cells. *Blood* 99, 1505–1511.

Zhang, H., Yang, X. Y., Hong, T., Feldman, T., and Bhattacharyya, P. K. (2010). Kaposi sarcoma-associated herpesvirus (human herpesvirus type 8)-associated extracavitary lymphoma: Report of a case in an HIV-positive patient with simultaneous kaposi sarcoma and a review of the literature. *Acta Haematol 123*, 237-241.

Zhu, X., Ma, Y., and Liu, D. (2010). Novel agents and regimens for acute myeloid leukemia: 2009 American Society of Hematology annual meeting highlights. *J Hematol Oncol*, 3-17.

Zur Hausen, H. (2009). The search for infectious causes of human cancers: where and why (Nobel lecture). *Angew Chem Int Ed Engl* 48(32), 5798-5808.

9

Roles of MicroRNA in T-Cell Leukemia

Mariko Tomita
Department Pathology and Oncology
Graduate School of Medical Science
University of the Ryukyus
Japan

1. Introduction

Previously, cancer researchers have been focused on the genes that code proteins. They have considered those effects on tumorigenesis. However, discoveries of microRNAs (miRNAs) have shed a light on the role of non-protein-coding RNAs in tumorigenesis. The first small non-coding RNA, named *lin-4* in *Caenorhabditis elegans* (*C. elegans*) was described by Lee et al in 1993 (Lee et al., 1993). *Lin-4* codes miRNA that regulates the timing of *C. elegans* larval development by translational repression (Ambros, 2000). Since then, many miRNAs in different organisms such as plants, *C. elegans*, Drosophila, and mammals including humans have been discovered substantially. Up to now, the human genome is predicted to encode as many as 1,000 miRNAs.

miRNAs belong to a class of regulatory genes that are single-stranded 19-25 nucleotides non-cording RNAs and are generated from endogenous hairpin-shaped transcripts (Kim, 2005). miRNA genes are located either within the introns or exons of protein-coding genes (70%) or in intergenic regions (30%). More than 50% of mammalian miRNAs are located within the intronic regions of protein-coding genes. Most of the intronic or exonic miRNAs are transcribed in parallel with their host genes, indicating that these miRNAs use their host genes transcriptional machinalies. On the other hand, miRNAs produced from intergenic regions are transcribed separately from internal promoters (Rodriguez et al., 2004).

The first step of miRNA synthesis is the transcription of primary miRNA (pri-miRNA) from *miRNA* genes (Fig.1). pri-miRNAs are transcribed in a RNA polymerase II (Pol II) - dependent manner as several hundreds or thousands of nucleotides long polyadenylated RNAs. In the nucleus, the pri-miRNA is processed to a precursor miRNA (pre-miRNA) of 60-100 nucleotides in length with a stem-loop structure by the nuclear protein Drosha that belongs to class II RNase III. Drosha interacts with its cofactor DGCR8 (the DiGeorge syndrome critical region gene 8 protein). Then, the pre-miRNA is exported from the nucleus to the cytoplasm by the Exportin 5/Ran-GTP complex. In the cytoplasm, the pre-miRNA is cleaved by class III RNase III, Dicer, which is a 200-kDa protein and miRNA is produced. Primary function of miRNAs in the cytoplasm is the negative regulation of gene expression by binding to complementary target sequences in the 3' untranslated region (UTR) of mRNA. Binding of a miRNA to the target mRNA typically leads to translational repression or degradation of mRNA, which means that miRNAs repress the expression of the target genes. In mammals, miRNAs guide the RNA induced silencing complex (RISC) to

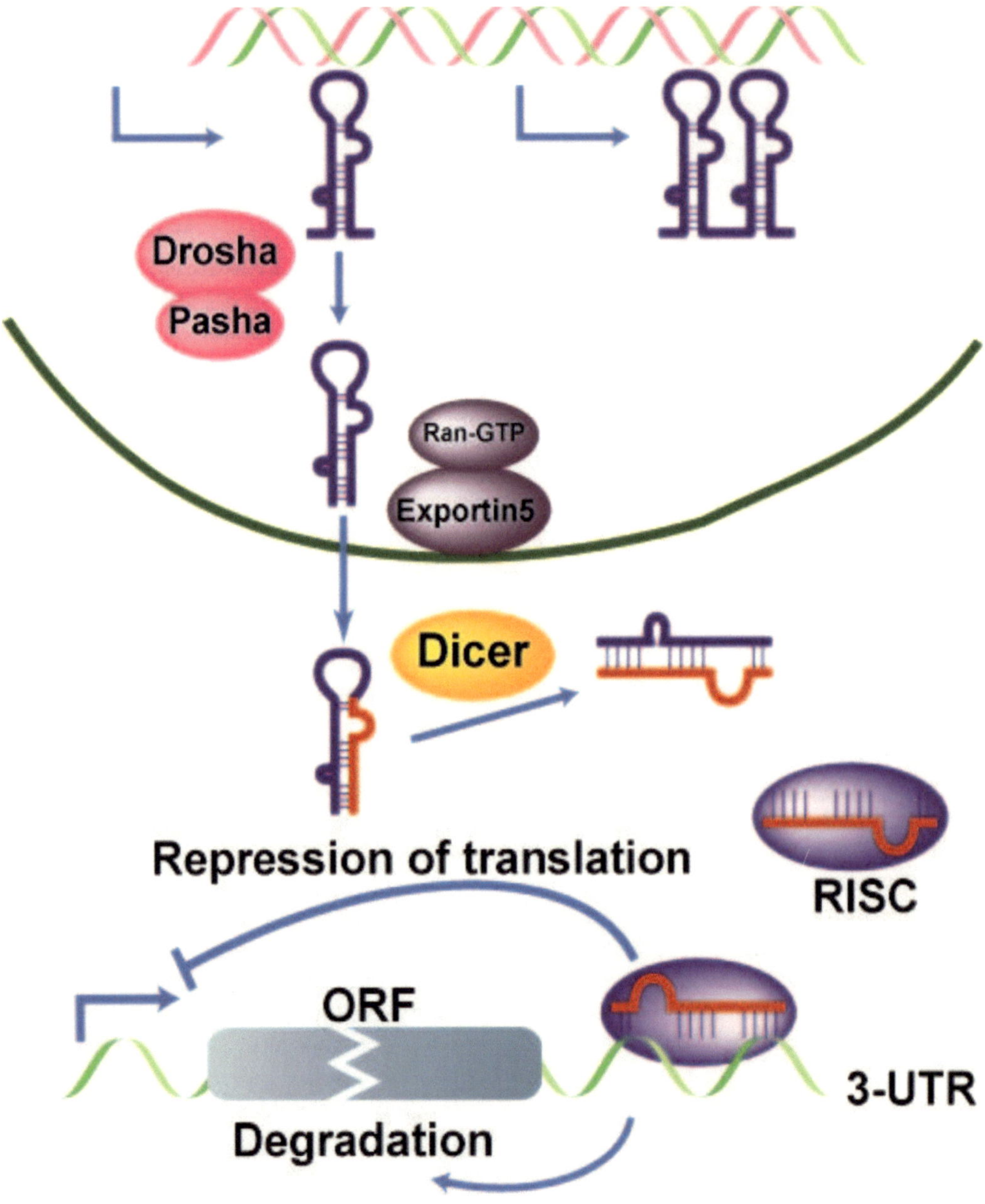

Fig. 1. miRNA biogenesis

complementary target sites of their specific target mRNAs, where endonucleolytically active Ago protein cleaves the mRNAs (Martinez et al., 2002). In contrast, other miRNAs predominantly bind to partially complementary target sites. Such imperfect binding between miRNAs and target mRNAs leads to repression of translation and/or deadenylation, followed by destabilization of the target mRNAs (Pillai et al., 2007). miRNAs are estimated to regulate more than 30% of mRNAs. Therefore, miRNAs have many roles in biological processes, such as development, differentiation, cell proliferation, apoptosis, and stress responses (Bartel, 2004). Moreover, one target gene usually contains binding sites for multiple miRNAs, allowing miRNAs to form more complex regulatory networks of gene expression (Lewis et al., 2003).

2. microRNA in cancer

Over the recent years, many miRNAs have been implicated in many human cancers. The first evidence for the importance of miRNAs in human cancer was the discovery of the loss of miR-15a/miR-16-1 cluster in chronic lymphocytic leukemia (CLL) (Calin et al., 2002). Since then, aberrant numerous miRNAs expression has been shown to be involved in the development of human cancers.

Many miRNAs have been shown to function as oncogenes in human cancers. Among them, miR-155, which is encoded by nucleotides 241 - 262 of B-cell integration cluster (*BIC*), is the first miRNAs linked with cancer (Metzler et al., 2004). After the discovery, many research groups have shown that *miR-155* is highly expressed in various human cancers, including childrend's Burkitt's lymphoma (Metzler et al., 2004), Hodgkin's lymphoma, CLL (Kluiver et al., 2005), primary mediastinal non-Hodgkin's lymphoma (Calin et al., 2005), acute myelogenous leukemia (Garzon et al., 2008), lung cancer, breast cancer (Volinia et al., 2006), and pancreatic cancer (Greither et al., 2010). *miR-155* transgenic mice develop acute lymphoblastic leukemia (ALL) and high-grade lymphoma (Costinean et al., 2009). These results support the idea that miR-155 plays a role as oncogene *in vivo*.

On the other hand, many miRNA encoding genes have been shown as tumor suppressor genes. As mentioned above, miR-15a/miR-16-1 cluster was the first to establish the link between miRNAs and cancer. This study showed loss of miR-15a/miR-16-1 cluster, which are located at chromosome 13q14, a region deleted in more than 65% of B cell CLL (Calin et al., 2002). These miRNAs induce apoptosis through the negative regulation of the anti-apoptotic gene *Bcl2* (Cimmino et al., 2005). Indeed, down-regulation of miR-15a/miR-16-1 has been associated with the pathogenesis of CLL (Calin et al., 2008). These data support the idea that miR-15a/miR-16-1 plays a role as tumor-suppressor genes.

In this review, we introduce the accumulating evidences for the central roles that miRNAs play in hematological malignancy, in particular focusing on their role in T-cell leukemia and lymphoma.

3. microRNA in T-cell leukemia and lymphoma

3.1 Acute lymphoblastic T-cell leukemia/lymphoma (T-ALL)

Acute lymphoblastic leukemia (ALL) is the most common neoplasm in children, while it is relatively rare in adults. Although ALL originates from either B or T-cell progenitors, most cases are of B-cell ALL (B-ALL) (Pui & Evans, 2006). The less common type, T-cell ALL (T-ALL) is induced by the transformation of T-cell progenitors, and is diagnosed in 10-15% of children and 25% of adults with ALL (Copelan & McGuire, 1995). Molecular mechanisms of leukemogenesis of T-ALL have been investigated intensively. Recent studies revealed that 50-70% of T-ALLs have gain-of-function mutations in *Notch1*, a gene that is essential for T-cell development (Ferrando, 2009). miRNAs expression profiles in T- and B-ALL are highly associated with the lineage from which the leukemia derived (Lu et al., 2005). Some miRNAs can be discriminative of T-ALL versus B-ALL (Fulci et al., 2009). Although miRNAs that associated with leukemogenesis of B-ALL have been well documented (Lawrie, 2008), a few studies have been demonstrated association between particular miRNA and pathogenesis of T-ALL.

Recently, Mavrakis et al. have revealed association between miR-19 and leukemogenesis in T-ALL (Mavrakis et al., 2010). miR-19 was identified within the miR-17-92 cluster. The cluster is located at human chromosome 13q31 in a genomic region that is often amplified in many human cancers (Lu et al., 2005; Nagel et al., 2009). This cluster is also implicated in human hematopoietic malignancies (He et al., 2005; Mendell, 2008; Xiao et al., 2008). Xiao et al. have shown that miR-17-92 cluster is highly expressed in hematopoietic tumors and promotes lymphomagenesis *in vivo* (Xiao et al., 2008). Indeed, retroviral expression of miR-17-92 cluster genes accelerates c-Myc-induced B-cell lymphoma (Mu et al., 2009). The miR-17-92 cluster encodes 15 miRNAs including miR-19 with overlapping functions in development (Ventura et al., 2008). More recently, Mavrakis et al. demonstrated that miR-19 expresses at levels seen in other human tumors, enhances lymphocyte survival and is sufficient to cooperate with Notch1 in T-ALL *in vivo*. They found a 5-17 fold increase in miR-19 expression in T-ALL, and less for other miRNAs in the miR-17-92 cluster. miR-19 has a distinct ability to enhance lymphocyte survival *in vitro*. miR-19 target genes were identified by a large-scale short hairpin RNA screening, including multiple negative regulators in PI3K pathway such as PTEN, Bim, AMP-activated kinase (Prkaa1), and PP2A (Mavrakis & Wendel, 2010). The expression of these genes is regulated by miR-19 in lymphocytes, indicating that miR-19 produces a coordinate clampdown on multiple negative regulators of PI3K-related survival signals (Mavrakis et al., 2010).

Bhatia et al. recently reported downregulation of the expression of miR-196b in the human T-cell leukemia cell line, and T-ALL patients samples (Bhatia et al., 2011). Same group has shown that miR-196b has the capacity to downregulation the overamplified *c-myc* gene, recognized as a common pathogenomic feature leading to many cancers including B-ALL (Bhatia et al., 2010). In addition, they have demonstrated that miR-196b downregulation several *c-myc* effector genes like human telomerase reverse transcriptase (hTERT), the catalytic component of telomerase enzyme responsible for unlimited proliferative potential of cancerous cells, Bcl-2, the anti-apoptotic protein involved in inhibition of cellular apoptosis, and apoptosis antagonizing transcription factor (AATF). Indeed, restoration of miR-196b in EB-3 cells derived from a Burkitt lymphoma leads to significant downregulation of *c-myc* and its effector genes and qualifies for tumor suppressor function in B-ALL (Bhatia et al., 2010). On the contrary, miR-196b loses its ability to down regulate *c-myc* gene in T-ALL as a consequence of mutations in its target binding region in 3'UTR of *c-myc* gene (Bhatia et al., 2011). Although miR-196b is implicated to have different functions in T-ALL from in B-ALL, the role of miR-196b on leukemogenesis of T-ALL is still unclear. Another group's recent study has shown that miR-196a and miR-196b as regulators of the oncogenic ETS transcription factor *ERG* (Coskun et al., 2011). *ERG* has been known as playing important physiological and oncogenic roles in hematopoiesis (Baldus et al., 2006). It is also a prognostic factor in a subset of adult patients with T-ALL (Baldus et al., 2006; Loughran et al., 2008). They found that miR-196a and miR-196b expression was associated with an immature immunophenotype (CD34 positive) in T-ALL patients (Coskun et al., 2011). These findings indicate miR-196a and miR-196b as *ERG* regulators and implicate a potential role for these miRNAs in T-ALL.

3.2 Adult T-cell leukemia/lymphoma (ATLL)

ATLL is an aggressive lymphoproliferative disorder that occurs in individuals infected with human T-cell leukemia virus type 1 (HTLV-1) (Matsuoka & Jeang, 2007). HTLV-1 causes ATLL in 3-5% of infected individuals after a long latent period of 40-60 years (Tajima, 1990). More than 20 million people are infected with HTLV-1 worldwide. ATLL occurs mainly in regions where HTLV-1 is endemic, mainly southern Japan, West Africa, and the Caribbean basin. ATLL is classified into four clinical subtypes termed acute, lymphoma, smoldering, and chronic. The prognosis of ATLL patients remains poor with a median survival time of 13 months in aggressive cases (Yamada et al., 2001). HTLV-1 encodes a protein Tax in its genome. The malignant growth and survival of HTLV-1-infected T-cells can be attributed to Tax, that is a modulator of many transcription factors and associations with molecules of signal transduction pathways that alter expression of host-cell genes involved in proliferation, apoptosis, and genetic stability (Marriott & Semmes, 2005; Boxus et al., 2008). Recent studies have shown the interactions between HTLV-1 and the miRNA regulatory network.

miRNA expression profiling studies in HTLV-1-infected T-cell lines and ATLL patients samples have been performed by some groups (Pichler et al., 2008; Yeung et al., 2008; Bellon et al., 2009). Pichler et al. demonstrated that 4 miRNAs (miR-21, miR-24, miR-146a, and miR-155) are upregulated and miR-223 is downregulated in HTLV-1-transfected cells by real-time RT-PCR to analyze selected sets of miRNAs that already been implicated in oncogenic transformation (Pichler et al., 2008). Bellon et al. idenentified aberrant expression of hematopoietic-specific miRNAs included miR-150, miR-155, miR-223, miR-142-3p, and miR142-5p (upregulated) and miR-181a, miR-132, miR-125a, and miR-146b (downregulated) in ATLL cells versus control peripheral blood mononuclear cells (PBMC) and CD4+ T-cells, and HTLV-1-infected cells lines *in vitro* and uncultured *ex vivo* ATLL cells (Bellon et al., 2009). These results were confirmed by real-time RT-PCR in additional ATLL cases and infected cell lines. They also demonstrated that treatment of HTLV-1-infected cell lines with an NF-κB inhibitor (pathenolide) or JNK inhibitor (JNK II) resulted in reduced levels of the miR-155 precursor (Bellon et al., 2009).

Moreover, Yeung et al. demonstrated that 6 miRNAs (miR-9, miR-17-3p, miR-20b, miR-93, miR-130b, and miR-18a) are upregulated and 9 mi-RNAs (miR-1, miR-144, miR-126, miR-130a, miR-199a*, miR-338, miR-432, miR-335, and miR-337) are downregulated both in HTLV-1-transformed cell lines and primary ATLL cells (Yeung et al., 2008). To distinguish miRNAs that are responding to proliferative stimuli, they also examined PBMC exposed to phorbol-12-myristate 13-acetate (PMA) compared to untreated PBMC. By these comparisons, they identified 3 miRNAs (miR-93, miR-130b, and miR-18a) that were upregulated in ATLL cells, HTLV-1-infected cell lines and PMA-treated cells, an additional miRNA, miR-335, was downregulated in all three cell types. Then they focused on miR-93 and miR-130b, those were confirmed increased expression in the ATLL samples by real-time RT-PCR. These miRNAs served to regulate tumor protein 53-induced nuclear protein 1 (TP53INP1), that is a cellular tumor suppressor protein whose activity governs cellular survival and proliferation (Yeung et al., 2008). Pichler et al. have shown that TP53INP1 is a potential mRNA target of miR-21, miR-24, miR-146a, and miR-155 (Pichler et al., 2008) .TP53INP1 is induced by the p53 response triggered by various stress treatments such as gamma irradiation, UV irradiation, and oxidative stress. Accumulation of TP53INP1 results in a block in the cell cycle at G_1 (Tomasini et al., 2003) and triggers apoptosis through increased phosphorylation of p53 on Ser46 (Okamura et al., 2001) and upregulation of selected p53-responsive genes such as p53AIP1 (Okamura et al., 2001), p21 and Bax (Tomasini et al., 2001). These results suggest that miRNAs enhance cell growth and suppress apoptosis through targeting TP53INP1.

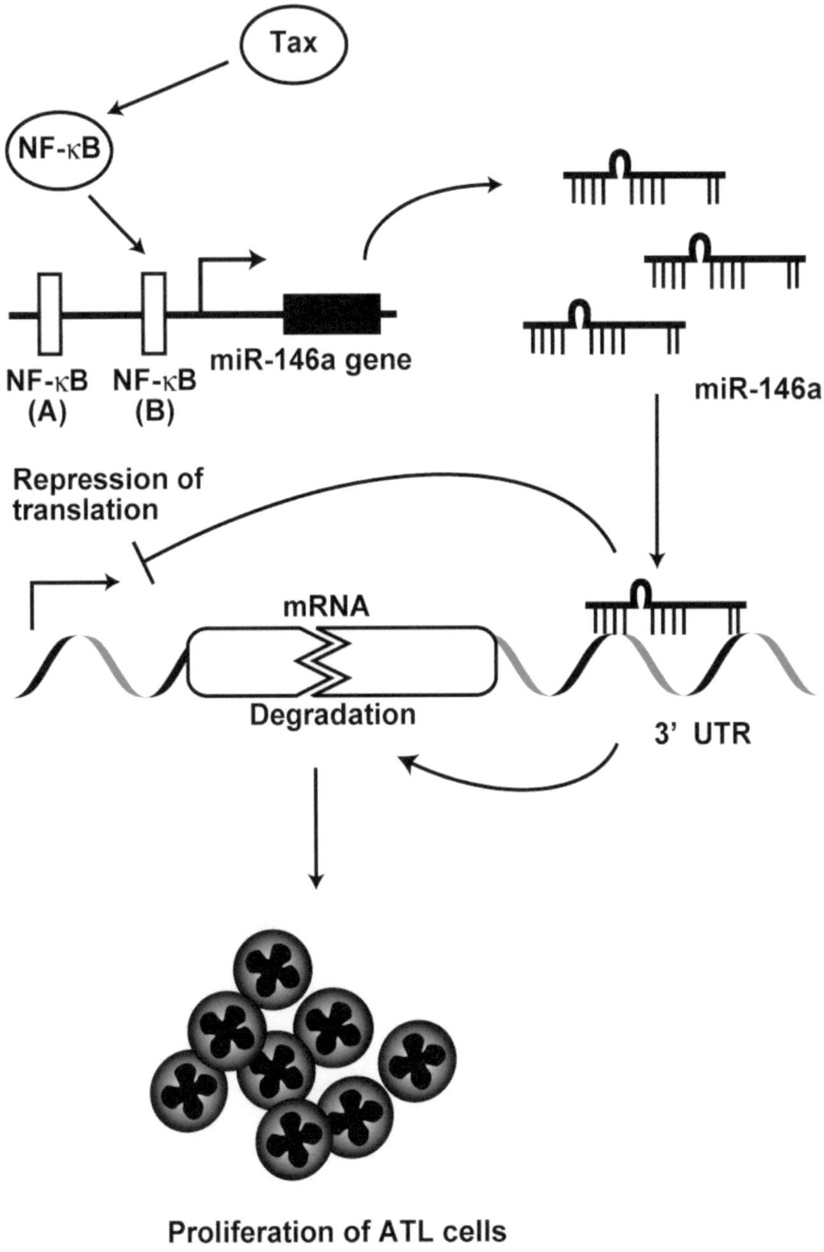

Fig. 2. Schematic representation of the effects of Tax on miR-146a expression (Tomita et al., 2011)

Although several miRNA profiling experiments accumulate miRNA subsets up or downregulated in HTLV-1-infected T-cell lines and ATLL patient's samples, data of miRNA expression profiles are not consistent in these reports. This inconsistency could be due to methodological differences in the techniques employed to prepare RNA from the cells and/or to hybridize probes to microarray.

Among the miRNA expression profilings, miR-146a was found to be activated by Tax in an NF-κB-dependent manner (Pichler et al., 2008). Two potential NF-κB binding sites were identified in the miR-146a promoter. They found that the proximal NF-κB binding site on the *miR-146a* gene is responsible for transcriptional activation by Tax (Pichler et al., 2008). Recently, our group demonstrated that *miR-146a* gene expression is activated by Tax in NF-κB-dependent manner (Tomita et al., 2011). We found that the miR-146a promoter was highly bound by NF-κB complexes in HTLV-1-infected cells, while treatment with the NF-κB inhibitor Bay11-7082 reduced binding and interfered with expression of the miR-146a (Tomita et al., 2011). In contrast to Picheler's results, we observed binding between NF-κB protein and distal NF-κB binding site, not proximal one (Fig. 2). Moreover, we observed that miR-146a plays an important role in the growth of HTLV-1-infected T-cells (Tomita et al., 2011). Treatment of HTLV-1-infected cell lines with an anti-miR-146a inhibitor interfered with their growth and increased the expression levels of TRAF6, a predicted target for miR-146a. On the other hand, a growth-enhancing effect was observed in HTLV-1-infected cell line forced to overexpress miR-146a. These results suggest that miR-146a might be a good therapeutic target in ATLL.

Recently, Sasaki et al. demonstrated that ATLL cells showed a decreased level of miR-101 and miR-128a expression compared with the cells from HTLV-1 carriers (Sasaki et al., 2011). Moreover, there was a clear inverse correlation between *Enhancer of zeste homolog 2* (EZH2) expression and miR-101 expression or *EZH2* expression and miR-128a expression, suggesting that increased EZH2 is caused by the decrease in these miRNAs expression (Sasaki et al., 2011). EZH2 is a critical component of polycomb repressive complex 2 (PRC2), which mediates epigenetic gene silencing through trimethylation of H3K27 (Cao et al., 2002; Czermin et al., 2002). ATLL patients with high *EZH2* expression showed shorter survival than patients with low *EZH2* expression (Sasaki et al., 2011), indicating that increased EZH2 plays a role in the process of ATLL progression.

3.3 Sézary syndrome and mycosis fungoides

Sézary syndrome is a rare aggressive form of primary cutaneous T-cell lymphoma characterized by erythroderma, generalized lymphadenopathy, and the presence of neoplastic cerebriform nucleated $CD4^+$ T-cells (Sézary cells) in peripheral blood. Patients with Sézary syndrome have a high leukemic burden and a poor prognostic outcome, with an estimated 5-year survival of only 24% (Willemze et al., 2005). Mycosis fungoides, the most common cutaneous T-cell lymphoma, is a malignancy of mature, skin-homing T-cells. Sézary syndrome is often considered to represent a leukemic phase of mycosis fungoides. Recently, Ballabio et al. performed miRNA profile of $CD4^+$ T-cells from Sézary syndrome patients. They identified 114 miRNAs specifically expressed in Sézary syndrome (Ballabio et al., 2010). They demonstrated that levels of 4 microRNAs (miR-150, miR-191, miR-15a, and miR-16) correctly predicted diagnosis of Sézary syndrome with 100% accuracy, whereas miR-223 and miR-17-5p were 96% accurate. Further analysis revealed that levels of miR-223 distinguished Sézary syndrome samples from healthy controls and patients with mycosis fungoides in more than 90% of samples (Ballabio et al., 2010). miR-342 expression in Sézary syndrome was negatively regulated by miR-199a* expression. Transfection with either miR-342 or miR-199a* inhibitor resulted in a significant increase in levels of apoptosis of SeAx cells, suggesting that downregulation of miR-342 plays an important role in the pathogenesis of Sézary syndrome by inhibiting apoptosis (Ballabio et al., 2010). These data indicate that miRNAs are important in the pathogenesis of Sézary syndrome and provide possibilities for the diagnosis and treatment of this disease.

3.4 Anaplastic large-cell lymphoma

Anaplastic large cell lymphoma (ALCL) with anaplastic lymphoma kinase (ALK)-positive is a T-cell lymphoma consisting of lymphoid cells that are usually large with abundant cytoplasm and pleomorphic, often horseshoe-shaped nuclei, with *ALK* gene rearrangements. It tends to occur in children or young adults. The most commonly involved extranodal sites are skin, bone, soft tissues, lung and liver. The 5-year survival of ALCL with ALK-positive patients is about 70%, in contrast to ALCL with ALK-negative, which shows poor prognosis (Swerdlow et al., 2008). Recently, Merkel et al. demonstrated that five members of the miR-17–92 cluster were expressed more highly in ALCL with ALK-positive, whereas miR-155 was expressed more than 10-fold higher in ALCL with ALK-negative. Moreover, miR-101 was downregulated in all ALCL model systems, but forced expression of miR-101 attenuated cell proliferation only in ALK-positive and not in ALK-negative cell lines, suggesting different modes of ALK-dependent regulation of its target proteins (Merkel et al., 2010). For future therapeutical and diagnostic application, it will be interesting to study the physiological implications and prognostic value of the identified miRNA profiles.

4. Conclusion

Molecular targeting therapy based on miRNAs hold great promise for the development of more effective and less toxic personalized treatment strategies against cancer. Approach of targeting therapy needs deeper knowledge of the molecular changes that associate with development and progression of the diseases. The research on miRNAs is rapidly progressing from *in vitro* to *in vivo* and this becomes a powerful tool for molecular targeting therapy for human cancers. Although there is emerging evidence that miRNAs are involved in the pathogenesis of many cancers, including B-cell lymphomas, there are very little published data on the involvement of miRNAs in human T-cell leukemias/lymphomas that were discussed in this review. It is necessary to accumulate more molecular data that indicate association between miRNAs and T-cell leukemia/lymphoma.

5. Acknowledgment

I appreciate Dr. Shuji Tomita for valuable discussions and critical reading.

6. References

Ambros, V. (2000). Control of developmental timing in Caenorhabditis elegans. Current Opinion in Genetics & Development 10(4): 428-433.

Baldus, CD., Burmeister, T., Martus, P., Schwartz, S., Gokbuget, N., Bloomfield, CD., Hoelzer, D., Thiel, E. & Hofmann, WK. (2006). High expression of the ETS transcription factor ERG predicts adverse outcome in acute T-lymphoblastic leukemia in adults. Journal of Clinical Oncology 24(29): 4714-4720.

Ballabio, E., Mitchell, T., van Kester, MS., Taylor, S., Dunlop, HM., Chi, J., Tosi, I., Vermeer, MH., Tramonti, D., Saunders, NJ., Boultwood, J., Wainscoat, JS., Pezzella, F., Whittaker, SJ., Tensen, CP., Hatton, CS. & Lawrie, CH. (2010). MicroRNA expression in Sezary syndrome: identification, function, and diagnostic potential. Blood 116(7): 1105-1113.

Bartel, DP. (2004). MicroRNAs: Genomics, Biogenesis, Mechanism, and Function. Cell 116(2): 281-297.

Bellon, M., Lepelletier, Y., Hermine, O. & Nicot, C. (2009). Deregulation of microRNA involved in hematopoiesis and the immune response in HTLV-I adult T-cell leukemia. Blood 113(20): 4914-4917.

Bhatia, S., Kaul, D. & Varma, N. (2010). Potential tumor suppressive function of miR-196b in B-cell lineage acute lymphoblastic leukemia. Molecular and Cellular Biochemistry 340(1-2): 97-106.

Bhatia, S., Kaul, D. & Varma, N. (2011). Functional genomics of tumor suppressor miR-196b in T-cell acute lymphoblastic leukemia. Molecular and Cellular Biochemistry 346(1-2): 103-116.

Boxus, M., Twizere, J-C., Legros, S., Dewulf, J-F., Kettmann, R. & Willems, L. (2008). The HTLV-1 Tax interactome. Retrovirology 5(1): 76.

Calin, GA., Cimmino, A., Fabbri, M., Ferracin, M., Wojcik, SE., Shimizu, M., Taccioli, C., Zanesi, N., Garzon, R., Aqeilan, RI., Alder, H., Volinia, S., Rassenti, L., Liu, X., Liu, CG., Kipps, TJ., Negrini, M. & Croce, CM. (2008). MiR-15a and miR-16-1 cluster functions in human leukemia. Proceedings of the National Academy of Sciences the United States of America 105(13): 5166-5171.

Calin, GA., Dumitru, CD., Shimizu, M., Bichi, R., Zupo, S., Noch, E., Aldler, H., Rattan, S., Keating, M., Rai, K., Rassenti, L., Kipps, T., Negrini, M., Bullrich, F. & Croce, CM. (2002). Frequent deletions and down-regulation of micro- RNA genes miR15 and miR16 at 13q14 in chronic lymphocytic leukemia. Proceedings of the National Academy of Sciences the United States of America 99(24): 15524-15529.

Calin, GA., Ferracin, M., Cimmino, A., Di Leva, G., Shimizu, M., Wojcik, SE., Iorio, MV., Visone, R., Sever, NI., Fabbri, M., Iuliano, R., Palumbo, T., Pichiorri, F., Roldo, C., Garzon, R., Sevignani, C., Rassenti, L., Alder, H., Volinia, S., Liu, CG., Kipps, TJ., Negrini, M. & Croce, CM. (2005). A MicroRNA signature associated with prognosis and progression in chronic lymphocytic leukemia. New England Journal of Medicine 353(17): 1793-1801.

Cao, R., Wang, L., Wang, H., Xia, L., Erdjument-Bromage, H., Tempst, P., Jones, RS. & Zhang, Y. (2002). Role of histone H3 lysine 27 methylation in Polycomb-group silencing. Science 298(5595): 1039-1043.

Cimmino, A., Calin, GA., Fabbri, M., Iorio, MV., Ferracin, M., Shimizu, M., Wojcik, SE., Aqeilan, RI., Zupo, S., Dono, M., Rassenti, L., Alder, H., Volinia, S., Liu, C., Kipps, TJ., Negrini, M. & Croce, CM. (2005). miR-15 and miR-16 induce apoptosis by targeting BCL2. Proceedings of the National Academy of Sciences the United States of America 102(39): 13944-13949.

Copelan, EA. & McGuire, EA. (1995). The biology and treatment of acute lymphoblastic leukemia in adults. Blood 85(5): 1151-1168.

Coskun, E., von der Heide, EK., Schlee, C., Kuhnl, A., Gokbuget, N., Hoelzer, D., Hofmann, WK., Thiel, E. & Baldus, CD. (2011). The role of microRNA-196a and microRNA-

196b as ERG regulators in acute myeloid leukemia and acute T-lymphoblastic leukemia. Leukemia Research 35(2): 208-213.

Costinean, S., Sandhu, SK., Pedersen, IM., Tili, E., Trotta, R., Perrotti, D., Ciarlariello, D., Neviani, P., Harb, J., Kauffman, LR., Shidham, A. & Croce, CM. (2009). Src homology 2 domain-containing inositol-5-phosphatase and CCAAT enhancer-binding protein beta are targeted by miR-155 in B cells of Emicro-MiR-155 transgenic mice. Blood 114(7): 1374-1382.

Czermin, B., Melfi, R., McCabe, D., Seitz, V., Imhof, A. & Pirrotta, V. (2002). Drosophila enhancer of Zeste/ESC complexes have a histone H3 methyltransferase activity that marks chromosomal Polycomb sites. Cell 111(2): 185-196.

Ferrando, AA (2009). The role of NOTCH1 signaling in T-ALL. Hematology Am Soc Hematol Educ Program, United States.

Fulci, V., Colombo, T., Chiaretti, S., Messina, M., Citarella, F., Tavolaro, S., Guarini, A., Foa, R. & Macino, G. (2009). Characterization of B- and T-lineage acute lymphoblastic leukemia by integrated analysis of MicroRNA and mRNA expression profiles. Genes Chromosomes Cancer 48(12): 1069-1082.

Garzon, R., Volinia, S., Liu, CG., Fernandez-Cymering, C., Palumbo, T., Pichiorri, F., Fabbri, M., Coombes, K., Alder, H., Nakamura, T., Flomenberg, N., Marcucci, G., Calin, GA., Kornblau, SM., Kantarjian, H., Bloomfield, CD., Andreeff, M. & Croce, CM. (2008). MicroRNA signatures associated with cytogenetics and prognosis in acute myeloid leukemia. Blood 111(6): 3183-3189.

Greither, T., Grochola, LF., Udelnow, A., Lautenschlager, C., Wurl, P. & Taubert, H. (2010). Elevated expression of microRNAs 155, 203, 210 and 222 in pancreatic tumors is associated with poorer survival. International Journal of Cancer 126(1): 73-80.

He, L., Thomson, JM., Hemann, MT., Hernando-Monge, E., Mu, D., Goodson, S., Powers, S., Cordon-Cardo, C., Lowe, SW., Hannon, GJ. & Hammond, SM. (2005). A microRNA polycistron as a potential human oncogene. Nature 435(7043): 828-833.

Kim, VN. (2005). MicroRNA biogenesis: coordinated cropping and dicing. Nature Reviews Molecular Cell Biology 6(5): 376-385.

Kluiver, J., Poppema, S., de Jong, D., Blokzijl, T., Harms, G., Jacobs, S., Kroesen, BJ. & van den Berg, A. (2005). BIC and miR-155 are highly expressed in Hodgkin, primary mediastinal and diffuse large B cell lymphomas. Journal of Pathology 207(2): 243-249.

Lawrie, CH. (2008). MicroRNA expression in lymphoid malignancies: new hope for diagnosis and therapy? Journal of Cellular and Molecular Medicine 12(5A): 1432-1444.

Lee, RC., Feinbaum, RL. & Ambros, V. (1993). The C. elegans heterochronic gene lin-4 encodes small RNAs with antisense complementarity to lin-14. Cell 75(5): 843-854.

Lewis, BP., Shih, IH., Jones-Rhoades, MW., Bartel, DP. & Burge, CB. (2003). Prediction of mammalian microRNA targets. Cell 115(7): 787-798.

Loughran, SJ., Kruse, EA., Hacking, DF., de Graaf, CA., Hyland, CD., Willson, TA., Henley, KJ., Ellis, S., Voss, AK., Metcalf, D., Hilton, DJ., Alexander, WS. & Kile, BT. (2008). The transcription factor Erg is essential for definitive hematopoiesis and the function of adult hematopoietic stem cells. Nature Immunology 9(7): 810-819.

Lu, J., Getz, G., Miska, EA., Alvarez-Saavedra, E., Lamb, J., Peck, D., Sweet-Cordero, A., Ebert, BL., Mak, RH., Ferrando, AA., Downing, JR., Jacks, T., Horvitz, HR. & Golub, TR. (2005). MicroRNA expression profiles classify human cancers. Nature 435(7043): 834-838.

Marriott, SJ. & Semmes, OJ. (2005). Impact of HTLV-I Tax on cell cycle progression and the cellular DNA damage repair response. Oncogene 24(39): 5986-5995.

Martinez, J., Patkaniowska, A., Urlaub, H., Luhrmann, R. & Tuschl, T. (2002). Single-stranded antisense siRNAs guide target RNA cleavage in RNAi. Cell 110(5): 563-574.

Matsuoka, M. & Jeang, KT. (2007). Human T-cell leukaemia virus type 1 (HTLV-1) infectivity and cellular transformation. Nature Reviews Cancer 7(4): 270-280.

Mavrakis, KJ. & Wendel, HG. (2010). TargetScreen: An unbiased approach to identify functionally important microRNA targets. Cell Cycle 9(11).

Mavrakis, KJ., Wolfe, AL., Oricchio, E., Palomero, T., de Keersmaecker, K., McJunkin, K., Zuber, J., James, T., Khan, AA., Leslie, CS., Parker, JS., Paddison, PJ., Tam, W., Ferrando, A. & Wendel, HG. (2010). Genome-wide RNA-mediated interference screen identifies miR-19 targets in Notch-induced T-cell acute lymphoblastic leukaemia. Nature Cell Biology 12(4): 372-379.

Mendell, JT. (2008). miRiad roles for the miR-17-92 cluster in development and disease. Cell 133(2): 217-222.

Merkel, O., Hamacher, F., Laimer, D., Sifft, E., Trajanoski, Z., Scheideler, M., Egger, G., Hassler, MR., Thallinger, C., Schmatz, A., Turner, SD., Greil, R. & Kenner, L. (2010). Identification of differential and functionally active miRNAs in both anaplastic lymphoma kinase (ALK)+ and ALK- anaplastic large-cell lymphoma. Proceedings of the National Academy of Sciences the United States of America 107(37): 16228-16233.

Metzler, M., Wilda, M., Busch, K., Viehmann, S. & Borkhardt, A. (2004). High expression of precursor microRNA-155/BIC RNA in children with Burkitt lymphoma. Genes Chromosomes Cancer 39(2): 167-169.

Mu, P., Han, YC., Betel, D., Yao, E., Squatrito, M., Ogrodowski, P., de Stanchina, E., D'Andrea, A., Sander, C. & Ventura, A. (2009). Genetic dissection of the miR-17~92 cluster of microRNAs in Myc-induced B-cell lymphomas. Genes & Development 23(24): 2806-2811.

Nagel, S., Venturini, L., Przybylski, GK., Grabarczyk, P., Schmidt, CA., Meyer, C., Drexler, HG., Macleod, RA. & Scherr, M. (2009). Activation of miR-17-92 by NK-like homeodomain proteins suppresses apoptosis via reduction of E2F1 in T-cell acute lymphoblastic leukemia. Leukemia & Lymphoma 50(1): 101-108.

Okamura, S., Arakawa, H., Tanaka, T., Nakanishi, H., Ng, CC., Taya, Y., Monden, M. & Nakamura, Y. (2001). p53DINP1, a p53-inducible gene, regulates p53-dependent apoptosis. Molecular Cell 8(1): 85-94.

Pichler, K., Schneider, G. & Grassmann, R. (2008). MicroRNA miR-146a and further oncogenesis-related cellular microRNAs are dysregulated in HTLV-1-transformed T lymphocytes. Retrovirology 5: 100.

Pillai, RS., Bhattacharyya, SN. & Filipowicz, W. (2007). Repression of protein synthesis by miRNAs: how many mechanisms? Trends in Cell Biology 17(3): 118-126.

Pui, CH. & Evans, WE. (2006). Treatment of acute lymphoblastic leukemia. New England Journal of Medicine 354(2): 166-178.

Rodriguez, A., Griffiths-Jones, S., Ashurst, JL. & Bradley, A. (2004). Identification of mammalian microRNA host genes and transcription units. Genome Research 14(10A): 1902-1910.

Sasaki, D., Imaizumi, Y., Hasegawa, H., Osaka, A., Tsukasaki, K., Choi, YL., Mano, H., Marquez, VE., Hayashi, T., Yanagihara, K., Moriwaki, Y., Miyazaki, Y., Kamihira, S. & Yamada, Y. (2011). Overexpression of enhancer of zeste homolog 2 with trimethylation of lysine 27 on histone H3 in adult T-cell leukemia/lymphoma as a target for epigenetic therapy. Haematologica 96(5): 712-719.

Swerdlow, S., Campo, E., Harris, N., Jaffe, E., Pileri, S., Stein, H., Thiele, J. & Vardiman, J. (2008). WHO Classification of Tumours of Haematopoietic and Lymphoid Tissues, Fourth Edition. Lyon, IARC.

Tajima, K. (1990). The 4th nation-wide study of adult T-cell leukemia/lymphoma (ATL) in Japan: estimates of risk of ATL and its geographical and clinical features. The T- and B-cell Malignancy Study Group. International Journal of Cancer 45(2): 237-243.

Tomasini, R., Samir, AA., Carrier, A., Isnardon, D., Cecchinelli, B., Soddu, S., Malissen, B., Dagorn, JC., Iovanna, JL. & Dusetti, NJ. (2003). TP53INP1s and homeodomain-interacting protein kinase-2 (HIPK2) are partners in regulating p53 activity. Journal of Biological Chemistry 278(39): 37722-37729.

Tomasini, R., Samir, AA., Vaccaro, MI., Pebusque, MJ., Dagorn, JC., Iovanna, JL. & Dusetti, NJ. (2001). Molecular and functional characterization of the stress-induced protein (SIP) gene and its two transcripts generated by alternative splicing. SIP induced by stress and promotes cell death. Journal of Biological Chemistry 276(47): 44185-44192.

Tomita, M., Tanaka, Y. & Mori, N. (2011). MicroRNA miR-146a is induced by HTLV-1 tax and increases the growth of HTLV-1-infected T-cells. International Journal of Cancer 129(n/a).

Ventura, A., Young, AG., Winslow, MM., Lintault, L., Meissner, A., Erkeland, SJ., Newman, J., Bronson, RT., Crowley, D., Stone, JR., Jaenisch, R., Sharp, PA. & Jacks, T. (2008). Targeted deletion reveals essential and overlapping functions of the miR-17 through 92 family of miRNA clusters. Cell 132(5): 875-886.

Volinia, S., Calin, GA., Liu, CG., Ambs, S., Cimmino, A., Petrocca, F., Visone, R., Iorio, M., Roldo, C., Ferracin, M., Prueitt, RL., Yanaihara, N., Lanza, G., Scarpa, A., Vecchione, A., Negrini, M., Harris, CC. & Croce, CM. (2006). A microRNA expression signature of human solid tumors defines cancer gene targets. Proceedings of the National Academy of Sciences the United States of America 103(7): 2257-2261

Willemze, R., Jaffe, ES., Burg, G., Cerroni, L., Berti, E., Swerdlow, SH., Ralfkiaer, E., Chimenti, S., Diaz-Perez, JL., Duncan, LM., Grange, F., Harris, NL., Kempf, W., Kerl, H., Kurrer, M., Knobler, R., Pimpinelli, N., Sander, C., Santucci, M., Sterry, W., Vermeer, MH., Wechsler, J., Whittaker, S. & Meijer, CJ. (2005). WHO-EORTC classification for cutaneous lymphomas. Blood 105(10): 3768-3785.Xiao, C., Srinivasan, L., Calado, DP., Patterson, HC., Zhang, B., Wang, J., Henderson, JM., Kutok, JL. & Rajewsky, K. (2008). Lymphoproliferative disease and autoimmunity in mice with increased miR-17-92 expression in lymphocytes. Nature Immunology 9(4): 405-414.

Yamada, Y., Tomonaga, M., Fukuda, H., Hanada, S., Utsunomiya, A., Tara, M., Sano, M., Ikeda, S., Takatsuki, K., Kozuru, M., Araki, K., Kawano, F., Niimi, M., Tobinai, K., Hotta, T. & Shimoyama, M. (2001). A new G-CSF-supported combination chemotherapy, LSG15, for adult T-cell leukaemia-lymphoma: Japan Clinical Oncology Group Study 9303. British Journal of Haematology 113(2): 375-382.

Yeung, ML., Yasunaga, J., Bennasser, Y., Dusetti, N., Harris, D., Ahmad, N., Matsuoka, M. & Jeang, KT. (2008). Roles for microRNAs, miR-93 and miR-130b, and tumor protein 53-induced nuclear protein 1 tumor suppressor in cell growth dysregulation by human T-cell lymphotrophic virus 1. Cancer Research 68(21): 8976-8985.

10

Mechanisms of Humoral Hypercalcemia of Malignancy in Leukemia/Lymphoma

Sherry T. Shu, Wessel P. Dirksen,
Katherine N. Weibaecher and Thomas J. Rosol
Ohio State University and Washington University (KNW)
United States of America

1. Introduction

Hypercalcemia is one of the most common paraneoplastic syndromes. The incidence of hypercalcemia is 50-90% in adult T-cell leukemia/lymphoma (ATLL), 27-35% in lung cancer, 25-30% in breast cancer, 7-30% in multiple myeloma, and less than 10% in other types of cancer patients (Mundy & Martin, 1982; Roodman, 1997). Patients with severe hypercalcemia (>12 mg/dL; > 6.0 mM) usually develop neuromuscular, gastrointestinal and renal symptoms including lethargy, depression, anorexia, nausea, vomiting, polyuria and polydipsia. Patients with serum calcium concentrations >15 mg/dL (7.6 mM) can develop renal failure or cardiovascular abnormalities with arrhythmias and coma (Mundy & Martin, 1982). Depending on the sources of the stimulating factors, hypercalcemia in cancer can be divided into 3 types: (1) humoral hypercalcemia of malignancy (HHM) in which humoral factors secreted by tumor cells directly or indirectly affect cells in the target organs including bone, kidney and intestine that regulate calcium homeostasis; (2) local osteolytic hypercalcemia in which factors secreted by either primary or metastatic tumor cells locally in the bone microenvironment stimulate osteoclastic bone resorption; and (3) primary hyperparathyroidism that coexists with the malignancy (Stewart, 2005). This review will focus on HHM, although some types of cancers may induce both HHM and local osteolytic hypercalcemia, since several factors can function both systemically and locally.

2. Overview of humoral hypercalcemia of malignancy

Humoral hypercalcemia of malignancy (HHM) is characterized by (1) circulating humoral factors derived from cancer cells; (2) uncoupling of bone formation and bone resorption; (3) increased renal calcium reabsorption even though there is hypercalciuria caused by increased Ca^{2+} in the glomerular filtrate. In contrast to HHM in primary hyperparathyroidism, bone formation and resorption are both increased resulting in fibrous osteodystrophy in patients with longstanding disease.

HHM is a common complication of certain lymphoma/leukemias; squamous cell carcinomas (e.g., of the lung or other organs); renal and breast carcinomas, and occasionally other tumors (Stewart, 2002). Factors secreted by the cancer cells (see Table 1 below) stimulate osteoclastic bone resorption (directly or indirectly through osteoblasts) by increasing the activity and/or survival of osteoclast precursors or mature osteoclasts. Most cancer-derived hypercalcemic factors stimulate osteoclastic bone resorption indirectly by inducing osteoclast-stimulating factors from osteoblasts or bone stromal cells. Under normal physiological conditions, increased serum calcium concentration can be compensated for by decreasing the intestinal calcium absorption, increasing renal calcium excretion, decreasing PTH secretion from the parathyroid glands, and decreasing bone resorption. However, secretion of the cancer-related factor, parathyroid hormone-related protein (PTHrP), also increases renal calcium reabsorption in the kidney through the activation of parathyroid hormone receptor 1 (PTH1R), which facilitates the development of HHM.

Factors	Origin	Target cells/molecule	Function in bone
PTHrP	Cancer cells	Osteoblast	Catabolic and anabolic
RANKL	Osteoblast, cancer cells	Osteoclast	Catabolic
OPG	Osteoblast	RANKL	Inhibit RANKL
MIP-1α	Cancer cells	Osteoblast	Catabolic
Calcitriol	Kidney, cancer cells, tumor-associated macrophages	Intestines, kidney, osteoclast, osteoblast, parathyroid chief cells	Increases calcium in blood
TNF-α, IL-1, IL-6, IL-17	T-cells	Osteoclast	Catabolic
OPG, IL-3, IL-4, IL-10, IL-13, IFN-β, IFN-γ, GM-CSF, and sFRPs	T-cells	Osteoclast	Inhibit osteoclast formation and/or function
Calcium (Ca^{+2})	Bone Kidney Intestinal tract	Calcium-sensing receptor (CaR) on bone and cancer cells and parathyroid chief cells	Anabolic (bone cells) Catabolic (cancer cells) Decreases PTH secretion

Table 1. Factors associated with HHM that cause bone formation (anabolic action) or resorption (catabolic action) in bone.

3. Factors involved in the pathogenesis of HHM

3.1 Parathyroid hormone-related protein (PTHrP)

PTHrP was first cloned by Suva et al. (Suva et al., 1987) and purified by Broadus et al. (Broadus et al., 1988). PTHrP is widely expressed in normal tissues and functions as an endocrine, autocrine, paracrine and intracrine hormone. PTHrP is a polyhormone that results from alternative mRNA splicing and post-translational proteolytic processing. During development, PTHrP is essential for the growth and regulation of endochondral bone (Karaplis et al., 1994; Wysolmerski et al., 1998), epithelial-mesenchymal interactions in mammary gland (Wysolmerski et al., 1998), and has important functions in many other tissues. PTHrP knockout mice die soon after birth due to asphyxia caused by developmental abnormalities of bones in the thorax (Karaplis et al., 1994). PTHrP has been shown to be the principal factor in most cases of cancer-induced HHM. The expression of PTHrP is up-

regulated by NF-κB, TGF-β, and/or Ras-MAPK signaling (Nadella et al., 2007; Richard et al., 2005). In adult T-cell leukemia/lymphoma, the promoter of PTHrP can be activated by the binding of HTLV-1 oncoprotein, Tax (Ejima et al., 1993; Watanabe et al., 1990).
The functions of PTHrP depend on the activation of different signal transduction pathways, including cyclic adenosine monophosphate/protein kinase A (cAMP/PKA) and protein lipase C/protein kinase C (PLC/PKC) cascades. In addition, PTHrP fragments have different functions that depend on the tissue-specific expression of distinct receptors. Activation of the cAMP-PKA pathway is required for PTHrP to induce bone resorption through the PTH1R, which recognizes both PTH and PTHrP (Greenfield et al., 1995).
Besides the catabolic effect of PTHrP on bone, intermittent administration or pulsatile secretion of the N-terminal fragment of PTH (1-34) and PTHrP (1-36) by a neuroendocrine tumor, such as islet cell carcinoma, can induce bone anabolic effects (Takeuchi et al., 2002). When osteoblastic cells were transiently exposed to the C-terminus of PTHrP (107-139), anabolic effects were induced by the upregulation of vascular endothelial growth factor receptor 2 (VEGFR2) through PKC/ERK activation (de Gortazar et al., 2006).

3.2 Receptor activator of nuclear kappa-B ligand (RANKL) and osteoprotegerin (OPG)

RANKL belongs to the tumor necrosis factor (TNF) family and represents one of the most common mediators for inducing osteoclastic bone resorption. Mature osteoblasts produce two forms of RANKL, a membrane-bound and secreted form. Both are important for osteoclast stimulation (Leibbrandt & Penninger, 2008). The expression of RANKL in osteoblasts and stromal cells is activated by the RUNX2 transcriptional factor under the regulation of PTHrP, 1,25-dihydroxyvitamin D_3, and prostaglandins (Lipton et al., 2009). RANKL binds and activates its receptor, RANK, which is expressed on the surface of osteoclasts. The binding of RANKL to RANK activates at least three major signaling pathways, NFAT, p38 and JNK, resulting in up-regulation of genes that are required for induction of osteoclast fusion, differentiation, activation and survival (Leibbrandt & Penninger, 2008). The secreted form of RANKL is important for the recruitment of osteoclast precursors and osteoclastogenesis. RANKL is an essential activator for normal bone remodeling. RANKL knockout mice have severe osteopetrosis (Lomaga et al., 1999).
OPG, or osteoclastogenesis inhibitory factor (OCIF), is a secreted member of the tumor necrosis receptor superfamily that is expressed by osteoblasts and functions as a RANKL 'decoy receptor' (Simonet et al., 1997). OPG binds to RANKL and blocks its interaction with RANK on osteoclast precursors (Lacey et al., 1998); therefore, it is a potent inhibitor of osteoclast formation and bone resorption. OPG knockout mice have early-onset osteopenia (Bucay et al., 1998; Mizuno et al., 1998), whereas OPG overexpressing mice develop osteopetrosis that results from the failure to form osteoclasts (Simonet et al., 1997). PTH and PTHrP suppress OPG expression by downregulating the promoter of OPG through activation of the cAMP/PKA pathway (Yang et al., 2002). PTHrP, on the other hand, stimulates RANKL expression to induce bone resorption. The ratio between RANKL and OPG levels in osteoblasts is a key factor in the regulation of osteoclast activity (Horwood et al., 1998).
In ATLL, the expression of RANKL in tumor cells correlated with hypercalcemia in patients. RANKL on the surface of leukemia cells induced osteoclastogenesis through direct contact with precursor cells (Nosaka et al., 2002). The direct activation of osteoclasts by tumor cells may play a key role in the decoupling of bone formation and bone resorption in HMM.

Therefore, RANKL from either osteoblasts or tumor cells is an important mediator of bone resorption in many forms of HHM.

3.3 Cytokines

The increased secretion of inflammatory cytokines from cancer cells, such as tumor necrosis factor-α (TNF-α), IL-1, IL-6, IL-8, M-CSF, CCL2 and CXCL12, is one of the key mechanisms by which NF-κB is constitutively activated in tumor cells (Lu & Stark, 2004). The proinflammatory cytokine, TNF-α, is a critical factor in the pathogenesis of many inflammatory and non-inflammatory diseases which are characterized by increased osteoclastic bone resorption including rheumatoid arthritis (Chu et al., 1991), osteoporosis (Horowitz, 1993), osteomyelitis (Meghji et al., 1998) and aseptic loosening (an osteolysis syndrome caused by macrophages in joint replacements) (Merkel et al., 1999). TNF-α mediates lipopolysaccharide-stimulated osteoclastogenesis through the p55 receptor expressed on bone marrow macrophages and activation of NF-κB (Abu-Amer et al., 1997; Abu-Amer et al., 1998). Whether osteoclastogenesis induced by TNF-α depends on RANKL or not remains controversial. Some studies have shown that without exogenous RANKL, TNF-α is sufficient to induce osteoclast differentiation (Kudo et al., 2002), and the increase of osteoclastogenesis was inhibited by OPG (Hounoki et al., 2008). However, Boyle et al. have shown that administration of TNF-α to RANK-deficient mice failed to induce osteoclastogenesis and restore hypocalcemia, suggesting that TNF-α cannot substitute for RANKL (Li et al., 2000). Teitelbaum et al. have reported that TNF-α alone was not able to induce osteoclastogenesis in murine osteoclast precursors; rather, RANKL was required for TNF-α to stimulate osteoclast precursors to form osteoclasts (Lam et al., 2000). Regardless, TNF-α has shown its potential to be a therapeutic target for bone resorption. Increased TNF-α levels have been found in patients with advanced chronic lymphocytic leukemia (CLL) and acute nonlymphocytic leukemia with HHM (Ferrajoli et al., 2002).

Increased plasma IL-6 has been found in cancer patients with HHM, including patients with multiple myeloma, squamous cell carcinoma of the liver, acute nonlymphocytic leukemia, and adult T-cell leukemia/lymphoma (Asanuma et al., 2002; Kounami et al., 2004; Roodman, 1997). IL-6 increases osteoclast recruitment by binding to its receptor on osteoblasts and inducing the signal of transducer and activator of transcription (STAT)-1/3 and mitogen-activated protein kinase (MAPK) signaling pathways (Sims et al., 2004). It also enhances the effects of PTH and PTHrP and mediates the effects of inflammatory cytokines, such as IL-1 and TNF-α, on osteoclast formation (Roodman, 2001). IL-6 does not directly increase RANKL expression; therefore, its osteoclastogenic effect is RANKL-independent (Hofbauer et al., 2000). However, there is no correlation between serum IL-6 and HHM in cancer patients, suggesting that IL-6 functions additively or synergistically with other factors and may be a redundant factor for development of HHM (Vanderschueren et al., 1994).

Granulocyte macrophage-colony stimulating factor (GM-CSF) also plays a role in osteoclastogenesis and it has two distinct effects on osteoclast activity depending upon the presence of RANKL. GM-CSF increases the proliferation of osteoclast progenitors when RANKL is absent. On the other hand, it induces osteoclast progenitors to differentiate into dendritic cells when RANKL is present (Gillespie, 2007).

Macrophage colony-stimulating factor (M-CSF) is essential for osteoclast differentiation and proliferation of osteoclast progenitor cells (Tanaka et al., 1993). Increased serum M-CSF concentration has been reported in acute nonlymphocytic leukemia patients with HHM (Kounami et al., 2004).

Interferon (IFN)-γ disrupts JAK/STAT signaling in osteoblasts to induce the expression of OPG and Wnt, causing decreased cathepsin K and tartrate-resistant acid phosphatase (TRAP) in mature osteoclasts (Gallo et al., 2008; Gillespie, 2007). Transgenic mice with the HTLV-1 viral oncoprotein, Tax, and knockout of IFN-γ developed more severe osteolytic bone lesions and increased osteoclast activity. Administration of IFN-γ to mice transplanted with Tax-positive tumors inhibited tumor growth and decreased hypercalcemia, suggesting a protective role for IFN-γ in HHM development (Xu and Hurchla et al., 2009).

Cytokines have been shown to play a more important role in the pathogenesis of HHM in patients with lymphoma and leukemia compared to patients with carcinoma. However, further investigation is needed to clarify the additive and synergistic roles of cytokines in causing hypercalcemia because multiple cytokines are often produced by the tumor cells.

3.4 Macrophage inflammatory protein-1 alpha (MIP-1α)

MIP-1α is a pro-inflammatory chemokine expressed by many different cell types including macrophages, dendritic cells and lymphocytes. It normally functions as a chemoattractant for T-cells, macrophages, and other proinflammatory cells at the site of inflammation. It also regulates the transendothelial migration of NK cells, monocytes and dendritic cells (Maurer & von, 2004). Therefore, it plays an important role in autoimmune and inflammatory diseases, such as multiple sclerosis, rheumatoid arthritis, asthma, and organ transplant rejection (Maurer & von, 2004). MIP-1α binds to several chemokine (c-c motif) G-protein-coupled receptors including CCR1, CCR5 and CCR9, which are expressed in lymphocytes and monocytes/macrophages. It activates several signaling pathways, including PI3K, PLC, PKC, MAP kinase and JAK/STAT pathways (Tsubaki et al., 2007). MIP-1α can potently inhibit the binding of HIV to CCR5 on macrophages (Baba et al., 1999; Maurer & von, 2004).

Both CCR1 and CCR5 are expressed in bone marrow stromal cells. MIP-1α is chemotactic for osteoclasts and osteoclast precursors (Fuller et al., 1995). MIP-1α was first identified as a putative osteoclastogenic factor in a human myeloma cDNA expression library derived from marrow samples of myeloma patients (Zlotnik & Yoshie, 2000). Subsequently, CCR1 and CCR5 expression was demonstrated in human and murine multiple myeloma cell lines (Menu et al., 2006). Furthermore, MIP-1α enhances osteoclast formation induced by IL-6, PTHrP and RANKL in multiple myeloma (Han et al., 2001) and increases adhesion of myeloma cells to bone marrow cells through its binding to both CCR1 and CCR5 receptors (Oba et al., 2005). *In vivo,* mice bearing Chinese hamster ovary cells that overexpress MIP-1α develop more severe osteolytic lesions after intramuscular inoculation (Oyajobi et al., 2003).

The mechanisms by which MIP-1α induces osteoclastic bone resorption are controversial. One study demonstrated that a RANKL-dependent pathway was responsible for activation of osteoclasts (Tsubaki et al., 2007). MIP-1α enhances RANKL expression in mouse bone marrow stromal cells and osteoblasts through the MAPK and PI3K/Akt signaling pathways. On the other hand, RANK-Fc did not block the activation of osteoclasts by MIP-1α, indicating that MIP-1α used a RANKL-independent pathway to increase bone resorption (Han et al., 2001). Therefore, it has been suggested that MIP-1α is a RANKL-independent osteoclastogenic factor that acts directly on osteoclast precursors (Choi et al., 2000). In any case, it is apparent that MIP-1α is a significant osteoclast activator. The role of MIP-1α in

HHM is highlighted by the fact that HTLV-1 infected T-cells express and secrete MIP-1α (Shu et al., 2007; Shu et al., 2010), and the increased serum levels of MIP-1α correlated well with the development of HHM in HTLV-1-infected patients (Okada et al., 2004).

3.5 1α,25-Dihydroxyvitamin D (Calcitriol)

Vitamin D is an essential hormone for calcium homeostasis. Its active form, 1α,25-dihydroxyvitamin D_3 or calcitriol, is synthesized by hydroxylation of vitamin D in the kidney. The renal 25-hydroxyvitamin D 1-α hydroxylase is the rate limiting enzyme for production of calcitriol. Calcitriol increases calcium absorption from the intestinal tract, increases osteoclastic bone resorption, and decreases PTH gene expression in the parathyroid glands (Guise et al., 2005). Calcitriol is an uncommon primary cause of HHM in patients with leukemia or lymphoma even though serum calcitriol concentrations may be increased in up to 50% of patients (Seymour & Gagel, 1993). Some lymphomas or tumor-associated macrophages express 25-hydroxyvitamin D 1-α hydroxylase, which is responsible for the increased production of calcitriol (Hewison et al., 2003).

3.6 Cell membrane calcium-sensing receptor (CaR)

CaR is expressed on multiple cell types including the chief cells of the parathyroid gland where it regulates PTH expression and secretion. Under normal conditions, CaR, a G protein-coupled receptor, senses extracellular calcium concentrations and activates downstream signaling pathways, such as the PLC/inositol trisphosphate (IP3) and ERK1/2 pathways, in a tissue-specific manner (Saidak et al., 2009). In bone, CaR is expressed in osteoblasts, osteoclasts, stromal cells, monocytes-macrophages, and chondrocytes. CaR promotes osteoblast proliferation, differentiation and mineralization (Sharan et al., 2008). It also mediates osteoclast differentiation and apoptosis. Therefore, CaR in bone cells promotes the bone formation phase of bone remodeling (Yamaguchi, 2008). CaR is also expressed in some cancer cells, such as breast and prostate cancers (Liao et al., 2006). However, in these cells, increased extracellular calcium leads to increased PTHrP expression (Chattopadhyay, 2006). Increased PTHrP induces osteoclastic bone resorption and renal calcium reabsorption, resulting in HHM. The positive feedback loop formed by PTHrP, calcium and CaR is a unique phenomena in HHM. In addition to the specific activation of PTHrP expression, gain-of-function mutations in CaR have been demonstrated in breast cancer. Lorch *et al.* have found single nucleotide polymorphisms in CaR in human lung squamous cell carcinoma (Lorch et al., 2011). Functional evaluation of a nonconservative amino acid substitution (R990G) in CaR induced HHM in patients with lung squamous cell carcinoma. Dysregulation of PTHrP expression and HHM caused by CaR signaling has been demonstrated in breast and prostate cancer (Saidak et al., 2009). However, the role of CaR in HHM induced by lymphoma/leukemia remains to be determined.

3.7 Role of T cells in calcium homeostasis

The skeletal and immune systems share many regulatory molecules and systems. An interdisciplinary research area called "Osteoimmunology" has been developed recently to understand the interplay between these two systems. Cytokines, receptors, signaling molecules and transcriptional factors, and their signaling pathways are comprehensively reviewed by Takayanagi (Takayanagi, 2007). T-cells have both pro- and antiresorptive effects on osteoclasts. The proresorptive effect is present in osteoclast-stimulating T-cells, which secrete a soluble form of RANKL. TNF-α is also expressed by activated T-cells to act in concert with RANKL. IL-1, IL-6 and IL-17 secreted from T-cells increase RANKL expression in osteoblasts. This mechanism is important for rheumatoid arthritis where TH17 cells have been shown to be an immunomodulator of osteoclastic bone resorption (Sato et al., 2006). In addition, T-cells produce IL-7 which increase bone resorption in a RANKL-independent mechanism (Weitzmann & Pacifici, 2005). T-cells also play a major role in postmenopausal osteoporosis induced by decreased estrogen levels and decreased transforming growth factor (TGF)-β expression in bone cells (Gillespie, 2007).

In contrast, T-cells can also exert an antiresorptive effect directly by secreting OPG, IL-3, IL-4, IL-10, IL-13, IFN-β, IFN-γ, GM-CSF, and secreted frizzled-related proteins (sFRPs) to inhibit osteoclastogenesis (Quinn & Gillespie, 2005). In addition, T-cells can inhibit osteoclast formation and activity indirectly by expressing GM-CSF (induced by the upregulation of IL-18 in bone microenvironment), IFN-γ (by IL-12) and OPG (by leptin) (Horwood et al., 2001). It will be important to understand the effects of T-cells on osteoblast and stromal cell function, as well as signaling in the immune response to further understand the interactions between the immune system and bone biology.

4. HHM in leukemia/lymphoma in humans and animals

4.1 Adult T-cell leukemia lymphoma (ATLL)

50-90% of ATLL patients develop HHM and osteolytic lesions in the long bones and calvaria (Olivo et al., 2008). Bone resorption may act as a 'vicious cycle' for ATLL growth in bone, since factors released by resorbing bone increased the growth of ATLL and HTLV-1-infected T-cells *in vitro* (Shu et al., 2010). The mechanisms by which HTLV-1 induces HHM are not completely known. We and others have demonstrated that ATLL primary cell lines (T-cell lines derived from leukemic ATLL patients) and *in vitro* HTLV-1 transformed T-cell lines express and secrete PTHrP, particularly transcripts from the P3 promoter (Nadella et al., 2007; Richard et al., 2005; Shu et al., 2010) (Figure 1). The expression of PTHrP was upregulated by both oncoviral protein Tax-dependent and -independent pathways. Tax cooperates with Ets to activate the P3 promoter of PTHrP, while constitutive activation of NF-κB in ATLL cells contributes to expression of the PTHrP P2 promoter (Nadella et al., 2007; Richard et al., 2005). Despite the essential role of PTHrP in HHM in carcinomas (such as lung, breast and prostate cancers), the correlation between the plasma PTHrP and HHM in ATLL patients has been controversial. It has been concluded that PTHrP is not the sole factor that induces HHM in ATLL, but it likely plays an important cooperative or synergistic role with other humoral factors (Figure 1).

In ATLL, there were increased plasma MIP-1α concentrations in mice with human ATLL cells and HHM (Shu et al., 2007). In a human clinical study, plasma MIP-1α concentrations had a strong correlation with HHM in ATLL patients (Okada et al., 2004). MIP-1α expression in ATLL cells is induced by Tax and increased plasma calcium concentrations may further up-regulate MIP-1α expression through the calmodulin-dependent protein kinase kinase (CaM-KK) cascade (Matsumoto et al., 2008; Sharma & May, 1999). Treatment with a neutralizing MIP-1α antibody decreased osteoclast formation induced by ATLL cells *in vitro* (Okada et al., 2004).

The increase in RANKL expression observed in the ATL leukemic cells has been shown to correlate with the occurrence of HHM in ATLL patients (Nosaka et al., 2002). Although the levels of RANKL expression were not high in HTLV-1-infected cell lines *in vitro* (Shu et al.,

2010), leukemic cells isolated from ATLL patients did have up-regulation of RANKL expression (Nosaka et al., 2002). In addition, HTLV-1 infected leukocytes *in vitro* were able to convert 25-dihydroxyvitamin D_3 to its active form, 1α,25-dihydroxyvitamin D_3 or calcitriol (Fetchick et al., 1986). High levels of calcitriol have been found in ATLL patients with hypercalcemia (Johnston & Hammond, 1992; Seymour & Gagel, 1993)

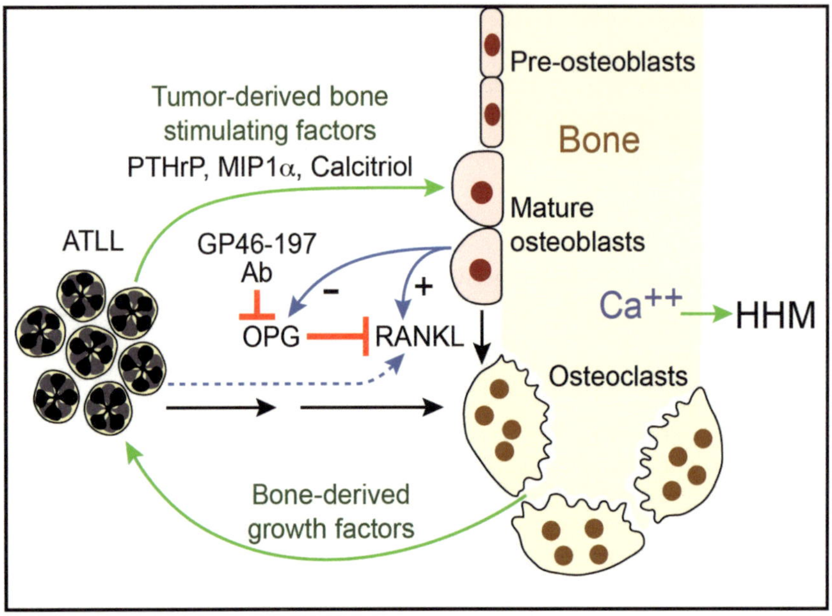

Fig. 1. HHM in ATLL is caused by increased osteoclastic bone resorption. Cancer cells secrete bone regulatory factors, including PTHrP, MIP-1α, calcitriol, and RANKL to increase osteoclast activity. The resorbing bone secretes bone-derived growth factors that increase ATLL cell growth. In osteoblasts, the RANKL/OPG expression ratio increases when cells are co-cultured with T-cell leukemia lines. Antibodies against HTLV-1 Gp46 can inhibit OPG and contributes to the pathogenesis of hypercalcemia.

In addition to the direct effects of factors secreted from ATLL cells on osteoclasts, we recently found decreased OPG expression and secretion in osteoblasts that were co-cultured with leukemic T-cell lines (Shu et al., 2010). This suggests that the regulation of gene expression in osteoblasts by leukemic T-cells plays an indirect role in HHM in ATLL.

Finally, an endogenous antibody recognizing the HTLV-1 viral envelope protein Gp46-197 can occur in ATLL patients, which correlated with disease progression. The amino acid sequence of Gp46-197 is homologous with the C-terminus of OPG. Rabbits immunized with the Gp46-197 peptide developed hypercalcemia and died. Sprague-Dawley rats injected with Gp46-197 peptide developed decreased bone mineral density and hypercalcemia. Administration of recombinant human OPG restored femoral bone growth. These data suggest that HTLV-1 Gp46 contributes to the pathogenesis of hypercalcemia due to cross-reactive antibodies in the patients that antagonize the action of OPG (Sagara et al., 2009).

Other factors proposed to be humoral factors for HHM in ATLL include TNF-β (lymphotoxin) (Ishibashi et al., 1992), IL-6 (Chiba et al., 2009), and IL-1 (Wano et al., 1987).

4.2 Other leukemias/lymphomas that develop HHM (Table 2)

4.2.1 De novo acute nonlymphocytic leukemia (ANLL)

Hypercalcemia in de novo ANLL patients can be caused by either local osteolytic hypercalcemia or HHM. Elevated circulating concentrations of several humoral factors, including PTHrP, TNF-α, IL-6, and M-CSF, in de novo ANLL patients with HHM have been reported supporting a role for HHM in ANLL (Kounami et al., 2004). Generalized osteoporosis with normal renal function was observed in these patients, indicating that the increased calcium was mainly from bone.

Cancer Type	Incidence of HHM	Humoral factor(s)
ATLL	50-90%	PTHrP, MIP-1α, RANKL, IL-1, TNF-β, IL-6
Diffuse large B cell lymphoma	Rare	PTHrP, IL-6, 1,25-dihydroxyvitamin D
Acute nonlymphocytic leukemia	Rare	PTHrP, IL-6, TNF-α, M-CSF
Primary cutaneous B-cell lymphoma	Rare	1,25-dihydroxyvitamin D
Canine T-cell lymphoma	40% in mediastinal lymphoma; 10-20% in multicentric lymphoma	PTHrP, 1,25-dihydroxyvitamin D
Feline lymphoma	Has been reported	PTHrP
Feline leukemia virus associated leukemia/lymphoma	Has been reported	Unknown
Avain malignant lymphoma	Has been reported	Unknown

Table 2. Incidence and humoral factors of HHM in leukemia/lymphoma in humans and animals. Other undefined factors or cytokines may also be involved.

4.2.2 Diffuse large B-cell lymphoma

Increased PTHrP, IL-6, and 1,25-dihydroxyvitamin D concentrations have been reported in the serum from patients with diffuse large B cell lymphoma that developed hypercalcemia (Amezyane et al., 2008; Chang et al., 2008). Diffuse osteolytic lesions and nephrocalcinosis also occurred in these patients.

4.2.3 Primary cutaneous B-cell lymphoma

Hypercalcemia has been reported in patients with primary cutaneous B-cell lymphoma (Habra et al., 2007; Narimatsu et al., 2003). Increased serum 1,25-dihydroxyvitamin D and undetectable PTH and PTHrP levels were found in one patient. The pathogenesis of hypercalcemia in these patients has not been determined.

4.2.4 HHM in animals with leukemia/lymphoma

HHM occurs in 10-40% of dogs with T-cell lymphoma (Fournel-Fleury et al., 2002). Increased circulating PTHrP and 1,25-dihydroxyvitamin D were found in dogs with lymphoma and HHM, but the serum concentrations did not always correlate with hypercalcemia. Therefore, it was speculated that additional cytokines are involved in the pathogenesis of HHM in dogs with lymphoma (Mellanby et al., 2006; Rosol et al., 1992). In a xenograft mouse model of canine lymphoma, there was increased expression of TNF-α in the tumor *in vivo* (Nadella et al., 2008). Bone histomorphometry indicated that increased osteoclastic bone resorption was the major cause of HHM in these mice. Increased circulating PTHrP has also been reported in cats with lymphoma and HHM (Bolliger et al., 2002). Cats may also develop HHM due to unknown humoral factors induced by feline leukemia virus infection (Engelman et al., 1985). Hypercalcemia has also been reported in an Amazon parrot with lymphoma (de Wit et al., 2003).

5. Therapy of HHM in leukemia/lymphoma

For urgent care, saline hydration is the first step to correct hypercalcemia by diluting the serum calcium concentration and increasing the clearance of calcium by the kidneys. Treatment of the underlying leukemia/lymphoma, including chemotherapy and radiation therapy, is necessary. Several drugs have been used for long-term management of hypercalcemia associated with HHM.

5.1 Bisphosphonates

Bisphosphonates are structural analogs of pyrophosphoric acid and have been widely used to treat cancer patients with hypercalcemia, heritable skeletal disorders in children, and postmenopausal and glucocorticoid-induced osteoporosis patients with significant bone loss (Fleisch, 1997). Intravenous aminobisphosphonates are a standard of care for the treatment of HHM. The newest generation of bisphosphonates, nitrogen-containing aminobisphosphonates, inhibits farnesyl pyrophosphate (FPP) and geranylgeranyl pyrophosphate (GGPP) synthetases in the mevalonic acid metabolic pathway resulting in decreased prenylation of low-molecular-weight G proteins including Ras. Functional Ras signaling is necessary for osteoclast activity and survival (Fleisch, 1998). It also has been suggested that bisphosphonates exert a cytotoxic effect on HTLV-1-infected T-cells. However, high doses of bisphosphonates were needed for cytotoxic effects *in vitro* and *in vivo* (Gao et al, 2005; Ishikawa et al., 2007; Shu et al., 2007; Hirbe et al., 2009). The clinical relevance of a direct effect of bisphosphonates on ATLL cells needs to be further evaluated. Bisphosphonates have a high affinity for bone mineral and bind to hydroxyapatite crystals *in vivo*. Therefore, bisphosphonates are rapidly depleted from the circulation and extracellular fluid and become highly concentrated in bone. Bisphosphonate therapy may have complications including hypocalcemia, osteonecrosis of the jaw, low bone turnover with pathologic fractures, and increased incidence of atrial fibrillation (Drake et al., 2008). In addition to the effects on osteoclasts, a new bisphosphonate, YM527/ONO-5920, decreased MIP-1α expression and secretion through inhibition of the transient increase of phosphorylated ERK1/2 and Akt in mouse myeloma cells after lipopolysaccharide (LPS) stimulation (Drake & Rajkumar, 2009). Since MIP-1α has been shown to play an important role in cancer cell growth and osteolysis in multiple myeloma, bisphosphonates may be useful for inhibiting the growth of myeloma cells and to prevent osteolysis by decreasing MIP-1α expression. This may also apply to ATLL. Commonly used bisphosphonates include pamidronate and zoledronic acid.

5.2 Calcitonin

Calcitonin is a 32-amino acid peptide secreted by thyroid C-cells. It inhibits calcium absorption in the intestine and reabsorption of calcium and phosphate in renal tubules. It is a potent (but transient) inhibitor of osteoclastic bone resorption. The mechanisms of action have been shown to involve several signaling pathways including cAMP/PKA, PKC, and pyk2/src activity. It has also been shown that calcitonin up-regulates renal 1α-hydroxylase, an important enzyme for the synthesis of calcitriol, through the binding of C/EBPβ and brahma-related gene 1 (BRG1), an ATPase in the SWItch/Sucrose NonFermentable (SWI/SNF) chromatin remodeling complex, on the 1α-hydroxylase promoter (Zhong et al., 2009). Because of its potent inhibitory effect on bone resorption, calcitonin has clinical applications in the treatment of Paget's disease, osteoporosis, and hypercalcemia. However, due to its short duration of action, calcitonin may not be suitable for treatment of chronic hypercalcemia. Salmon calcitonin is used clinically due to its greater potency compared to human calcitonin (Zaidi et al., 2002).

5.3 Corticosteroids

Corticosteroids have been used for the treatment of hypercalcemia induced by multiple myeloma and certain types of lymphoma. Corticosteroids act by decreasing calcium absorption in gastrointestinal tract, decreasing bone resorption, and increasing renal calcium excretion (Unal et al., 2008; Yarbro et al., 2003). Corticosteroids generally are not effective in patients with HHM induced by solid tumors.

5.4 Bortezomib (PS-341)

Bortezomib is a selective proteasome inhibitor that decreases the ubiquination of IκB, the inhibitor for NF-κB, thereby stabilizing IκB and inhibiting NF-κB. NF-κB is necessary for osteoclast function and constitutively activated NF-κB plays an important role in ATLL cells. Bortezomib has been shown to inhibit tumor growth in models of ATLL (Mitra-Kaushik et al., 2004b; Nasr et al., 2005; Satou et al., 2004; Shu et al., 2007; Tan & Waldmann, 2002). Shu et al. reported that bortezomib not only decreased tumor burden in mice bearing ATLL cells, but also decreased the severity of HHM (Shu et al., 2007). Although the decrease in serum calcium concentrations was mainly due to the decreased tumor burden, several studies have shown that bortezomib inhibited osteoclastogenesis by decreasing p38, AP-1 and NF-κB activity in osteoclasts (von Metzler et al., 2007) and increased bone formation by decreasing the expression of Dkk-1, a potent osteoblast inhibitor (Drake & Rajkumar, 2009; Heider et al., 2009; Pennisi et al., 2009; Qiang et al., 2009; Terpos et al., 2006). Bortezomib is now a standard of care for treatment of multiple myeloma patients. Several clinical trials involving bortezomib are ongoing for the treatment of prostate cancer, nonsmall cell lung cancer, acute myelogenous leukemia, and other cancers.

5.5 Humanized anti-parathyroid hormone-related protein antibody and small molecule antagonists of the PTH/PTHrP receptor (PTH1R)

Although bisphophonates have been widely used for treatment of HHM to inhibit osteoclastic bone resorption, they do not function on the kidney to decrease renal calcium reabsorption. To eliminate the actions of PTHrP in bone and kidney, an anti-PTHrP antibody has been developed and tested (Sato et al., 2003). Anti-PTHrP antibody prevented hypercalcemia and skeletal metastasis, but not visceral metastasis, induced by PTHrP-producing cancer cells in mice (Guise & Mundy, 1996; Sato et al., 2003). Although it has been difficult to identify small molecule antagonists for type B G-protein-coupled receptors, including the PTH1R, two compounds have been recently developed that antagonize PTH1R. SW106 was discovered by Bristol-Myers-Squibb Company by screening compounds that inhibited targets downstream of the PTHR1 (Carter et al., 2007). The benzoxazepinone non-peptide inhibits the cAMP response induced by a PTH1R agonist. The pharmacological behavior of SW106 is not yet completely understood. A similar compound, 1,3,4-benzotriazepine was identified and serves as a base molecule to develop non-peptide PTH1R antagonist derivatives (McDonald et al., 2007). Using a radioligand binding assay that measures cAMP production, N-1 anilino-substituted compounds were identified that have up to a 1000-fold more potency at inhibiting PTH1R compared to the original compound. Efforts are ongoing to determine the effects of these compounds on bone metastasis, hypercalcemia and hyperparathyroidism.

5.6 RANKL inhibitors

Ever since RANKL and OPG were discovered to be major regulators of osteoclastic bone resorption, RANK-Fc, Fc-OPG, antibodies targeting RANKL or inhibitors imitating OPG function have been developed for the treatment of osteolytic bone diseases (Schwarz & Ritchlin, 2007). RANK-Fc was generated by combining the carboxyl-terminus of RANK with the Fc portion of human IgG1. It has been shown to decrease tumor burden in two multiple myeloma mouse models, inhibit prostate cancer bone metastasis, and decrease the incidence of lung metastasis and bone lysis in a osteosarcoma mouse model (Lamoureux et al., 2008; Sordillo & Pearse, 2003; Zhang et al., 2003). Fc-OPG was generated by combining the Fc portion of the immunoglobulin heavy chain to the amino-terminus of OPG. The inhibitory effect of Fc-OPG on bone resorption is similar to pamidronate (Bekker et al., 2001; Body et al., 2003). However, Fc-OPG and RANK-Fc have been replaced by denosumab (Amgen), which is a fully human monoclonal antibody developed using the xenomouse technology that specifically inhibits primate RANKL (Green, 1999). Denosumab does not bind to murine RANKL, human TRAIL, or other TNF family proteins and has a longer half-life than Fc-OPG (Kostenuik et al., 2009). Denosumab has been tested in patients with varying diseases/conditions, including osteoporosis, treatment-induced bone loss, bone metastases, multiple myeloma and rheumatoid arthritis, and is now a standard of care for patients with solid tumor bone metastases (Schwarz & Ritchlin, 2007). Denosumab can significantly delay or prevent skeleton-related events (SREs), including hypercalcemia, in patients with bone metastasis (Castellano et al., 2011). Due to its longer half life, higher specificity and lower toxicity, the therapeutic potential of denosumab is superior to that of Fc-OPG and RANK-Fc (Schwarz & Ritchlin, 2007).

6. Development of *in vivo* models of HHM in leukemia/lymphoma

6.1 Mouse models of HHM and ATLL

Animal models of ATLL are divided into infectious models, which are useful to study viral infection, viral transmission and the immune response, and pathogenesis models, which are useful for preclinical therapy studies. Pathogenesis models, including tumor xenografts and transgenic mice that develop tumors, are useful to study the development and treatment of HHM in ATLL. Unfortunately, there are few animal models of ATLL that develop HHM. The following animal models are currently available for studying HHM in ATLL.

6.1.1 Human RV-ATL xenograft mouse model of ATLL

The RV-ATL model was first developed by the laboratory of Dr. Irvin Chen by injecting RV-ATL cells, derived from an ATLL patient, into severe combined immunodeficient (SCID) mice (Feuer et al., 1993). Richard et al. characterized the tumorigenesis and HHM of this cell line in SCID/beige mice (Richard et al., 2001). SCID/beige mice developed severe hypercalcemia one month after intraperitoneal injection of RV-ATL cells. The mice had bone loss due to increased osteoclastic bone resorption. Shu et al. introduced the luciferase gene into the RV-ATL cells by lentiviral infection and developed a bioluminescent model of HHM in ATLL for preclinical studies (Shu et al., 2007). It was found that both zoledronic acid, a nitrogen-containing bisphosphonate, and PS-341, a selective proteasome inhibitor, decreased tumor burden and HHM in mice. No complication of using the combination of PS-341 and zoledronic acid was observed in this preclinical study (Shu et al., 2007).

6.1.2 Uchiyama human xenograft mouse model of ATLL

The laboratory of Dr. Takashi Uchiyama developed a mouse xenograft model by injecting cells from the lymph node of a lymphoma-type ATLL patient intraperitoneally into SCID mice (Imada et al., 1996). The mice developed tumors and hypercalcemia within three weeks. There was a marked increase in serum C-terminal PTHrP concentrations with decreased bone formation rates reported in the mice (Takaori-Kondo et al., 1998). However, no significant increase in bone resorption measured by bone histomorphometry was observed in the mice, which is in contrast to ATLL patients with HHM.

6.1.3 Human MET-1 xenograft mouse model of ATLL

Recently, a NOD/SCID mouse model using human ATLL MET-1 cells has been developed (Phillips et al., 2000). The mice developed leukemia and HHM after intraperitoneal injection. Marked infiltration of tumor cells in multiple organs including spleen, lungs, liver, lymph nodes was observed. Increased plasma PTHrP concentrations in the mice and expression of PTHrP and RANKL in MET-1 cells were reported (Parrula et al., 2009). It is not known whether the HHM in this model was caused by an increase in bone resorption or other mechanisms.

6.1.4 HTLV-1 LTR-Tax transgenic model

Transgenic mice have been used to study the pathogenesis and role of the HTLV-1 viral oncoprotein, Tax. Several Tax transgenic mice have been developed using different promoters. A transgenic mouse model overexpressing Tax under the regulation of the HTLV-1 long terminal repeat (LTR) was generated (Ruddle et al., 1993). These mice developed neurofibromas and adrenal medullary tumors, but did not develop leukemia or lymphoma. Unexpectedly, a significant increase in bone remodeling with a net increase in bone volume was observed. This was surprising because the authors also demonstrated that osteoclasts were increased in number, size and degree of multinucleation, which would have been expected to lead to a net decrease in bone volume. It was not reported whether HHM developed in the mice.

6.1.5 Human granzyme B-Tax transgenic mice

The laboratory of Dr. Lee Ratner developed a tissue-specific Tax overexpressing mouse model (Grossman et al., 1995). Tax expression in the mice was under the regulation of the human granzyme B promoter, which limited Tax expression primarily to activated $CD4^+$ and $CD8^+$ T-cells and NK cells. The mice developed mild hypercalcemia and multifocal osteolytic bone lesions, especially in the tail, with increased osteoclastic bone resorption (Gao et al., 2005). The mice have increased serum IL-6 concentrations, which is a potent osteoclast activator. When the mice were crossed to mice that overexpressed OPG, they were protected from the development of osteolytic lesions and soft tissue tumors, indicating that increased bone resorption in Tax transgenic mice was induced, at least in part, through a RANKL-dependent pathway. The mouse model also has been used for preclinical studies and zoledronic acid not only prevented the osteolytic bone lesions but also decreased tumor burden. After crossing the mice with IFN-γ knockout mice, the resulting $Tax^{+}IFN\text{-}\gamma^{-/-}$ mice had accelerated tumor formation, dissemination, and death, when compared with $Tax^{+}IFN\text{-}\gamma^{+/-}$ or $Tax^{+}IFN\text{-}\gamma^{+/+}$ mice (Mitra-Kaushik et al., 2004a). The mice also develop increased osteolytic bone lesions, increased osteoclast formation and more severe hypercalcemia compared to $Tax^{+}IFN\text{-}\gamma^{+/+}$ mice (Xu et al., 2009). These data indicate that IFN-γ may contribute to the host defense systems that prevent HTLV-1-induced malignancy, bone metastasis and HHM.

6.2 Mouse model of canine lymphoma and HHM

A bioluminescent NOD/SCID mouse model of canine T-cell lymphoma and HHM has been developed (Nadella et al., 2008). The mice developed multicentric lymphoma in the mesenteric lymph nodes after intraperitoneal injection of tumor cells. Moderate to marked splenomegaly and enlarged thymuses were observed. There was increased osteoclastic bone resorption in trabecular bone in mice with lymphoma. HHM developed 6-8 weeks after injection of tumor cells. The increase in plasma PTHrP concentrations likely played a central role in HHM in the mice. The cause of canine T-cell lymphoma is unknown and retroviruses have not been identified as a cause of lymphoma in dogs (in contrast to humans and cats).

7. Conclusion

HHM is a life-threatening complication in certain patients with lymphoma or leukemia. As outlined in this review, progress has been made in elucidating the mechanisms by which humoral factors from neoplastic lymphocytes induce HHM, including increased osteoclastic bone resorption and renal calcium reabsorption. However, further efforts are needed to fully understand the pathogenesis of HHM, including the endocrine or paracrine role of interactions between tumor-associated and host-produced cytokines. PTHrP plays a major endocrine and paracrine role in HHM, but the effects of other factors secreted from tumor cells or host cells cannot be neglected. For example, the expression of RANKL in ATLL cells suggests that ATLL cells may function directly as inducers of osteoclastic bone resorption. Additional effective treatments are needed for this paraneoplastic syndrome. Small molecules or humanized antibodies targeting essential factors or their receptors may be an attractive future therapeutic strategy for treatment of HHM.

8. Acknowledgements

This work was supported by the National Cancer Institute (P01 CA100730) and the National Center for Research Resources (T32 RR07073). We thank Tim Vojt for the illustrations.

9. References

Abu-Amer, Y.; Ross, F. P.; Edwards, J. & Teitelbaum, S. L. (1997). Lipopolysaccharide-stimulated osteoclastogenesis is mediated by tumor necrosis factor via its P55 receptor. J.Clin.Invest, 100, No.6, pp. 1557-1565, 0021-9738

Abu-Amer, Y.; Ross, F. P.; McHugh, K. P.; Livolsi, A.; Peyron, J. F. & Teitelbaum, S. L. (1998). Tumor necrosis factor-alpha activation of nuclear transcription factor-kappaB in marrow macrophages is mediated by c-Src tyrosine phosphorylation of Ikappa Balpha. J.Biol.Chem., 273, No.45, pp. 29417-29423, 0021-9258

Amezyane, T.; Lecoules, S.; Bordier, L.; Blade, J. S.; Desrame, J.; Bechade, D.; Coutant, G. & Algayres, J. P. (2008). [Humoral hypercalcemia revealing a malignant non hodgkin lymphoma]. Ann.Endocrinol.(Paris), 69, No.1, pp. 58-62, 0003-4266

Asanuma, N.; Hagiwara, K.; Matsumoto, I.; Matsuda, M.; Nakamura, F.; Kouhara, H.; Miyamoto, M.; Miyashita, Y.; Noguchi, S. & Morimoto, Y. (2002). PTHrP-producing tumor: squamous cell carcinoma of the liver accompanied by humoral hypercalcemia of malignancy, increased IL-6 and leukocytosis. Intern.Med., 41, No.5, pp. 371-376, 0918-2918

Baba, M.; Nishimura, O.; Kanzaki, N.; Okamoto, M.; Sawada, H.; Iizawa, Y.; Shiraishi, M.; Aramaki, Y.; Okonogi, K.; Ogawa, Y.; Meguro, K. & Fujino, M. (1999). A small-molecule, nonpeptide CCR5 antagonist with highly potent and selective anti-HIV-1 activity. Proc.Natl.Acad.Sci.U.S.A, 96, No.10, pp. 5698-5703, 0027-8424

Bekker, P. J.; Holloway, D.; Nakanishi, A.; Arrighi, M.; Leese, P. T. & Dunstan, C. R. (2001). The effect of a single dose of osteoprotegerin in postmenopausal women. J.Bone Miner.Res., 16, No.2, pp. 348-360, 0884-0431

Body, J. J.; Greipp, P.; Coleman, R. E.; Facon, T.; Geurs, F.; Fermand, J. P.; Harousseau, J. L.; Lipton, A.; Mariette, X.; Williams, C. D.; Nakanishi, A.; Holloway, D.; Martin, S. W.; Dunstan, C. R. & Bekker, P. J. (2003). A phase I study of AMGN-0007, a recombinant osteoprotegerin construct, in patients with multiple myeloma or breast carcinoma related bone metastases. Cancer, 97, No.3 Suppl, pp. 887-892, 0008-543X

Bolliger, A. P.; Graham, P. A.; Richard, V.; Rosol, T. J.; Nachreiner, R. F. & Refsal, K. R. (2002). Detection of parathyroid hormone-related protein in cats with humoral hypercalcemia of malignancy. Vet.Clin.Pathol., 31, No.1, pp. 3-8, 0275-6382

Broadus, A. E.; Mangin, M.; Ikeda, K.; Insogna, K. L.; Weir, E. C.; Burtis, W. J. & Stewart, A. F. (1988). Humoral hypercalcemia of cancer. Identification of a novel parathyroid hormone-like peptide. N.Engl.J.Med., 319, No.9, pp. 556-563, 0028-4793

Bucay, N.; Sarosi, I.; Dunstan, C. R.; Morony, S.; Tarpley, J.; Capparelli, C.; Scully, S.; Tan, H. L.; Xu, W.; Lacey, D. L.; Boyle, W. J. & Simonet, W. S. (1998). Osteoprotegerin-deficient mice develop early onset osteoporosis and arterial calcification. Genes Dev., 12, No.9, pp. 1260-1268, 0890-9369

Carter, P. H.; Liu, R. Q.; Foster, W. R.; Tamasi, J. A.; Tebben, A. J.; Favata, M.; Staal, A.; Cvijic, M. E.; French, M. H.; Dell, V.; Apanovitch, D.; Lei, M.; Zhao, Q.; Cunningham, M.; Decicco, C. P.; Trzaskos, J. M. & Feyen, J. H. (2007). Discovery of a small molecule antagonist of the parathyroid hormone receptor by using an N-terminal parathyroid hormone peptide probe. Proc.Natl.Acad.Sci.U.S.A, 104, No.16, pp. 6846-6851, 0027-8424

Castellano, D.; Sepulveda, J. M.; Garcia-Escobar, I.; Rodriguez-Antolin, A.; Sundlov, A. & Cortes-Funes, H. (2011). The role of RANK-ligand inhibition in cancer: the story of denosumab. Oncologist., 16, No.2, pp. 136-145, 1083-7159

Chang, P. Y.; Lee, S. H.; Chao, T. K. & Chao, T. Y. (2008). Acute renal failure due to hypercalcemia-related nephrocalcinosis in a patient of non-Hodgkin's lymphoma featuring swelling of bilateral kidneys. Ann.Hematol., 87, No.6, pp. 489-490, 0939-5555

Chattopadhyay, N. (2006). Effects of calcium-sensing receptor on the secretion of parathyroid hormone-related peptide and its impact on humoral hypercalcemia of malignancy. Am.J.Physiol Endocrinol.Metab, 290, No.5, p. E761-E770, 0193-1849

Chiba, K.; Hashino, S.; Izumiyama, K.; Toyoshima, N.; Suzuki, S.; Kurosawa, M. & Asaka, M. (2009). Multiple osteolytic bone lesions with high serum levels of interleukin-6 and CCL chemokines in a patient with adult T cell leukemia. Int.J.Lab Hematol., 31, No.3, pp. 368-371, 1751-5521

Choi, S. J.; Cruz, J. C.; Craig, F.; Chung, H.; Devlin, R. D.; Roodman, G. D. & Alsina, M. (2000). Macrophage inflammatory protein 1-alpha is a potential osteoclast stimulatory factor in multiple myeloma. Blood, 96, No.2, pp. 671-675, 0006-4971

Chu, C. Q.; Field, M.; Feldmann, M. & Maini, R. N. (1991). Localization of tumor necrosis factor alpha in synovial tissues and at the cartilage-pannus junction in patients with rheumatoid arthritis. Arthritis Rheum., 34, No.9, pp. 1125-1132, 0004-3591

de Gortazar, A. R.; Alonso, V.; Alvarez-Arroyo, M. V. & Esbrit, P. (2006). Transient exposure to PTHrP (107-139) exerts anabolic effects through vascular endothelial growth factor receptor 2 in human osteoblastic cells in vitro. Calcif.Tissue Int., 79, No.5, pp. 360-369, 0171-967X

de Wit, M.; Schoemaker, N. J.; Kik, M. J. & Westerhof, I. (2003). Hypercalcemia in two Amazon parrots with malignant lymphoma. Avian Dis., 47, No.1, pp. 223-228, 0005-2086

Drake, M. T.; Clarke, B. L. & Khosla, S. (2008). Bisphosphonates: mechanism of action and role in clinical practice. Mayo Clin.Proc., 83, No.9, pp. 1032-1045, 0025-6196

Drake, M. T. & Rajkumar, S. V. (2009). Effects of bortezomib on bone disease in multiple myeloma. Am.J.Hematol., 84, No.1, pp. 1-2, 0361-8609

Ejima, E.; Rosenblatt, J. D.; Massari, M.; Quan, E.; Stephens, D.; Rosen, C. A. & Prager, D. (1993). Cell-type-specific transactivation of the parathyroid hormone-related protein gene promoter by the human T-cell leukemia virus type I (HTLV-I) tax and HTLV-II tax proteins. Blood, 81, No.4, pp. 1017-1024, 0006-4971

Engelman, R. W.; Tyler, R. D.; Good, R. A. & Day, N. K. (1985). Hypercalcemia in cats with feline-leukemia-virus-associated leukemia-lymphoma. Cancer, 56, No.4, pp. 777-781, 0008-543X

Ferrajoli, A.; Keating, M. J.; Manshouri, T.; Giles, F. J.; Dey, A.; Estrov, Z.; Koller, C. A.; Kurzrock, R.; Thomas, D. A.; Faderl, S.; Lerner, S.; O'Brien, S. & Albitar, M. (2002). The clinical significance of tumor necrosis factor-alpha plasma level in patients having chronic lymphocytic leukemia. Blood, 100, No.4, pp. 1215-1219, 0006-4971

Fetchick, D. A.; Bertolini, D. R.; Sarin, P. S.; Weintraub, S. T.; Mundy, G. R. & Dunn, J. F. (1986). Production of 1,25-dihydroxyvitamin D3 by human T cell lymphotrophic virus-I-transformed lymphocytes. J.Clin.Invest, 78, No.2, pp. 592-596, 0021-9738

Feuer, G.; Zack, J. A.; Harrington, W. J., Jr.; Valderama, R.; Rosenblatt, J. D.; Wachsman, W.; Baird, S. M. & Chen, I. S. (1993). Establishment of human T-cell leukemia virus type

I T-cell lymphomas in severe combined immunodeficient mice. Blood, 82, No.3, pp. 722-731, 0006-4971

Fleisch, H. (1997). Mechanisms of action of the bisphosphonates. Medicina (B Aires), 57 Suppl 1, pp. 65-75, 0025-7680

Fleisch, H. (1998). Bisphosphonates: mechanisms of action. Endocr.Rev., 19, No.1, pp. 80-100, 0163-769X

Fournel-Fleury, C.; Ponce, F.; Felman, P.; Blavier, A.; Bonnefont, C.; Chabanne, L.; Marchal, T.; Cadore, J. L.; Goy-Thollot, I.; Ledieu, D.; Ghernati, I. & Magnol, J. P. (2002). Canine T-cell lymphomas: a morphological, immunological, and clinical study of 46 new cases. Vet.Pathol., 39, No.1, pp. 92-109, 0300-9858

Fuller, K.; Owens, J. M. & Chambers, T. J. (1995). Macrophage inflammatory protein-1 alpha and IL-8 stimulate the motility but suppress the resorption of isolated rat osteoclasts. J.Immunol., 154, No.11, pp. 6065-6072, 0022-1767

Gallo, J.; Raska, M.; Mrazek, F. & Petrek, M. (2008). Bone remodeling, particle disease and individual susceptibility to periprosthetic osteolysis. Physiol Res., 57, No.3, pp. 339-349, 0862-8408

Gao, L.; Deng, H.; Zhao, H.; Hirbe, A.; Harding, J.; Ratner, L. & Weilbaecher, K. (2005). HTLV-1 Tax transgenic mice develop spontaneous osteolytic bone metastases prevented by osteoclast inhibition. Blood, 106, No.13, pp. 4294-4302, 0006-4971

Gillespie, M. T. (2007). Impact of cytokines and T lymphocytes upon osteoclast differentiation and function. Arthritis Res.Ther., 9, No.2, p. 103, 1478-6354

Green, L. L. (1999). Antibody engineering via genetic engineering of the mouse: XenoMouse strains are a vehicle for the facile generation of therapeutic human monoclonal antibodies. J.Immunol.Methods, 231, No.1-2, pp. 11-23, 0022-1759

Greenfield, E. M.; Shaw, S. M.; Gornik, S. A. & Banks, M. A. (1995). Adenyl cyclase and interleukin 6 are downstream effectors of parathyroid hormone resulting in stimulation of bone resorption. J.Clin.Invest, 96, No.3, pp. 1238-1244, 0021-9738

Grossman, W. J.; Kimata, J. T.; Wong, F. H.; Zutter, M.; Ley, T. J. & Ratner, L. (1995). Development of leukemia in mice transgenic for the tax gene of human T-cell leukemia virus type I. Proc.Natl.Acad.Sci.U.S.A, 92, No.4, pp. 1057-1061, 0027-8424

Guise, T. A.; Kozlow, W. M.; Heras-Herzig, A.; Padalecki, S. S.; Yin, J. J. & Chirgwin, J. M. (2005). Molecular mechanisms of breast cancer metastases to bone. Clin.Breast Cancer, 5 Suppl, No.2, p. S46-S53, 1526-8209

Guise, T. A. & Mundy, G. R. (1996). Physiological and pathological roles of parathyroid hormone-related peptide. Curr.Opin.Nephrol.Hypertens., 5, No.4, pp. 307-315, 1062-4821

Habra, M. A.; Weaver, E. J. & Prewitt, P. V., III (2007). Primary cutaneous large B-cell lymphoma of the leg and acute hypercalcemia. J.Clin.Oncol., 25, No.36, pp. 5825-5826, 0732-183X

Han, J. H.; Choi, S. J.; Kurihara, N.; Koide, M.; Oba, Y. & Roodman, G. D. (2001). Macrophage inflammatory protein-1alpha is an osteoclastogenic factor in myeloma that is independent of receptor activator of nuclear factor kappaB ligand. Blood, 97, No.11, pp. 3349-3353, 0006-4971

Heider, U.; Kaiser, M.; Mieth, M.; Lamottke, B.; Rademacher, J.; Jakob, C.; Braendle, E.; Stover, D. & Sezer, O. (2009). Serum concentrations of DKK-1 decrease in patients with multiple myeloma responding to anti-myeloma treatment. Eur.J.Haematol., 82, No.1, pp. 31-38, 0902-4441

Hewison, M.; Kantorovich, V.; Liker, H. R.; Van Herle, A. J.; Cohan, P.; Zehnder, D. & Adams, J. S. (2003). Vitamin D-mediated hypercalcemia in lymphoma: evidence for hormone production by tumor-adjacent macrophages. J.Bone Miner.Res., 18, No.3, pp. 579-582, 0884-0431

Hirbe, A.C., Roelofs, A.J., Floyd, D.H., Deng, H., Becker, S.N., Lanigan, L.G., Apicelli, A.J., Xu, Z., Prior, J.L., Eagleton, M.C., Piwnica-Worms, D., Rogers, M.J., & Weilbaecher, K. (2009). The bisphosphonate zoledronic acid decreases tumor growth in bone in mice with defective osteoclasts. Bone, 44, No. 5, pp. 908-916, 8756-3282

Hofbauer, L. C.; Khosla, S.; Dunstan, C. R.; Lacey, D. L.; Boyle, W. J. & Riggs, B. L. (2000). The roles of osteoprotegerin and osteoprotegerin ligand in the paracrine regulation of bone resorption. J.Bone Miner.Res., 15, No.1, pp. 2-12, 0884-0431

Horowitz, M. C. (1993). Cytokines and estrogen in bone: anti-osteoporotic effects. Science, 260, No.5108, pp. 626-627, 0036-8075

Horwood, N. J.; Elliott, J.; Martin, T. J. & Gillespie, M. T. (1998). Osteotropic agents regulate the expression of osteoclast differentiation factor and osteoprotegerin in osteoblastic stromal cells. Endocrinology, 139, No.11, pp. 4743-4746, 0013-7227

Horwood, N. J.; Elliott, J.; Martin, T. J. & Gillespie, M. T. (2001). IL-12 alone and in synergy with IL-18 inhibits osteoclast formation in vitro. J.Immunol., 166, No.8, pp. 4915-4921, 0022-1767

Hounoki, H.; Sugiyama, E.; Mohamed, S. G.; Shinoda, K.; Taki, H.; Abdel-Aziz, H. O.; Maruyama, M.; Kobayashi, M. & Miyahara, T. (2008). Activation of peroxisome proliferator-activated receptor gamma inhibits TNF-alpha-mediated osteoclast differentiation in human peripheral monocytes in part via suppression of monocyte chemoattractant protein-1 expression. Bone, 42, No.4, pp. 765-774, 8756-3282

Imada, K.; Takaori-Kondo, A.; Sawada, H.; Imura, A.; Kawamata, S.; Okuma, M. & Uchiyama, T. (1996). Serial transplantation of adult T cell leukemia cells into severe combined immunodeficient mice. Jpn.J.Cancer Res., 87, No.9, pp. 887-892, 0910-5050

Ishibashi, K.; Kodama, M.; Hanada, S. & Arima, T. (1992). Tumor necrosis factor-beta and hypercalcemia. Leuk.Lymphoma, 7, No.5-6, pp. 409-417, 1042-8194

Ishikawa, C.; Matsuda, T.; Okudaira, T.; Tomita, M.; Kawakami, H.; Tanaka, Y.; Masuda, M.; Ohshiro, K.; Ohta, T. & Mori, N. (2007). Bisphosphonate incadronate inhibits growth of human T-cell leukaemia virus type I-infected T-cell lines and primary adult T-cell leukaemia cells by interfering with the mevalonate pathway. Br.J.Haematol., 136, No.3, pp. 424-432, 0007-1048

Johnston, S. R. & Hammond, P. J. (1992). Elevated serum parathyroid hormone related protein and 1,25-dihydroxycholecalciferol in hypercalcaemia associated with adult T-cell leukaemia-lymphoma. Postgrad.Med.J., 68, No.803, pp. 753-755, 0032-5473

Karaplis, A. C.; Luz, A.; Glowacki, J.; Bronson, R. T.; Tybulewicz, V. L.; Kronenberg, H. M. & Mulligan, R. C. (1994). Lethal skeletal dysplasia from targeted disruption of the parathyroid hormone-related peptide gene. Genes Dev., 8, No.3, pp. 277-289, 0890-9369

Kostenuik, P. J.; Nguyen, H. Q.; McCabe, J.; Warmington, K. S.; Kurahara, C.; Sun, N.; Chen, C.; Li, L.; Cattley, R. C.; Van, G.; Scully, S.; Elliott, R.; Grisanti, M.; Morony, S.; Tan, H. L.; Asuncion, F.; Li, X.; Ominsky, M. S.; Stolina, M.; Dwyer, D.; Dougall, W. C.; Hawkins, N.; Boyle, W. J.; Simonet, W. S. & Sullivan, J. K. (2009). Denosumab, a fully human monoclonal antibody to RANKL, inhibits bone resorption and increases BMD in knock-in mice that express chimeric (murine/human) RANKL. J.Bone Miner.Res., 24, No.2, pp. 182-195, 0884-0431

Kounami, S.; Yoshiyama, M.; Nakayama, K.; Hiramatsu, C.; Aoyagi, N. & Yoshikawa, N. (2004). Severe hypercalcemia in a child with acute nonlymphocytic leukemia: the role of parathyroid hormone-related protein and proinflammatory cytokines. Acta Haematol., 112, No.3, pp. 160-163, 0001-5792

Kudo, O.; Fujikawa, Y.; Itonaga, I.; Sabokbar, A.; Torisu, T. & Athanasou, N. A. (2002). Proinflammatory cytokine (TNFalpha/IL-1alpha) induction of human osteoclast formation. J.Pathol., 198, No.2, pp. 220-227, 0022-3417

Lacey, D. L.; Timms, E.; Tan, H. L.; Kelley, M. J.; Dunstan, C. R.; Burgess, T.; Elliott, R.; Colombero, A.; Elliott, G.; Scully, S.; Hsu, H.; Sullivan, J.; Hawkins, N.; Davy, E.; Capparelli, C.; Eli, A.; Qian, Y. X.; Kaufman, S.; Sarosi, I.; Shalhoub, V.; Senaldi, G.; Guo, J.; Delaney, J. & Boyle, W. J. (1998). Osteoprotegerin ligand is a cytokine that regulates osteoclast differentiation and activation. Cell, 93, No.2, pp. 165-176, 0092-8674

Lam, J.; Takeshita, S.; Barker, J. E.; Kanagawa, O.; Ross, F. P. & Teitelbaum, S. L. (2000). TNF-alpha induces osteoclastogenesis by direct stimulation of macrophages exposed to permissive levels of RANK ligand. J.Clin.Invest, 106, No.12, pp. 1481-1488, 0021-9738

Lamoureux, F.; Picarda, G.; Rousseau, J.; Gourden, C.; Battaglia, S.; Charrier, C.; Pitard, B.; Heymann, D. & Redini, F. (2008). Therapeutic efficacy of soluble receptor activator of nuclear factor-kappa B-Fc delivered by nonviral gene transfer in a mouse model of osteolytic osteosarcoma. Mol.Cancer Ther., 7, No.10, pp. 3389-3398, 1535-7163

Leibbrandt, A. & Penninger, J. M. (2008). RANK/RANKL: regulators of immune responses and bone physiology. Ann.N.Y.Acad.Sci., 1143, pp. 123-150, 0077-8923

Li, J.; Sarosi, I.; Yan, X. Q.; Morony, S.; Capparelli, C.; Tan, H. L.; McCabe, S.; Elliott, R.; Scully, S.; Van, G.; Kaufman, S.; Juan, S. C.; Sun, Y.; Tarpley, J.; Martin, L.; Christensen, K.; McCabe, J.; Kostenuik, P.; Hsu, H.; Fletcher, F.; Dunstan, C. R.; Lacey, D. L. & Boyle, W. J. (2000). RANK is the intrinsic hematopoietic cell surface receptor that controls osteoclastogenesis and regulation of bone mass and calcium metabolism. Proc.Natl.Acad.Sci.U.S.A, 97, No.4, pp. 1566-1571, 0027-8424

Liao, J.; Schneider, A., Datta N.S., & McCauley, L.K. (2006). Extracellular calcium as a candidate mediator of prostate cancer skeletal metastasis. Cancer Res., 66, No. 18, pp. 9065-9073, 0008-5472

Lipton, A.; Uzzo, R.; Amato, R. J.; Ellis, G. K.; Hakimian, B.; Roodman, G. D. & Smith, M. R. (2009). The science and practice of bone health in oncology: managing bone loss and metastasis in patients with solid tumors. J.Natl.Compr.Canc.Netw., 7 Suppl 7, pp. S1-29, 1540-1405

Lomaga, M. A.; Yeh, W. C.; Sarosi, I.; Duncan, G. S.; Furlonger, C.; Ho, A.; Morony, S.; Capparelli, C.; Van, G.; Kaufman, S.; van der Heiden, A.; Itie, A.; Wakeham, A.; Khoo, W.; Sasaki, T.; Cao, Z.; Penninger, J. M.; Paige, C. J.; Lacey, D. L.; Dunstan, C. R.; Boyle, W. J.; Goeddel, D. V. & Mak, T. W. (1999). TRAF6 deficiency results in osteopetrosis and defective interleukin-1, CD40, and LPS signaling. Genes Dev., 13, No.8, pp. 1015-1024, 0890-9369

Lorch, G.; Viatchenko-Karpinski, S.; Ho, H. T.; Dirksen, W. P.; Toribio, R. E.; Foley, J.; Györke, S. & Rosol, T. J. (2011). The calcium-sensing receptor is necessary for the rapid development of hypercalcemia in human lung squamous cell carcinoma. Neoplasia, 13, No.5, pp. 428-438, 1522-8802

Lu, T. & Stark, G. R. (2004). Cytokine overexpression and constitutive NFkappaB in cancer. Cell Cycle, 3, No.9, pp. 1114-1117, 1538-4101

Matsumoto, K.; Murao, K.; Imachi, H.; Nishiuchi, T.; Cao, W.; Yu, X.; Li, J.; Ahmed, R. A.; Iwama, H.; Kobayashi, R.; Tokumitsu, H. & Ishida, T. (2008). The role of calcium/calmodulin-dependent protein kinase cascade on MIP-1alpha gene expression of ATL cells. Exp.Hematol., 36, No.4, pp. 390-400, 0301-472X

Maurer, M. & von, S. E. (2004). Macrophage inflammatory protein-1. Int.J.Biochem.Cell Biol., 36, No.10, pp. 1882-1886, 1357-2725

McDonald, I. M.; Austin, C.; Buck, I. M.; Dunstone, D. J.; Gaffen, J.; Griffin, E.; Harper, E. A.; Hull, R. A.; Kalindjian, S. B.; Linney, I. D.; Low, C. M.; Patel, D.; Pether, M. J.; Raynor, M.; Roberts, S. P.; Shaxted, M. E.; Spencer, J.; Steel, K. I.; Sykes, D. A.; Wright, P. T. & Xun, W. (2007). Discovery and characterization of novel, potent, non-peptide parathyroid hormone-1 receptor antagonists. J.Med.Chem., 50, No.20, pp. 4789-4792, 0022-2623

Meghji, S.; Crean, S. J.; Hill, P. A.; Sheikh, M.; Nair, S. P.; Heron, K.; Henderson, B.; Mawer, E. B. & Harris, M. (1998). Surface-associated protein from Staphylococcus aureus stimulates osteoclastogenesis: possible role in S. aureus-induced bone pathology. Br.J.Rheumatol., 37, No.10, pp. 1095-1101, 0263-7103

Mellanby, R. J.; Craig, R.; Evans, H. & Herrtage, M. E. (2006). Plasma concentrations of parathyroid hormone-related protein in dogs with potential disorders of calcium metabolism. Vet.Rec., 159, No.25, pp. 833-838, 0042-4900

Menu, E.; De, L. E.; De, R. H.; Coulton, L.; Imanishi, T.; Miyashita, K.; Van, V. E.; Van, R., I; Van, C. B.; Horuk, R.; Croucher, P. & Vanderkerken, K. (2006). Role of CCR1 and CCR5 in homing and growth of multiple myeloma and in the development of osteolytic lesions: a study in the 5TMM model. Clin.Exp.Metastasis, 23, No.5-6, pp. 291-300, 0262-0898

Merkel, K. D.; Erdmann, J. M.; McHugh, K. P.; Abu-Amer, Y.; Ross, F. P. & Teitelbaum, S. L. (1999). Tumor necrosis factor-alpha mediates orthopedic implant osteolysis. Am.J.Pathol., 154, No.1, pp. 203-210, 0002-9440

Mitra-Kaushik, S.; Harding, J.; Hess, J.; Schreiber, R. & Ratner, L. (2004a). Enhanced tumorigenesis in HTLV-1 tax-transgenic mice deficient in interferon-gamma. Blood, 104, No.10, pp. 3305-3311, 0006-4971

Mitra-Kaushik, S.; Harding, J. C.; Hess, J. L. & Ratner, L. (2004b). Effects of the proteasome inhibitor PS-341 on tumor growth in HTLV-1 Tax transgenic mice and Tax tumor transplants. Blood, 104, No.3, pp. 802-809, 0006-4971

Mizuno, A.; Amizuka, N.; Irie, K.; Murakami, A.; Fujise, N.; Kanno, T.; Sato, Y.; Nakagawa, N.; Yasuda, H.; Mochizuki, S.; Gomibuchi, T.; Yano, K.; Shima, N.; Washida, N.; Tsuda, E.; Morinaga, T.; Higashio, K. & Ozawa, H. (1998). Severe osteoporosis in mice lacking osteoclastogenesis inhibitory factor/osteoprotegerin. Biochem.Biophys.Res.Commun., 247, No.3, pp. 610-615, 0006-291X

Mundy, G. R. & Martin, T. J. (1982). The hypercalcemia of malignancy: pathogenesis and management. Metabolism, 31, No.12, pp. 1247-1277, 0026-0495

Nadella, M. V.; Dirksen, W. P.; Nadella, K. S.; Shu, S.; Cheng, A. S.; Morgenstern, J. A.; Richard, V.; Fernandez, S. A.; Huang, T. H.; Guttridge, D. & Rosol, T. J. (2007). Transcriptional regulation of parathyroid hormone-related protein promoter P2 by NF-kappaB in adult T-cell leukemia/lymphoma. Leukemia, 21, No.8, pp. 1752-1762, 0887-6924

Nadella, M. V.; Kisseberth, W. C.; Nadella, K. S.; Thudi, N. K.; Thamm, D. H.; McNiel, E. A.; Yilmaz, A.; Boris-Lawrie, K. & Rosol, T. J. (2008). NOD/SCID mouse model of canine T-cell lymphoma with humoral hypercalcaemia of malignancy: cytokine gene expression profiling and in vivo bioluminescent imaging. Vet.Comp Oncol., 6, No.1, pp. 39-54, 1476-5810

Narimatsu, H.; Morishita, Y.; Shimada, K.; Ozeki, K.; Kohno, A.; Kato, Y. & Nagasaka, T. (2003). Primary cutaneous diffuse large B cell lymphoma: a clinically aggressive case. Intern.Med., 42, No.4, pp. 354-357, 0918-2918

Nasr, R.; El-Sabban, M. E.; Karam, J. A.; Dbaibo, G.; Kfoury, Y.; Arnulf, B.; Lepelletier, Y.; Bex, F.; de, T. H.; Hermine, O. & Bazarbachi, A. (2005). Efficacy and mechanism of action of the proteasome inhibitor PS-341 in T-cell lymphomas and HTLV-I associated adult T-cell leukemia/lymphoma. Oncogene, 24, No.3, pp. 419-430, 0950-9232

Nosaka, K.; Miyamoto, T.; Sakai, T.; Mitsuya, H.; Suda, T. & Matsuoka, M. (2002). Mechanism of hypercalcemia in adult T-cell leukemia: overexpression of receptor activator of nuclear factor kappaB ligand on adult T-cell leukemia cells. Blood, 99, No.2, pp. 634-640, 0006-4971

Oba, Y.; Lee, J. W.; Ehrlich, L. A.; Chung, H. Y.; Jelinek, D. F.; Callander, N. S.; Horuk, R.; Choi, S. J. & Roodman, G. D. (2005). MIP-1alpha utilizes both CCR1 and CCR5 to induce osteoclast formation and increase adhesion of myeloma cells to marrow stromal cells. Exp.Hematol., 33, No.3, pp. 272-278, 0301-472X

Okada, Y.; Tsukada, J.; Nakano, K.; Tonai, S.; Mine, S. & Tanaka, Y. (2004). Macrophage inflammatory protein-1alpha induces hypercalcemia in adult T-cell leukemia. J.Bone Miner.Res., 19, No.7, pp. 1105-1111, 0884-0431

Olivo, R. A.; Martins, F. F.; Soares, S. & Moraes-Souza, H. (2008). Adult T-cell leukemia/lymphoma: report of two cases. Rev.Soc.Bras.Med.Trop., 41, No.3, pp. 288-292, 0037-8682

Oyajobi, B. O.; Franchin, G.; Williams, P. J.; Pulkrabek, D.; Gupta, A.; Munoz, S.; Grubbs, B.; Zhao, M.; Chen, D.; Sherry, B. & Mundy, G. R. (2003). Dual effects of macrophage inflammatory protein-1alpha on osteolysis and tumor burden in the murine 5TGM1 model of myeloma bone disease. Blood, 102, No.1, pp. 311-319, 0006-4971

Parrula, C.; Zimmerman, B.; Nadella, P.; Shu, S.; Rosol, T.; Fernandez, S.; Lairmore, M. & Niewiesk, S. (2009). Expression of tumor invasion factors determines systemic engraftment and induction of humoral hypercalcemia in a mouse model of adult T-cell leukemia. Vet.Pathol., 46, No.5, pp. 1003-1014, 0300-9858

Pennisi, A.; Li, X.; Ling, W.; Khan, S.; Zangari, M. & Yaccoby, S. (2009). The proteasome inhibitor, bortezomib suppresses primary myeloma and stimulates bone formation in myelomatous and nonmyelomatous bones in vivo. Am.J.Hematol., 84, No.1, pp. 6-14, 0361-8609

Phillips, K. E.; Herring, B.; Wilson, L. A.; Rickford, M. S.; Zhang, M.; Goldman, C. K.; Tso, J. Y. & Waldmann, T. A. (2000). IL-2Ralpha-Directed monoclonal antibodies provide effective therapy in a murine model of adult T-cell leukemia by a mechanism other than blockade of IL-2/IL-2Ralpha interaction. Cancer Res., 60, No.24, pp. 6977-6984, 0008-5472

Qiang, Y. W.; Hu, B.; Chen, Y.; Zhong, Y.; Shi, B.; Barlogie, B. & Shaughnessy, J. D., Jr. (2009). Bortezomib induces osteoblast differentiation via Wnt-independent activation of beta-catenin/TCF signaling. Blood, 113, No.18, pp. 4319-4330, 0006-4971

Quinn, J. M. & Gillespie, M. T. (2005). Modulation of osteoclast formation. Biochem.Biophys.Res.Commun., 328, No.3, pp. 739-745, 0006-291X

Richard, V.; Lairmore, M. D.; Green, P. L.; Feuer, G.; Erbe, R. S.; Albrecht, B.; D'Souza, C.; Keller, E. T.; Dai, J. & Rosol, T. J. (2001). Humoral hypercalcemia of malignancy: severe combined immunodeficient/beige mouse model of adult T-cell lymphoma independent of human T-cell lymphotropic virus type-1 tax expression. Am.J.Pathol., 158, No.6, pp. 2219-2228, 0002-9440

Richard, V.; Nadella, M. V.; Green, P. L.; Lairmore, M. D.; Feuer, G.; Foley, J. G. & Rosol, T. J. (2005). Transcriptional regulation of parathyroid hormone-related protein promoter P3 by ETS-1 in adult T-cell leukemia/lymphoma. Leukemia, 19, No.7, pp. 1175-1183, 0887-6924

Roodman, G. D. (1997). Mechanisms of bone lesions in multiple myeloma and lymphoma. Cancer, 80, No.8 Suppl, pp. 1557-1563, 0008-543X

Roodman, G. D. (2001). Biology of osteoclast activation in cancer. J.Clin.Oncol., 19, No.15, pp. 3562-3571, 0732-183X

Rosol, T. J.; Nagode, L. A.; Couto, C. G.; Hammer, A. S.; Chew, D. J.; Peterson, J. L.; Ayl, R. D.; Steinmeyer, C. L. & Capen, C. C. (1992). Parathyroid hormone (PTH)-related protein, PTH, and 1,25-dihydroxyvitamin D in dogs with cancer-associated hypercalcemia. Endocrinology, 131, No.3, pp. 1157-1164, 0013-7227

Ruddle, N. H.; Li, C. B.; Horne, W. C.; Santiago, P.; Troiano, N.; Jay, G.; Horowitz, M. & Baron, R. (1993). Mice transgenic for HTLV-I LTR-tax exhibit tax expression in bone, skeletal alterations, and high bone turnover. Virology, 197, No.1, pp. 196-204, 0042-6822

Sagara, Y.; Inoue, Y.; Sagara, Y. & Kashiwagi, S. (2009). Involvement of molecular mimicry between human T-cell leukemia virus type 1 gp46 and osteoprotegerin in induction of hypercalcemia. Cancer Sci., 100, No.3, pp. 490-496, 1347-9032

Saidak, Z.; Mentaverri, R. & Brown, E. M. (2009). The role of the calcium-sensing receptor in the development and progression of cancer. Endocr.Rev., 30, No.2, pp. 178-195, 0163-769X

Sato, K.; Onuma, E.; Yocum, R. C. & Ogata, E. (2003). Treatment of malignancy-associated hypercalcemia and cachexia with humanized anti-parathyroid hormone-related protein antibody. Semin.Oncol., 30, No.5 Suppl 16, pp. 167-173, 0093-7754

Sato, K.; Suematsu, A.; Okamoto, K.; Yamaguchi, A.; Morishita, Y.; Kadono, Y.; Tanaka, S.; Kodama, T.; Akira, S.; Iwakura, Y.; Cua, D. J. & Takayanagi, H. (2006). Th17 functions as an osteoclastogenic helper T cell subset that links T cell activation and bone destruction. J.Exp.Med., 203, No.12, pp. 2673-2682, 0022-1007

Satou, Y.; Nosaka, K.; Koya, Y.; Yasunaga, J. I.; Toyokuni, S. & Matsuoka, M. (2004). Proteasome inhibitor, bortezomib, potently inhibits the growth of adult T-cell leukemia cells both in vivo and in vitro. Leukemia, 18, No.8, pp. 1357-1363, 0887-6924

Schwarz, E. M. & Ritchlin, C. T. (2007). Clinical development of anti-RANKL therapy. Arthritis Res.Ther., 9 Suppl 1, p. S7, 1478-6354

Seymour, J. F. & Gagel, R. F. (1993). Calcitriol: the major humoral mediator of hypercalcemia in Hodgkin's disease and non-Hodgkin's lymphomas. Blood, 82, No.5, pp. 1383-1394, 0006-4971

Sharan, K.; Siddiqui, J. A.; Swarnkar, G. & Chattopadhyay, N. (2008). Role of calcium-sensing receptor in bone biology. Indian J.Med.Res., 127, No.3, pp. 274-286, 0971-5916

Sharma, V. & May, C. C. (1999). Human T-cell lymphotrophic virus type-I tax gene induces secretion of human macrophage inflammatory protein-1alpha. Biochem.Biophys.Res.Commun., 262, No.2, pp. 429-432, 0006-291X

Shu, S. T.; Martin, C. K.; Thudi, N. K.; Dirksen, W. P. & Rosol, T. J. (2010). Osteolytic bone resorption in adult T-cell leukemia/lymphoma. Leuk.Lymphoma, 51, No.4, pp. 702-714, 1042-8194

Shu, S. T.; Nadella, M. V.; Dirksen, W. P.; Fernandez, S. A.; Thudi, N. K.; Werbeck, J. L.; Lairmore, M. D. & Rosol, T. J. (2007). A novel bioluminescent mouse model and effective therapy for adult T-cell leukemia/lymphoma. Cancer Res., 67, No.24, pp. 11859-11866, 0008-5472

Simonet, W. S.; Lacey, D. L.; Dunstan, C. R.; Kelley, M.; Chang, M. S.; Luthy, R.; Nguyen, H. Q.; Wooden, S.; Bennett, L.; Boone, T.; Shimamoto, G.; DeRose, M.; Elliott, R.; Colombero, A.; Tan, H. L.; Trail, G.; Sullivan, J.; Davy, E.; Bucay, N.; Renshaw-Gegg, L.; Hughes, T. M.; Hill, D.; Pattison, W.; Campbell, P.; Sander, S.; Van, G.; Tarpley, J.; Derby, P.; Lee, R. & Boyle, W. J. (1997). Osteoprotegerin: a novel secreted protein involved in the regulation of bone density. Cell, 89, No.2, pp. 309-319, 0092-8674

Sims, N. A.; Jenkins, B. J.; Quinn, J. M.; Nakamura, A.; Glatt, M.; Gillespie, M. T.; Ernst, M. & Martin, T. J. (2004). Glycoprotein 130 regulates bone turnover and bone size by distinct downstream signaling pathways. J.Clin.Invest, 113, No.3, pp. 379-389, 0021-9738

Sordillo, E. M. & Pearse, R. N. (2003). RANK-Fc: a therapeutic antagonist for RANK-L in myeloma. Cancer, 97, No.3 Suppl, pp. 802-812, 0008-543X

Stewart, A. F. (2002). Hyperparathyroidism, humoral hypercalcemia of malignancy, and the anabolic actions of parathyroid hormone and parathyroid hormone-related protein on the skeleton. J.Bone Miner.Res., 17, No.5, pp. 758-762, 0884-0431

Stewart, A. F. (2005). Clinical practice. Hypercalcemia associated with cancer. N.Engl.J.Med., 352, No.4, pp. 373-379, 0028-4793

Suva, L. J.; Winslow, G. A.; Wettenhall, R. E.; Hammonds, R. G.; Moseley, J. M.; Diefenbach-Jagger, H.; Rodda, C. P.; Kemp, B. E.; Rodriguez, H.; Chen, E. Y. & . (1987). A parathyroid hormone-related protein implicated in malignant hypercalcemia: cloning and expression. Science, 237, No.4817, pp. 893-896, 0036-8075

Takaori-Kondo, A.; Imada, K.; Yamamoto, I.; Kunitomi, A.; Numata, Y.; Sawada, H. & Uchiyama, T. (1998). Parathyroid hormone-related protein-induced hypercalcemia in SCID mice engrafted with adult T-cell leukemia cells. Blood, 91, No.12, pp. 4747-4751, 0006-4971

Takayanagi, H. (2007). Osteoimmunology: shared mechanisms and crosstalk between the immune and bone systems. Nat.Rev.Immunol., 7, No.4, pp. 292-304, 1474-1733

Takeuchi, Y.; Fukumoto, S.; Nakayama, K.; Tamura, Y.; Yanagisawa, A. & Fujita, T. (2002). Parathyroid hormone-related protein induced coupled increases in bone formation and resorption markers for 7 years in a patient with malignant islet cell tumors. J.Bone Miner.Res., 17, No.5, pp. 753-757, 0884-0431

Tan, C. & Waldmann, T. A. (2002). Proteasome inhibitor PS-341, a potential therapeutic agent for adult T-cell leukemia. Cancer Res., 62, No.4, pp. 1083-1086, 0008-5472

Tanaka, S.; Takahashi, N.; Udagawa, N.; Tamura, T.; Akatsu, T.; Stanley, E. R.; Kurokawa, T. & Suda, T. (1993). Macrophage colony-stimulating factor is indispensable for both proliferation and differentiation of osteoclast progenitors. J.Clin.Invest, 91, No.1, pp. 257-263, 0021-9738

Terpos, E.; Heath, D. J.; Rahemtulla, A.; Zervas, K.; Chantry, A.; Anagnostopoulos, A.; Pouli, A.; Katodritou, E.; Verrou, E.; Vervessou, E. C.; Dimopoulos, M. A. & Croucher, P. I. (2006). Bortezomib reduces serum dickkopf-1 and receptor activator of nuclear factor-kappaB ligand concentrations and normalises indices of bone remodelling in patients with relapsed multiple myeloma. Br.J.Haematol., 135, No.5, pp. 688-692, 0007-1048

Tsubaki, M.; Kato, C.; Manno, M.; Ogaki, M.; Satou, T.; Itoh, T.; Kusunoki, T.; Tanimori, Y.; Fujiwara, K.; Matsuoka, H. & Nishida, S. (2007). Macrophage inflammatory protein-1alpha (MIP-1alpha) enhances a receptor activator of nuclear factor kappaB ligand (RANKL) expression in mouse bone marrow stromal cells and osteoblasts through MAPK and PI3K/Akt pathways. Mol.Cell Biochem., 304, No.1-2, pp. 53-60, 0300-8177

Unal, S.; Durmaz, E.; Erkocoglu, M.; Bayrakci, B.; Bircan, O.; Alikasifoglu, A. & Cetin, M. (2008). The rapid correction of hypercalcemia at presentation of acute lymphoblastic leukemia using high-dose methylprednisolone. Turk.J.Pediatr., 50, No.2, pp. 171-175, 0041-4301

Vanderschueren, B.; Dumon, J. C.; Oleffe, V.; Heymans, C.; Gerain, J. & Body, J. J. (1994). Circulating concentrations of interleukin-6 in cancer patients and their pathogenic role in tumor-induced hypercalcemia. Cancer Immunol.Immunother., 39, No.5, pp. 286-290, 0340-7004

von Metzler, I.; Krebbel, H.; Hecht, M.; Manz, R. A.; Fleissner, C.; Mieth, M.; Kaiser, M.; Jakob, C.; Sterz, J.; Kleeberg, L.; Heider, U. & Sezer, O. (2007). Bortezomib inhibits human osteoclastogenesis. Leukemia, 21, No.9, pp. 2025-2034, 0887-6924

Wano, Y.; Hattori, T.; Matsuoka, M.; Takatsuki, K.; Chua, A. O.; Gubler, U. & Greene, W. C. (1987). Interleukin 1 gene expression in adult T cell leukemia. J.Clin.Invest, 80, No.3, pp. 911-916, 0021-9738

Watanabe, T.; Yamaguchi, K.; Takatsuki, K.; Osame, M. & Yoshida, M. (1990). Constitutive expression of parathyroid hormone-related protein gene in human T cell leukemia virus type 1 (HTLV-1) carriers and adult T cell leukemia patients that can be trans-activated by HTLV-1 tax gene. J.Exp.Med., 172, No.3, pp. 759-765, 0022-1007

Weitzmann, M. N. & Pacifici, R. (2005). The role of T lymphocytes in bone metabolism. Immunol.Rev., 208, pp. 154-168, 0105-2896

Wysolmerski, J. J.; Philbrick, W. M.; Dunbar, M. E.; Lanske, B.; Kronenberg, H. & Broadus, A. E. (1998). Rescue of the parathyroid hormone-related protein knockout mouse demonstrates that parathyroid hormone-related protein is essential for mammary gland development. Development, 125, No.7, pp. 1285-1294, 0950-1991

Xu, Z.; Hurchla, M. A.; Deng, H.; Uluckan, O.; Bu, F.; Berdy, A.; Eagleton, M. C.; Heller, E. A.; Floyd, D. H.; Dirksen, W. P.; Shu, S.; Tanaka, Y.; Fernandez, S. A.; Rosol, T. J. & Weilbaecher, K. N. (2009). Interferon-gamma targets cancer cells and osteoclasts to prevent tumor-associated bone loss and bone metastases. J.Biol.Chem., 284, No.7, pp. 4658-4666, 0021-9258

Yamaguchi, T. (2008). The calcium-sensing receptor in bone. J.Bone Miner.Metab, 26, No.4, pp. 301-311, 0914-8779

Yang, X.; Halladay, D.; Onyia, J. E.; Martin, T. J. & Chandrasekhar, S. (2002). Protein Kinase C is a mediator of the synthesis and secretion of osteoprotegerin in osteoblast-like cells. Biochem.Biophys.Res.Commun., 290, No.1, pp. 42-46, 0006-291X

Yarbro, C. E.; Frogge, M. H. & Goodman, M. (2003). Cancer Symptom Management, p. 455, 0763721425

Zaidi, M.; Inzerillo, A. M.; Moonga, B. S.; Bevis, P. J. & Huang, C. L. (2002). Forty years of calcitonin--where are we now? A tribute to the work of Iain Macintyre, FRS. Bone, 30, No.5, pp. 655-663, 8756-3282

Zhang, J.; Dai, J.; Yao, Z.; Lu, Y.; Dougall, W. & Keller, E. T. (2003). Soluble receptor activator of nuclear factor kappaB Fc diminishes prostate cancer progression in bone. Cancer Res., 63, No.22, pp. 7883-7890, 0008-5472

Zhong, Y.; Armbrecht, H. J. & Christakos, S. (2009). Calcitonin, a regulator of the 25-hydroxyvitamin D3 1alpha-hydroxylase gene. J.Biol.Chem., 284, No.17, pp. 11059-11069, 0021-9258

Zlotnik, A. & Yoshie, O. (2000). Chemokines: a new classification system and their role in immunity. Immunity., 12, No.2, pp. 121-127, 1074-7613

11

The Role of T-Cell Leukemia Translocation-Associated Gene (TCTA) Protein in Human Osteoclastogenesis

Shigeru Kotake, Toru Yago, Manabu Kawamoto and Yuki Nanke
Institute of Rheumatology, Tokyo Women's Medical University
Japan

1. Introduction

Synovial tissues of patients with rheumatoid arthritis (RA) include factors regulating bone resorption, such as receptor activator NF-κB ligand (RANKL), TNF-α, IL-6, IL-17, and IFN-γ. However, in addition to these cytokines, other factors expressed in synovial tissues may play a role in regulating bone resorption. In 2009, we demonstrated that novel peptides from T-cell leukemia translocation-associated gene (TCTA) protein expressed in synovial tissues from patients with RA inhibits human osteoclastogenesis, preventing cellular fusion via the interaction between TCTA protein and a putative counterpart molecule. Only a few studies on the role of TCTA protein have been reported. In the current review paper, we summarized papers on TCTA protein and our recent findings.

Synovial tissues of patients with rheumatoid arthritis (RA) include factors regulating bone resorption by expressing cytokines such as RANKL, TNFα, IL-6, IL-17, and IFNγ (Horwood et al. 1999; Kawai et al. 2006; Kobayashi et al. 2000; Kotake et al.1996; 1999; 2001; 2005; Takayanagi et al. 2000; Yago et al. 2007, Yago et al. 2009). In addition to these cytokines, however, other factors expressed in synovial tissues may play a role in resorbing bone. To identify novel peptides or proteins expressed in synovial tissues of patients with RA that regulate human osteoclastogenesis, we purified proteins from synovial tissues of patients with RA, using gel filtration chromatography, reverse-aspect HPLC, and mass spectrometry. We finally demonstrated that a peptide derived from the extra-cellular domain of T-cell leukemia translocation-associated gene (TCTA) protein inhibits both RANKL-induced human osteoclastogenesis and pit formation of mature human osteoclasts (Kotake et al. 2009b, 2009c).

In 1995, Aplan et al. cloned and characterized a novel gene at the site of a t(1;3)(p34;p21) translocation breakpoint in T-cell acute lymphoblastic leukemia, designating this gene as TCTA (Aplan et al. 1995). TCTA is also reported as T-cell leukemia translocation-altered gene. TCTA mRNA is expressed ubiquitously in normal tissues, with the highest levels of expression in the kidney. TCTA has been conserved throughout evolution in organisms ranging from *Drosophila* to humans. A short open reading frame encodes a protein of 103 amino acid residues, M_r 11,300, without strong homology to any previously reported proteins. Of note, genomic Southern blots demonstrated a reduced TCTA signal in three of four small cell lung cancer cell lines, suggesting the loss of one of the two copies of the gene

(Aplan et al. 1995). On the other hand, in 2005, it has been reported that TCTA interacts with SMA- and MAD- related protein 4 (SMAD4) in a proteome-scale map of the human protein-protein interaction network (Rual et al. 2005); however, the function of TCTA has not been clarified.

2. Osteoclast

2.1 Structure and function of osteoclasts

Osteoclasts are unique multinucleated cells whose specialized function is to resorb calcified tissues (Fig. 1) (Kotake et al. 2005). On the surface of bone, osteoclasts develop a specialized adhesion structure, the 'podosome', which subsequently undergoes reorganization into sealing zones (Luxenburg et al. 2007). These ring-like adhesion structures, i.e., actin rings, seal osteoclasts to the surface of bone. In the sealed resorption lacuna, localized acidification is driven by carbonic anhydrase II and vacuolar H(+)-ATPase in osteoclasts; carbonic anhydrase II produces protons and vacuolar H(+)-ATPase transfers them into the lacuna. In acidified lacuna, cathepsin-K and matrix metalloproteinase-9 (MMP-9) are released from osteoclasts to degrade calcified tissues (Fuller et al. 2007).

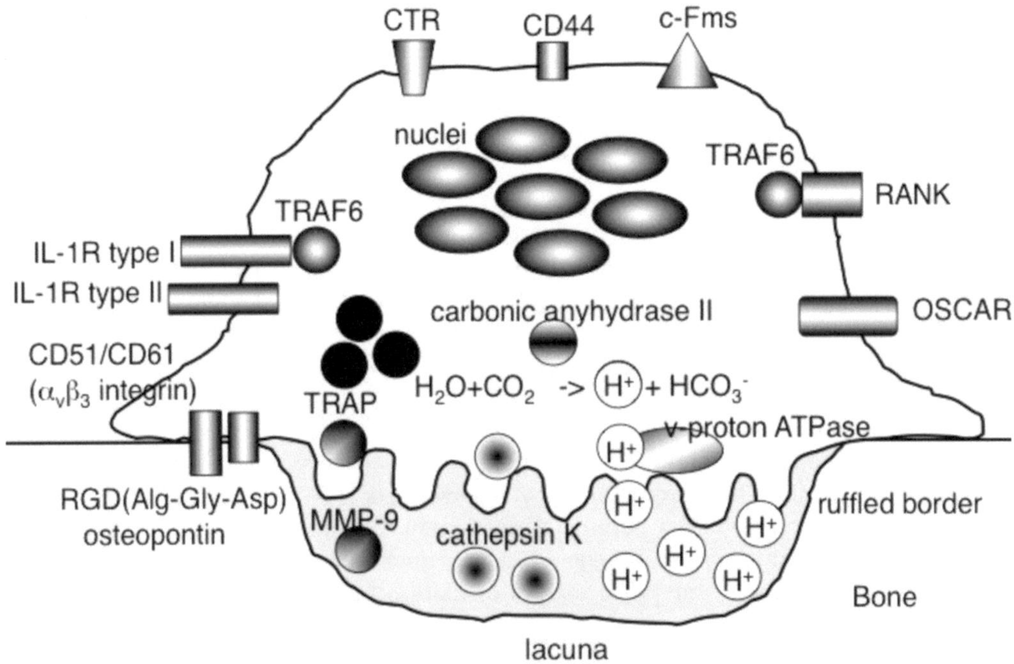

c-Fms, M-CSF receptor; CTR, calcitonin receptor; MMP, matrix metalloproteinase; OSCAR, osteoclast-associated receptor; RANK, receptor activator of NF κ B; TRAF, TNF receptor-associated factor; TRAP, tartrate-resistant acid phosphatase.

Fig. 1. Schematic structure of osteoclast

Osteoclasts express unique cell adhesion structures called podosomes, which contain actin filaments. Podosomes are organized differently depending on the activity of the osteoclast; in bone-resorbing osteoclasts, podosomes form the actin ring, representing a gasket-like structure, necessary for bone resorption, and in motile osteoclasts, podosomes are organized into lamellipodia (Latin lamella, a thin leaf; Greek pous, foot), the structure responsible for cell movement. Thus, the presence of actin rings and lamellipodia is mutually exclusive (Sarrazin et al. 2004). In 2004, Sarrazin et al. showed, using mature human osteoclasts extracted from the femurs and tibias of human fetuses, that osteoclasts have two subtypes of EP receptors, prostaglandin E_2 (PGE_2), EP_3 and EP_4, that mediate different actions of PGE_2 on these cells; activation of EP4 receptors inhibits actin ring formation and activation of EP3 receptors increases the number of lamellipodia (Sarrazin et al. 2004). Thus, PGE_2 directly inhibits bone resorption by human osteoclasts.

The cooperation of osteoclasts and osteoblasts is critical to maintain skeletal integrity in normal bones. After bone resorption by osteoclasts on normal bone tissues, osteoblasts subsequently rebuild bone in the lacunae resorbed by osteoclasts; this mechanism is called 'bone remodeling'. When the activity or number of osteoclasts is elevated compared with osteoblasts, the bone becomes fragile, that is, 'osteoporotic'. In addition, bone remodeling is disrupted in all bone diseases associated with changes in bone mass. Thus, bone remodeling is essential to retain both the structure and strength of normal bone.

2.2 Origin of osteoclasts

The origin of osteoclasts was unclear until the late 1980s. In 1988, Takahashi et al. established a co-culture system using mouse spleen cells and osteoblasts to induce osteoclastogenesis *in vitro*, demonstrating that the origin of osteoclasts is hematopoietic cells and that osteoblastic cells are required for the differentiation of osteoclast progenitors in splenic tissues into multinucleated osteoclasts (Takahashi et al. 1988b). The precursor of osteoclasts was then revealed to be colony-forming unit–macrophage (CFU–M) or CFU–granulocyte/macrophage (CFU–GM) in bone marrow or spleen in mice. In 1990, Udagawa et al. demonstrated that osteoclasts are formed from murine macrophages (Udagawa et al. 1990). From these findings, Suda et al. hypothesized that bone marrow hemopoietic cells differentiate into osteoclasts through the stimulation of 'osteoclast-differentiation factor (ODF)' expressed on osteoblasts (Suda et al. 1995).

Finally, ODF, now termed RANKL, which induces osteoclastogenesis from monocytes or macrophages, was independently cloned by three groups in 1997 (Fig. 2) (Udagawa et al. 2002). RANKL is a member of the TNF superfamily of cytokines. The protein constructs a trimeric complex to bind its receptor, receptor activator NF-κB (RANK)(Lam et al. 2001). A decoy receptor is also cloned, which is designated as 'osteoprotegerin (OPG)' (Udagawa et al. 2002). In 2000–2001, we and other groups showed that T cells expressing RANKL induce osteoclastogenesis (Kong et al. 1999; Horwood et al. 1999; Kotake et al. 2001); in particular, we demonstrated osteoclastogenesis using human cells (Kotake et al. 2001), whereas others used murine cells (Kong et al. 1999, Horwood et al. 1999). In addition, in 2009, we reported that, in human osteoclastogenesis induced by RANKL, T-cell leukemia translocation-associated gene (TCTA) protein is required for cellular fusion (Kotake et al. 2009b).

2.3 Development of culture systems to form osteoclasts *in vitro*

Culture systems were developed to form osteoclasts *in vitro* in 1981–1988. In 1981, Testa et al. first succeeded in forming osteoclast-like multinucleated cells from feline marrow cells in long-term Dexter cultures (Testa et al. 1981). In 1984, using this feline marrow culture system, Ibbotson et al. showed that the formation of osteoclast-like cells is greatly stimulated

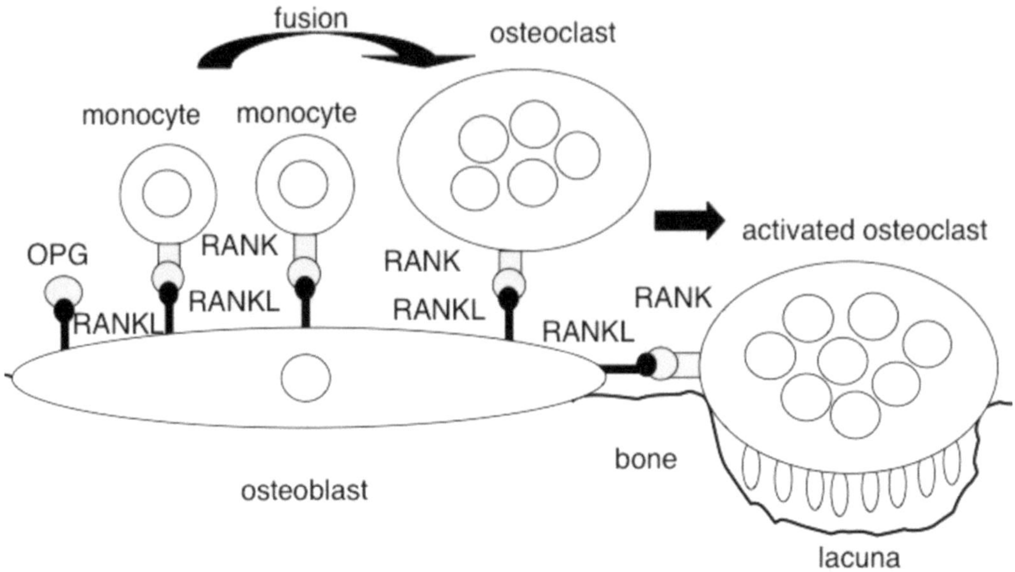

OPG, osteoprotegerin; RANK, receptor activator of NF κ B, RANKL, RANK ligand.

Fig. 2. Differentiation and activation of osteoclasts. A RANK-RANKL system induces both osteoclastogenesis from monocytes and the activation of mature osteoclasts.

by osteotropic hormones, such as $1,25(OH)_2D_3$, PTH, and PGE_2 (Ibbotson et al. 1984). In 1987, MacDonald et al. reported the formation of multinucleated cells that respond to osteotropic hormones in long-term human bone marrow cultures (MacDonald et al. 1987). In 1988, Takahashi et al. and in 1989, Hattersley et al. used marrow cells of mice to examine osteoclast-like cell formation from their progenitor cells (Takahashi et al. 1988a, Hattersley et al. 1989). Moreover, in 1988, Takahashi et al. established an innovative co-culture system using mouse spleen cells and osteoblasts to induce osteoclastogenesis *in vitro* (Takahashi et al. 1988b). Thus, since 1981, studies using osteoclastogenesis *in vitro* have been developed, and PGE_2 was shown to up-regulate murine osteoclastogenesis using the marrow culture system *in vitro*.

2.4 Role of osteoclasts in the pathogenesis of RA

Osteoclasts also play an important role in the pathogenesis of rheumatoid arthritis (RA). Since 1984, it has been reported that in bone destruction of RA, many activated osteoclasts are detected on the surface of eroded bone in the interface with synovial tissues (Shimizu et al. 1985). In addition, we have demonstrated that osteoclasts are detected in synovial tissues as well as eroded bone from patients with RA (Kotake et al. 1996). We have also reported that the number of precursor cells of osteoclasts increases in bone marrow adjacent to joints with arthritis (Kotake et al. 1992). Moreover, the amount of cytokines that induces osteoclastogenesis, such as IL-1, TNF-α and IL-6, is elevated in synovial tissues of patients with RA, while the amount of cytokines that induces osteoclastogenesis, such as IL-4 and IL-10, is decreased (Kotake et al. 1992; Kotake et al. 1996b; Kotake et al. 1997). Thus, patients with RA are likely to suffer from joint destruction as well as systemic osteoporosis, in which the number of osteoclasts increases, suggesting that osteoclasts play a critical role in the pathogenesis of RA.

2.5 Geranylgeranylacetone Inhibits the formation and function of human osteoclasts

The anti-ulcer drug geranylgeranylacetone (GGA), known as teprenon, is frequently used with nonstroidal anti-inflammatory drugs (NSAIDs) in Japan. In 2005, we demonstrated that GGA inhibits the formation and function of human osteoclasts and prevents bone loss in tail-suspended rats and ovariectomized rats (Nanke et al. 2005). Vitamin K is also used to protect against osteoporosis. It has been reported that the inhibitory effect of vitamin K2 (menatetrenone) on bone resorption may be related to its side chain. GGA has almost the same chemical structure as the side chain of menatetenone.

We hypothesized that GGA also has an inhibitory effect on osteoclastogenesis both *in vitro* and *in vivo*. GGA in pharmacological concentrations directly inhibited osteoclastogenesis from human monocytes induced by soluble RANKL. In addition, GGA induced the degradation of actin rings in mature osteoclasts, which was reversed by adding geranylgeranylpyrophosphatase. Moreover, GGA increased the bone mineral density of the total femur, proximal metaphysis, and diaphysis of femur in ovariectomized rats. GGA also prevented bone loss induced by hindlimb unloading in tail-suspended rats. These results indicate that GGA prevents bone loss by maintaining a positive balance of bone turnover through suppression of both the formation and activity of osteoclasts. In addition, in 2009, we also reported that GGA induces cell death in fibroblast-like synoviocytes from patients with RA (Nanke et al. 2009). Thus, GGA could be used to prevent and improve osteoporosis, especially in patients with RA.

3. 'Human osteoclastology' - Difference between human and mouse in immunology and cell biology

In basic science, murine cells are usually used, because these cells and experimental tools for them can be easily obtained. In addition, it is possible to create transgenic and knockout murine models. Indeed, biological science has made marked progress using murine cells and disease models. On the other hand, there are many disadvantages in studies using human cells, e.g., it is difficult to obtain human cells. In addition, it is impossible to perform an *in vivo* study.

However, to investigate the pathogenesis of RA, it is critical to investigate osteoclastogenesis using human cells. In bone cell biology, some cytokines show different functions between humans and mice. For example, M-CSF induces colony formation in mouse cells. In human cells, however, M-CSF usually induces the differentiation of progenitor cells of monocytes rather than colony formation, although Motoyoshi et al. initially reported that M-CSF induces colony formation in human macrophages in 1982 (Motoyoshi et al. 1982). On the other hand, some cytokines show different expressions between humans and mice; Kanamaru et al. reported that the expression of membrane-bound RANKL is limited in human T cells compared with mouse T cells (Kanamaru 2004). Moreover, the mouse $CD4^{+}CD25^{+}$ regulatory subset can be isolated from all $CD25^{+}$ T cells regardless of their level of CD25 expression; however, when similar criteria are followed to isolate these cells from human blood, $CD25^{+}$ cells (high and low together) do not exhibit an anergic phenotype or significant suppressive function. In 2001, Baecher-Allan et al. demonstrated that, in humans, $CD4^{+}$CD25**high** exhibit all the properties of regulatory T cells (Baecher-Allan et al. 2001). We also measured the percentages of $CD4^{+}$CD25**high** T cells as regulatory T cells in patients with Behcet's disease (Nanke et al. 2008). In addition, Amadi-Obi et al. reported that a major immunological difference between humans and mice is the presence of $CD4^{+}$T cells producing IL-17, Th17 cells, in the peripheral blood of healthy humans, but not mice (Amadi-Obi et al. 2007). Recently, several studies have also demonstrated the existence of substantial numbers of human CD4+ T cells that are able to produce both IL-17 and IFN-γ; the term "Th17/Th1" cells has been proposed (Annunziato et al. 2009).

In addition, two groups have reported the effects of PGE_2 on human osteoclastogenesis from monocytes alone stimulated by RANKL in the absence of osteoblasts, contrary to many reports on the stimulatory effects of PGE_2 on murine cells. In 1999, Itonaga et al. reported that PGE_2 inhibits osteoclast formation induced by RANKL in human peripheral blood mononuclear cell cultures (Itonaga et al. 1999). In 2005, Take et al. demonstrated that, unlike mouse macrophage cultures, PGE2 strongly inhibits RANKL-induced osteoclast formation in human $CD14^+$ cell cultures (Take et al. 2005). In addition, they showed that human osteoclast progenitors produce a soluble unidentified factor(s) in response to PGE_2 that strongly inhibits RANKL-induced osteoclast formation not only in human $CD14^+$ cell cultures but also in mouse macrophage cultures. They tried to identify the soluble factors, and concluded that $CD14^+$ cells produce an inhibitor(s) that does not correspond to known inhibitory factors, such as GM-CSF, IFN-γ, and IL-4. Thus, these reports demonstrated the possibility that PGE2 differently plays a direct role in osteoclastogenesis from monocytes alone in the absence of osteoblastic cells between humans and mice.

Thus, in the study of human diseases, it is essential to investigate human osteoclastogenesis using human cells; the differences in species used in studies are critical to discuss the function of cytokines. We suggest that the term 'human osteoclastology' be used to describe studies on human osteoclastogenesis (Kotake 2009a, Kotake 2010).

4. T-cell leukemia translocation-associated gene (TCTA)

In 1995, Aplan et al. cloned and characterized a novel gene at the site of a t(1;3)(p34;p21) translocation breakpoint in T-cell acute lymphoblastic leukemia, designating this gene as TCTA (Aplan et al. 1995). TCTA mRNA is expressed ubiquitously in normal tissues, with the highest levels of expression in the kidney. TCTA has been conserved throughout evolution in organisms ranging from *Drosophila* to humans. A short open reading frame encodes a protein of 103 amino acid residues, Mr 11,300, without strong homology to any previously reported proteins. Of note, genomic Southern blots demonstrated a reduced TCTA signal in three of four small cell lung cancer cell lines, suggesting the loss of one of the two copies of the gene (Aplan et al. 1995). On the other hand, in 2005, it has been reported that TCTA interacts with SMA- and MAD- related protein 4 (SMAD4) in a proteome-scale map of the human protein-protein interaction network (Supplementary Table S2, line 6175) (Rual et al. 2005); however, the function of TCTA has not been clarified.

5. Role of TCTA protein in human osteoclastogenesis

5.1 Hypothesis

Synovial tissues of patients with RA include factors regulating bone resorption by expressing cytokines such as RANKL, TNFα, IL-6, IL-17, and IFNγ as described in Introduction. In addition to these cytokines, however, other factors expressed in synovial tissues may play a role in resorbing bone. We hypothesized that a novel factor in synovial tissues of patients with RA regulates osteoclastogenesis. To test this hypothesis, we tried to identify novel peptides or proteins expressed in synovial tissues of patients with RA that regulate human osteoclastogenesis since 1996. We purified proteins from synovial tissues of patients with RA, using gel filtration chromatography, reverse-aspect HPLC, and mass spectrometry. We finally demonstrated that a peptide derived from the extra-cellular domain of TCTA protein inhibited both RANKL-induced human osteoclastogenesis and pit formation of mature human osteoclasts (Kotake et al. 2009b). We would like to present our findings as follows.

5.2 Purification of proteins from synovial tissues of patients with RA

Sixty-five grams of synovial tissues were obtained from 5 patients with RA at total knee replacement. The crude extract was obtained by homogenization of the synovial tissues. NH3Ac buffer was added to the freeze-dried crude extract. The supernatant was then applied to the column equilibrated with NH3Ac buffer and divided into two fractions, low molecular weight (MW) and high MW by first gel filtration chromatography. The low MW fraction was further applied to the column equilibrated with PBS by the second gel filtration chromatography. Proteins were eluted and protein concentration (A280) was monitored by UV absorption. Each fraction was added to the culture for human osteoclastogenesis to evaluate the activity on the osteoclastogenesis. Two fractions showed the inhibitory activity of osteoclastogenesis. These fractions were then subjected to ion-exchange chromatography. The "flow through" from the column showed the inhibitory activity on the osteoclastogenesis. The "flow through" was then applied to second gel filtration chromatography. Ten fractions from gel filtration chromatography showed the inhibitory activity on osteoclastogenesis. Thus, these fractions were applied to reverse-aspect HPLC. Thirty fractions were obtained by the reverse-aspect HPLC.

After each fraction obtained by reverse-aspect HPLC was concentrated, amino acid sequences were determined using a protein sequencer. Amino acid sequences (3-5 mers) were determined in 8 fractions. In addition, we tried to determine the sequence of each fraction by mass spectrometry; however, the sequences were not determined, although the total molecular weight of each peptide was speculated to be less than 1000 Da. Thus, we synthesized 8 peptides according to the sequences determined using the protein sequencer and evaluated the effect of each peptide on human osteoclastogenesis in vitro.

5.3 A small peptide including GQN inhibits human osteoclastogenesis

We finally revealed that the amino acid sequence of **Glycine-Glutamine-Asparagine (Gly-Gln-Asn; GQN)** alone in 8 synthesized peptides showed inhibitory activity in human osteoclastogenesis; **GQN** dose-dependently inhibited human osteoclastogenesis from peripheral monocytes by RANKL (IC50: around 30 μM)(Kotake et al. 2009b).

When searching for proteins that include **GQN** using FASTA search, we found only 2 proteins in human proteins, CDW52 antigen (CAMPATH-1 antigen) and TCTA. In the FASTA search, it was possible to identify 3 mer peptides, but we did not find any other human proteins. Using "PeptideCutter", by which it is possible to predict the site cleaved by enzymes in peptides, we synthesized 4 peptides from a sequence of CDW52 antigen and one peptide from a sequence of TCTA protein, which included **GQN**. A peptide from TCTA protein showed inhibitory activity on human osteoclastogenesis, but not peptides from CDW52 antigens.

5.4 Peptide A from TCTA strongly inhibits human, but not mouse, osteoclastogenesis

We then synthesized another 2 peptides, **GQN**GSTPDGSTHFPSWEMAANEPLKTHRE and **GQN**GSTPDGSTHFPSWEMAAN, using 'PeptideCutter', shown as "peptide A" (MW 3182.4) and "peptide A2", respectively, from a sequence of TCTA gene protein (Fig. 3). Osteoclastogenesis was more potently inhibited by these peptides than by **GQN** or **GQN**GST. Peptide A most strongly inhibited osteoclastogenesis; IC50 level was around 1.6 μM. Osteoclastogenesis induced by soluble RANKL (sRANKL) was not inhibited by adding 1.6 μM of a scrambled peptide, SPFTGTKGSWNETAHPDHGNEERQAPMSL (MW, 3182.4), randomly designed from the sequence of peptide A. We finally synthesized 3 more peptides from a sequence of TCTA protein, also using "PeptideCutter": "peptide B": **GQN**GSTPDGSTHF, "peptide C": PGLG**GQN**GSTPDGSTHF, and "peptide D": GFYGNTVTGLYHRPGLG**GQN**GSTPDGSTHFPSWEMAANEPLKTHRE, which is the whole of the human extra-cellular domain (Fig. 3). Sequences of both peptide B and peptide C are included in a human/mouse identical sequence of TCTA protein (Fig. 3).

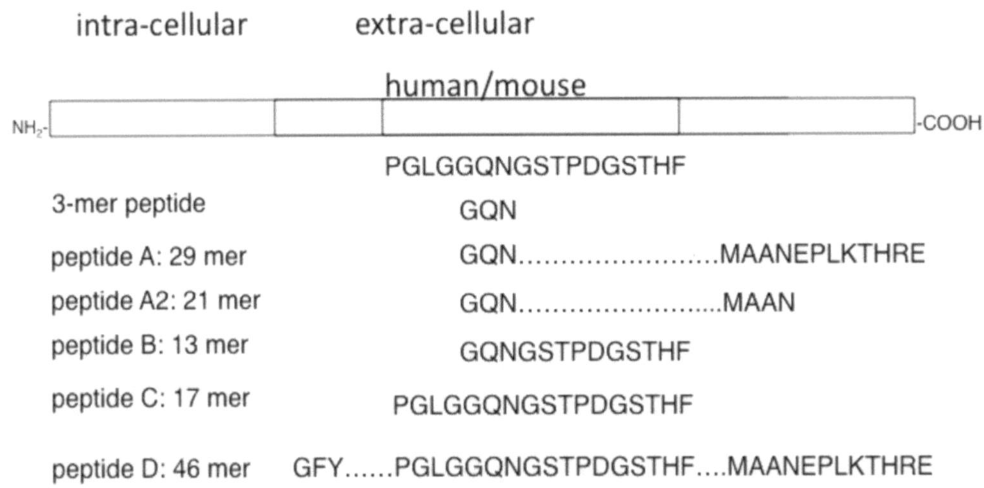

Structure of TCTA showing both intra-cellular (white bar) and extra-cellular (meshed bar) domains. Gray bar shows the human/mouse identical sequence in the extra-cellular domain.

Fig. 3. Structure of TCTA and sequences of peptides

Both peptide B and peptide C showed a weak inhibitory effect on human osteoclastogenesis from human peripheral monocytes. Peptide D did not show inhibitory activity. On the other hand, we also examined the effects of these peptides on mouse osteoclastogenesis; however, in contrast to our expectation, peptides B and C, which are included in the mouse sequence, did not inhibit ddY mouse osteoclastogenesis from mouse bone marrow cells stimulated by sRANKL and M-CSF. Peptides A and D did not show the inhibitory effects on mouse cells as we expected. Peptide A did not show cytotoxicity on human monocytes or cell proliferation on human monocytes (Kotake et al. 2009b).

5.5 Peptide A failed to inhibit the expression of protein and mRNA of NFATc1, and mRNA of cathepsin K

We then examined the effect of peptide A on the expression of both protein and mRNA of NFATc1, a key regulator of osteoclastogenesis under the signals of RANK-RANKL, in osteoclasts. Peptide A appeared to weakly inhibit the expression of protein of NFATc1 in osteoclasts in immunohistological staining for NFATc1. Peptide A (0.8 - 3.2 μM) also weakly, but not significantly, inhibited the expression of mRNA of NFATc1 in osteoclasts. In addition, peptide A did not inhibit the expression of mRNA of cathepsin K using the scrambled peptide as a control (Kotake et al. 2009b).

5.6 Peptide A inhibits pit formation of mature human osteoclasts in the culture of 3 days, but not 24 h

We then examined the effect of peptide A on pit formation of mature human osteoclasts on Osteologic^{R}. Mature osteoclasts formed from monocytes in culture with RANKL and M-CSF for 14 days were removed from plates. The mature osteoclasts then cultured on Osteologic^{R} discs with peptide A or a scrambled peptide in the presence of RANKL and M-CSF for 24 h or 3 days. Peptide A as well as a scrambled peptide did not inhibit pit formation for 24 h. However, peptide A significantly inhibited pit formation in the culture of 3 days, although a scrambled peptide did not inhibit pit formation at all. Thus, peptide A showed inhibitory activity on mature human osteoclasts in the culture of 3 days, but not 24 h (Kotake et al. 2009b).

5.7 Peptide A suppresses the formation of large osteoclasts in the culture of mature human osteoclasts

We then investigated the effects of peptide A on mature osteoclasts cultured with sRANKL and M-CSF for 3 days. In the control well with sRANKL alone in the absence of peptide A, larger osteoclasts were formed than osteoclasts cultured with sRANKL and peptide A. Huge osteoclasts were detected in the control well alone, but not in the well cultured with peptide A. Osteoclasts in the well cultured with peptide A showed usual size. The number of huge osteoclasts in the control well cultured without peptide A was significantly higher than in the well cultured with peptide A. Thus, we hypothesized that TCTA plays a role in the fusion of monocytes/macrophages, preosteoclasts and osteoclasts (Kotake et al. 2009b).

5.8 Polyclonal antibodies against TCTA inhibit both human osteoclastogenesis from monocytes and fusion of mature osteoclasts

We constructed indirect competitive enzyme-linked immunosorbent assay (ELISA) using 2 polyclonal antibodies against TCTA protein. Standard curves showed specificity and high affinity of the antibodies against TCTA protein. To investigate our hypothesis further, we cultured monocytes with M-CSF and sRANKL in the presence of the polyclonal antibody, #1 or #2, both of which significantly inhibited human osteoclastogenesis, reducing the size of osteoclasts. In addition, polyclonal antibody #2 inhibited the fusion of mature osteoclasts (Kotake et al. 2009b).

5.9 TCTA protein is immunohistologically detected on human osteoclasts and macrophages

Using antibody #1, TCTA protein was immunohistologically detected on human osteoclasts induced by sRANKL and M-CSF. TCTA protein was detected in the central area of cells or in the peripheral area of cells. TCTA protein stained in the peripheral area of cells was observed in both a pre-osteoclast with 2 nuclei and an osteoclast with 4 nuclei, using fluorescent microscopy. TCTA protein also detected human macrophages cultured with M-CSF (Kotake et al. 2009b).

5.10 Other findings on Peptide A

Peptide A as well as a scrambled peptide failed to disrupt the structure of actin rings of mature osteoclasts in the culture of 24h and 3 days. The amount of TCTA mRNA was significantly lower in human osteoclasts induced by sRANKL and M-CSF than in human macrophages cultured with M-CSF alone. Peptide A or the scrambled peptide, did not reduce the amount of TCTA mRNA in osteoclasts. TCTA mRNA was detected in human osteoclasts, monocytes, fibroblast-like synoviocytes, T cells, and PBMC by RT-PCR. TCTA protein was immunohistologically detected in cultured fibroblast-like synoviocytes using polyclonal anti-TCTA antibodies #1. TCTA protein was also immunohistologically detected in synovial tissues using polyclonal anti-TCTA antibodies #1. TCTA protein-positive cells were detected in synovial lining cells, but not in lymphoid folliculi with many lymphocytes. TCTA protein was significantly detected in human monocytes by flow cytometry using polyclonal anti-TCTA antibody #1 (Kotake et al. 2009b).

6. A novel hypothesis

We demonstrated that a novel peptide derived from the amino acid sequence of the extra-cellular domain of TCTA protein inhibited not only RANKL-induced human osteoclastogenesis from monocytes but also fusion of activated mature human osteoclasts (Kotake et al. 2009b). In the culture of mature osteoclasts, peptide A suppressed the formation of large mature osteoclasts after 3 days in the presence of sRANKL. In addition, although peptide A inhibited human osteoclastogenesis from monocytes with sRANKL, peptide A did not show significant inhibition of both protein and mRNA of NFATc1. The inhibitory effects of peptide A were not different among early, middle, and late phases of culture. In addition, the structure of actin rings of mature osteoclasts was not disrupted by peptide A. Thus, taken together, our findings suggest that the extracelluler domain of TCTA may play a role in the fusion of osteoclast precursors and mature osteoclasts, and that peptide A may block the interaction of TCTA and a putative counterpart of TCTA (Fig. 4). Supporting our putative mechanism, Saginario et al. reported that, because the soluble extracellular domain of macrophage fusion receptor (MFR) prevents the fusion of macrophages *in vitro*, MFR belongs to the fusion machinery of macrophages (Sarginario et al. 1998).

Several studies have reported that peptides inhibit osteoclastogenesis (Choi et al, 2001; Ikeda et al. 2004; Jimi et al. 2004). Jimi et al. reported that, using a cell-permeable peptide inhibitor of the I-κB-kinase complex, the peptide inhibits RANKL-stimulated NF-κB activation and osteoclastogenesis both *in vitro* and *in vivo*. They also showed that this peptide significantly reduces the severity of collagen-induced arthritis in mice by reducing levels of TNFα and IL-1β, abrogating joint swelling and reducing the destruction of bone and cartilage (Jimi et al. 2004). They used 20 μM of peptides to inhibit RANKL-induced mice osteoclastogenesis, whereas our peptide A inhibited RANKL-induced human osteoclastogenesis at 1.6 μM of IC50. Thus, our peptide more effectively inhibits osteoclastogenesis, although the different efficacy of the peptides may be derived from the different species used: humans and mice.

The reasons why peptides B and C, included in the mouse sequence, did not inhibit the osteoclastogenesis from mouse bone marrow cells remain unclear. We used only 3 peptides, peptide B, peptide C, and mouse "peptide A", in the culture of mouse cells. The other peptides, including GQN, may inhibit mouse osteoclastogenesis. On the other hand, even if TCTA protein plays a role in fusion as discussed above, TCTA protein in mice may be less important than the other molecules for fusion, such as, dendritic cell-specific transmembrane protein (DC-STAMP) (Kukita et al. 2004; Yagi et al. 2005), CD9 (Yi et al. 2006), CD47 (Lundberg et al. 2007; Yago et al. 2006), macrophage fusion protein (MFR)(Lundberg et al. 2007; Saginario et al. 1998; Yago et al. 2006), E-cadherin (Mbalaviele et al. 1995; Vignery 2000; Vignery 2005), meltrin-α (ADAM12) (Abe et al. 1999), or CD44 (Suzuki et al. 2002). These findings also underline the difference of differentiation of osteoclasts between human and mice, supporting the importance of the term, 'Human osteoclastology', as mentioned in section 3 in this article.

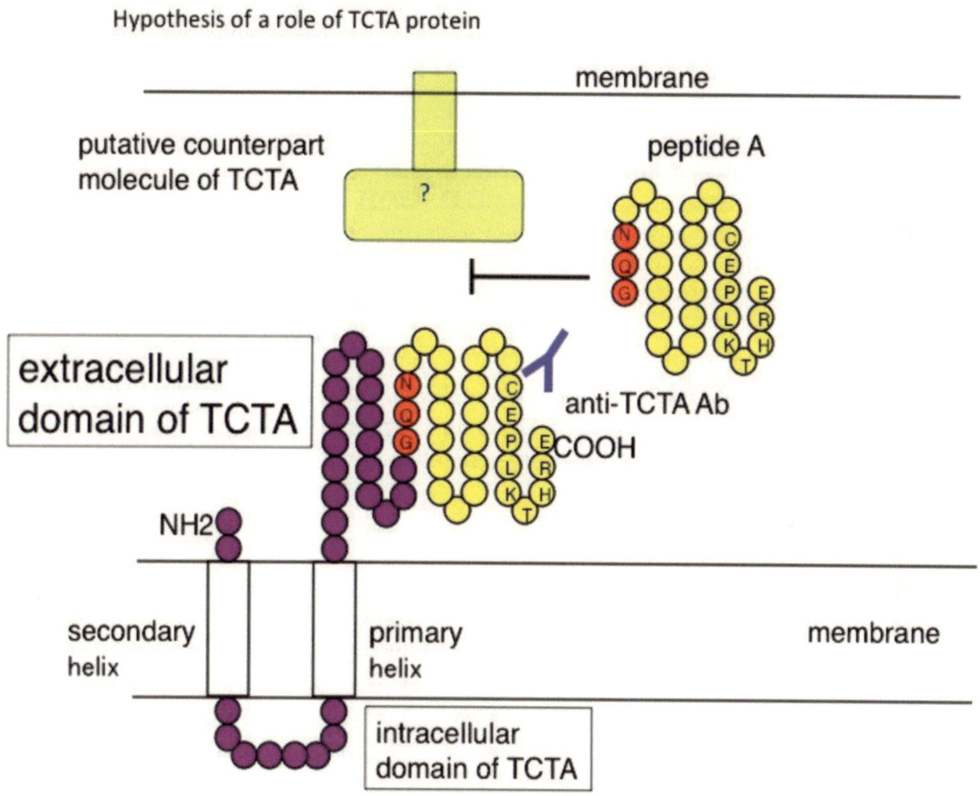

TCTA protein plays an important role in cellular fusion in human osteoclastogenesis from monocytes and mature osteoclasts. Both peptide A and antibodies block the interaction between TCTA protein and a putative counterpart of TCTA protein.

Fig. 4. Possible mechanism of human osteoclastogenesis by peptide A and antibodies against TCTA protein. (Structure of TCTA is derived from SOSUI; http://sosui.proteome.bio.tuat.ac.jp)

In conclusion, we demonstrated that peptide A and polyclonal antibody against TCTA protein inhibited not only human osteoclastogenesis from monocytes but also the further maturation of mature human osteoclasts *in vitro* (Kotake et al. 2009b). Our findings suggest that TCTA protein plays an important role in cellular fusion in human osteoclastogenesis from monocytes and mature osteoclasts. Thus, peptide A may show the same inhibitory function *in vivo*, offering an effective therapeutic approach for inhibiting bone resorption.

7. References

Abe, E., Mocharla, H., Yamate, T., Taguchi, Y., & Manolagas, S.C. (1999). Meltrin-alpha, a fusion protein involved in multinucleated giant cell and osteoclast formation. *Calcif Tissue Int* Vol.64:508-515.

Amadi-Obi, A.,Yu, CR., Liu, X., Mahdi, R.M., Clarke, G.L., Nussenblatt, R.B., Gery, I., Lee, Y.S., & Egwuagu, C.E. (2007). TH17 cells contribute to uveitis and scleritis and are expanded by IL-2 and inhibited by IL-27/STAT1. *Nat Med* Vol.13:711–718.

Annunziato, F., Cosmi L, Liotta F, Maggi E, & Romagnani S. Human Th17 cells: are they different from murine Th17 cells? (2009). *Eur J Immunol* Vol.39:637–640.

Aplan, P.D., Johnson, B.E., Russell, E., Chervinsky, D.S., & Kirsch, I.R. (1995). Cloning and characterization of TCTA, a gene located at the site of at (1;3) translocation. *Cancer Res* Vol.55:1917-1921.

Baecher-Allan, C., Brown, J.A., Freeman, G.J., & Hafler, D.A. (2001). CD4+CD25high regulatory cells in human peripheral blood. *J Immunol*, Vol.167:1245–1253.

Choi, S.J., Kurihara, N., Oba, Y., & Roodman, G.D. (2001). Osteoclast inhibitory peptide 2 inhibits osteoclast formation via its C-terminal fragment. *J Bone Miner Res* Vol.16:1804-1811.

Fuller, K., & Chambers, T.J. (1989). Effect of arachidonic acid metabolites on bone resorption by isolated rat osteoclasts. *J Bone Mines Res* Vol.4:209–215.

Fuller, K., Kirstein, B., & Chambers, T.J. (2007). Regulation and enzymatic basis of bone resorption by human osteoclasts. *Clin Sci (Lond)* Vol.112:567–575.

Hattersley, G., & Chambers, T.J. (1989). Calcitonin receptors as markers for osteoclastic differentiation: correlation between generation of bone-resorptive cells and cells that express calcitonin receptors in mouse bone marrow cultures. *Endocrinology* Vol.125:1606–1612.

Horwood, N.J., Kartsogiannis, V., Quinn, J.M., Romas, E., Martin, T.J., & Gillespie, M.T. (1999). Activated T lymphocytes support osteoclast formation in vitro. *Biochem Biophys Res Commun* Vol. 265:144-150.

Ibbotson, K.J., Roodman, G.D., McManus, L.M., & Mundy, G.R. (1984). Identification and characterization of osteoclast-like cells and their progenitors in cultures of feline marrow mononuclear cells. *J Cell Biol* 1984 Vol.? :471–480.

Ikeda, F., Nishimura, R., Matsubara, T., Tanaka, S., Inoue, J., Reddy, S.V., Hata, K., Yamashita, K., Hiraga, T., Watanabe, T., Kukita, T., Yoshioka, K., Rao, A., & Yoneda, T. (2004). Critical roles of c-Jun signaling in regulation of NFAT family and RANKL-regulated osteoclast differentiation. *J Clin Invest* Vol.114:475-84.

Itonaga, I., Sabokbar, A., Neale, S.D., & Athanasou, N.A. (1999) 1,25-Dihydroxyvitamin D(3) and prostaglandin E(2) act directly on circulating human osteoclast precursors. *Biochem Biophys Res Commun* Vol.264:590–595.

Jimi, E., Aoki, K., Saito, H., D'Acquisto, F., May, M.J., Nakamura, I., Sudo, T., Kojima, T., Okamoto, F., Fukushima, H., Okabe, K., Ohya, K., & Ghosh, S. (2004). Selective inhibition of NF-kappa B blocks osteoclastogenesis and prevents inflammatory bone destruction in vivo. *Nat Med* Vol.10:617–624.

Kanamaru, F., Iwai, H., Ikeda, T., Nakajima, A., Ishikawa, I., & Azuma, M. (2004). Expression of membrane-bound and soluble receptor activator of NF- B ligand (RANKL) in human T cells. *Immunol Lett* Vol.94: 239–246.

Kawai, T., Matsuyama, T., Hosokawa, Y., Makihira, S., Seki, M., Karimbux, N.Y., Goncalves, R.B., Valverde, P., Dibart, S., Li, Y.P., Miranda, L.A., Ernst, C.W., Izumi, Y., & Taubman, M.A. (2006). B and T lymphocytes are the primary sources of RANKL in the bone resorptive lesion of periodontal disease. *Am J Pathol* Vol.169:987-998.

Kobayashi, K., Takahashi, N., Jimi, E., Udagawa, N., Takami, M., Kotake, S., Nakagawa, N., Kinosaki, M., Yamaguchi, K., Shima, N., Yasuda, H., Morinaga, T., Higashio, K., Martin, T.J., & Suda, T. (2000). Tumor necrosis factor alpha stimulates osteoclast differentiation by a mechanism independent of the ODF/RANKL-RANK interaction. *J Exp Med* Vol.191:275-286.

Kong, Y.Y., Feige, U., Sarosi, I., Bolon, B., Tafuri, A., Morony, S., Capparelli, C., Li, J., Elliott, R., McCabe, S., Wong, T., Campagnuolo, G., Moran, E., Bogoch, E.R., Van, G., Nguyen, L.T., Ohashi, P.S., Lacey, D.L., Fish, E., Boyle, W.J., & Penninger, J.M. (1999). Activated T cells regulate bone loss and joint destruction in adjuvant arthritis through osteoprotegerin ligand. *Nature* Vol.402:304–309.

Kotake, S., Higaki, M., Sato, K., Himeno, S., Morita, H., Kim, K.J., Nara, N., Miyasaka, N., Nishioka, K., & Kashiwazaki, S. (1992). Detection of myeloid precursors (granulocyte/macrophage colony forming units) in the bone marrow adjacent to rheumatoid arthritis joints. *J Rheumatol* Vol.19:1511–1516

Kotake, S., Sato, K., Kim, K.J., Takahashi, N., Udagawa, N., Nakamura, I., Yamaguchi, A., Kishimoto, T., Suda, T., & Kashiwazaki, S. (1996a). Interleukin-6 and soluble interleukin-6 receptors in the synovial fluids from rheumatoid arthritis patients are responsible for osteoclast-like cell formation. *J Bone Miner Res* Vol.11:88–95.

Kotake, S., Schumacher, H.R. Jr., & Wilder, R.L. (1996b). A simple nested RT-PCR method for quantitation of the relative amounts of multiple cytokine mRNAs in small tissue samples. *J Immunol Methods.* Vol.199:193–203.

Kotake, S., Schumacher, H.R. Jr, Yarboro, C.H., Arayssi, T.K., Pando, J.A., Kanik, K.S., Gourley, M.F., Klippel, J.H., & Wilder, R.L. (1997). In vivo gene expression of type 1 and type 2 cytokines in synovial tissues from patients in early stages of rheumatoid, reactive, and undifferentiated arthritis. *Proc Assoc Am Physicians*, Vol.109:286–301.

Kotake, S., Schumacher, H.R. Jr., Arayssi, T.K., Gerard, H.C., Branigan, P.J., Hudson, A.P., Yarboro, C.H., Klippel, J.H. & Wilder, R.L. (1999). Gamma interferon and interleukin-10 gene expression in synovial tissues from patients with early stages of Chlamydia-associated arthritis and undifferentiated oligoarthritis and from healthy volunteers. *Infect Immun* Vol.67:2682–2686.

Kotake, S., Udagawa, N., Takahashi, N., Matsuzaki, K., Itoh, K., Ishiyama, S., Saito, S., Inoue, K., Kamatani, N., Gillespie, M.T., Martin, T.J, & Suda T. (1999). IL-17 in synovial fluids from patients with rheumatoid arthritis is a potent stimulator of osteoclastogenesis. *J Clin Invest* Vol.103:1345–1352.

Kotake, S., Udagawa, N., Hakoda, M., Mogi, M., Yano, K., Tsuda, E., Takahashi, K., Furuya, T., Ishiyama, S., Kim, K.J., Saito, S., Nishikawa, T., Takahashi, N., Togari, A., Tomatsu, T., Suda, T., & Kamatani, N. (2001). Activated human T cells directly induce osteoclastogenesis from human monocytes: possible role of T cells in bone destruction in rheumatoid arthritis patients. *Arthritis Rheum* Vol.44:1003–1012.

Kotake, S., Nanke, Y., Mogi, M., Kawamoto, M., Furuya, T., Yago, T., Kobashigawa, T., Togari, A., & Kamatani, N. (2005). IFN-gamma-producing human T cells directly induce osteoclastogenesis from human monocytes via the expression of RANKL. *Eur J Immunol* Vol.35:3353–3363.

Kotake, S., Nanke, Y., Yago, T., Kawamoto, M., & Yamanaka, H. (2009a). Human osteoclastogenic T cells and human osteoclastology (Editorial). *Arthritis Rheum* Vol.60:3158–3163.

Kotake, S., Nanke, Y., Kawamoto, M., Yago, T., Udagawa, N., Ichikawa, N., Kobashigawa. T., Saito. S., Momohara, S., Kamatani, N., & Yamanaka, H. (2009b). T-cell leukemia translocation-associated gene (TCTA) protein is required for human osteoclastogenesis. *Bone* Vol.45:627–639.

Kotake, S., Yago, T., Kawamoto, M., & Nanke, Y. (2009c) The role of T-cell leukemia translocation-associated gene (TCTA) protein in human osteoclastogenesis. *Jpn J Clin Immunol* Vol.32:466-471

Kukita, T., Wada, N., Kukita, A, Kakimoto, T., Sandra, F., Toh, K., Nagata, K., Iijima, T., Horiuchi, M., Matsusaki, H., Hieshima, K., Yoshie, O., & Nomiyama, H. (2004). RANKL-induced DC-STAMP is essential for osteoclastogenesis. *J Exp Med* Vol.200:941-946.

Lam, J., Nelson, C.A., Ross, F.P., Teitelbaum, S.L., & Fremont, D.H. (2001). Crystal structure of the TRANCE/RANKL cytokine reveals determinants of receptor-ligand specificity. *J Clin Invest* Vol.108:971–979.

Lundberg, P., Koskinen, C., Baldock, P.A., Löthgren, H., Stenberg, A., Lerner, U.H., & Oldenborg, P.A. (2007). Osteoclast formation is strongly reduced both in vivo and in vitro in the absence of CD47/SIRPalpha-interaction. *Biochem Biophys Res Commun* Vol.352:444-448.

Luxenburg, C., Geblinger, D., Klein, E., Anderson, K., Hanein, D., Geiger, B., & Addadi, L. (2007). The architecture of the adhesive apparatus of cultured osteoclasts: From podosome formation to sealing zone assembly. *PLoS ONE* Vol. 2, e179.

MacDonald, B.R., Takahashi, N., McManus, L.M., Holahan, J., Mundy, G.R., & Roodman, G.D. (1987). Formation of multinucleated cells that respond to osteotropic hormones in long term human bone marrow cultures. *Endocrinology* Vol.120: 2326-2333.

Mbalaviele, G., Chen, H., Boyce, B.F., Mundy, G.R., & Yoneda, T. (1995). The role of cadherin in the generation of multinucleated osteoclasts from mononuclear precursors in murine marrow. *J Clin Invest* Vol.95:2757-2765.

Motoyoshi, K., Suda, T., Kusumoto, K., Takaku, F., & Miura, Y. (1982). Granulocyte-macrophage colony-stimulating and binding activities of purified human urinary colony-stimulating factor to murine and human bone marrow cells. *Blood* Vol.60:1378–1386.

Nanke, Y., Kotake, S., Ninomiya, T., Furuya, T., Ozawa, H., & Kamatani, N. (2005). Geranylgeranylacetone inhibits formation and function of human osteoclasts and prevents bone loss in tail-suspended rats and ovariectomized rats. *Calcif Tissue Int* Vol.77:376–385.

Nanke, Y., Kotake, S., Goto, M., Ujihara, H., Matsubara, M., & Kamatani, N. (2008). Decreased percentages of regulatory T cells in peripheral blood of patients with Behcet's disease before ocular attack: a possible predictive marker of ocular attack. *Mod Rheumatol* Vol.18:354–358.

Nanke, Y., Kawamoto, M., Yago, T., Chiba, J., Yamanaka, H., & Kotake, S. (2009). Geranylgeranylacetone, a non-toxic inducer of heat shock protein, induces cell death in fibroblast-like synoviocytes from patients with rheumatoid arthritis. *Mod Rheumatol* Vol.19:379–383.

Rual, J.F., Venkatesan, K., Hao, T., Hirozane-Kishikawa, T., Dricot, A., Li, N., Berriz, G.F., Gibbons, F.D., Dreze, M., Ayivi-Guedehoussou, N., Klitgord, N., Simon, C., Boxem, M., Milstein, S., Rosenberg, J., Goldberg, D.S., Zhang, L.V., Wong, S.L., Franklin, G., Li, S., Albala, J.S., Lim, J., Fraughton, C., Llamosas, E., Cevik, S., Bex, C., Lamesch, P., Sikorski, R.S., Vandenhaute, J., Zoghbi, H.Y., Smolyar, A., Bosak, S., Sequerra, R., Doucette-Stamm, L., Cusick, M.E., Hill, D.E., Roth, F.P., & Vidal, M. (2005). Towards a proteome-scale map of the human protein-protein interaction network. *Nature* Vol.437:1173-1178.

Saginario, C., Sterling, H., Beckers, C., Kobayashi, R., Solimena, M., Ullu, E., & Vignery, A. (1998). MFR, a putative receptor mediating the fusion of macrophages. *Mol Cell Biol* Vol.18:6213-6223.

Sarrazin, P., Hackett, J.A., Fortier, I., Gallant, M.A., & de Brum-Fernandes, A. (2004). Role of EP3 and EP4 prostaglandin receptors in reorganization of the cytoskeleton in mature human osteoclasts. *J Rheumatol* Vo.31:1598–1606.

Shimizu, S., Shiozawa, S., Shiozawa, K., Imura, S., & Fujita, T. (1985). Quantitative histologic studies on the pathogenesis of periarticular osteoporosis in rheumatoid arthritis. *Arthritis Rheum* Vol.28:25–31.

Suda, T., Udagawa, N., Nakamura, I., Miyaura, C., & Takahashi, N. (1985). Modulation of osteoclast differentiation by local factors. *Bone* Vol.17(2 Suppl.1), 87S–91S.

Suzuki, K., Zhu, B., Rittling, S.R., Denhardt, D.T., Goldberg, H.A., McCulloch, C.A., & Sodek, J. (2002). Colocalization of intracellular osteopontin with CD44 is associated with migration, cell fusion, and resorption in osteoclasts. *J Bone Miner Res* Vol.17:1486-1497.

Takahashi, N., Yamana, H., Yoshiki, S., Roodman, G.D., Mundy, G.R., Jones, S.J., Boyde, A., & Suda, T. (1988a). Osteoclast-like cell formation and its regulation by osteotropic hormones in mouse bone marrow cultures. *Endocrinology*Vol.122:1373–1382.

Takahashi, N., Akatsu, T., Udagawa, N., Sasaki, T., Yamaguchi, A., Moseley, J.M., Martin, T.J., & Suda, T. (1988b). Osteoblastic cells are involved in osteoclast formation. *Endocrinology* Vol.123:2600–2602.

Takayanagi, H., Ogasawara, K., Hida, S., Chiba, T., Murata, S., Sato, K., Takaoka, A., Yokochi, T., Oda, H., Tanaka, K., Nakamura, K., & Taniguchi, T. (2000). T-cell-mediated regulation of osteoclastogenesis by signalling cross-talk between RANKL and IFN-gamma. *Nature* Vol.408:600-605.

Take, I., Kobayashi, Y., Yamamoto, Y., Tsuboi, H., Ochi, T., Uematsu, S., Okafuji, N., Kurihara, S., Udagawa, N., & Takahashi, N. (2005). Prostaglandin E2 strongly inhibits human osteoclast formation. *Endocrinology* Vol.146:5204–5214.

Testa, N.G., Allen, T.D., Lajtha, L.G., Onions, D., & Jarret, O. (1981). Generation of osteoclasts in vitro. *J Cell Sci* Vol.47:127–137.

Udagawa, N., Takahashi, N., Akatsu, T., Tanaka, H., Sasaki, T., Nishihara, T., Koga, T., Martin, T.J., & Suda, T. (1990). Origin of osteoclasts: Mature monocytes and macrophages are capable of differentiating into osteoclasts under a suitable microenvironment prepared by bone marrow-derived stromal cells. *Proc Natl Acad Sci USA* Vol.87:7260–7264.

Udagawa, N., Kotake, S., Kamatani, N., Takahashi, N., & Suda, T. (2002). The molecular mechanism of osteoclastogenesis in rheumatoid arthritis. *Arthritis Res* Vol.4:281–289.

Yagi, M., Miyamoto, T., Sawatani, Y., Iwamoto, K., Hosogane, N., Fujita, N., Morita, K., Ninomiya, K., Suzuki, T., Miyamoto, K., Oike, Y., Takeya, M., Toyama, Y., & Suda, T. (2005). DC-STAMP is essential for cell-cell fusion in osteoclasts and foreign body giant cells. *J Exp Med* Vol.202:345-351.

Yago, T., Nanke, Y., Kawamoto, M., Furuya, T., Kobashigawa, T., Kamatani, N., Kotake, S. (2006). Antibodies against CD47 expressed on monocytes in rheumatoid arthritis patients inhibits human osteoclastogenesis by blocking fusion of monocytes. *Arthritis Rheum* Vol.50 (supple):1394, S354 (abst).

Yago, T., Nanke, Y., Kawamoto, M., Furuya, T., Kobashigawa, T., Kamatani, N., Kotake, S. (2007). IL-23 induces human osteoclastogenesis via IL-17 in vitro, and anti-IL-23 antibody attenuates collagen-induced arthritis in rats. *Arthritis Res Ther* Vol.9:R96.

Yago, T., Nanke, Y., Ichikawa, N., Kobashigawa, T., Mogi, M., Kamatani, N., & Kotake, S. (2009). IL-17 induces osteoclastogenesis from human monocytes alone in the absence of osteoblasts, which is potently inhibited by anti-TNF-alpha antibody: a novel mechanism of osteoclastogenesis by IL-17. *J Cell Biochem* Vol.108:947–955.

Yi, T., Kim, H.J., Cho, J.Y., Woo, K.M., Ryoo, H.M., Kim, G.S., & Baek, J.H. (2006). Tetraspanin CD9 regulates osteoclastogenesis via regulation of p44/42 MAPK activity. *Biochem Biophys Res Commun* Vol.347:178-184.

Vignery A. (2000). Osteoclasts and giant cells: macrophage-macrophage fusion mechanism. *Int J Exp Pathol* Vol.81:291-304.

Vignery, A. (2005). Macrophage fusion: the making of osteoclasts and giant cells. *J Exp Med* Vol.202:337-340.

12

Retrovirus Infection and Retinoid

Yasuhiro Maeda[1], Masaya Kawauchi[1,2], Chikara Hirase[2], Terufumi Yamaguchi[2], Jun-ichi Miyatake[1,2] and Itaru Matsumura[2]
[1]*Department of Hematology, National Hospital Organization Osaka Minami Medical Center*
[2]*Department of Hematology, Kinki University School of Medicine Japan*

1. Introduction

Human T cell leukemia virus type I (HTLV-I) is a human retrovirus that is an etiologic agent of adult T cell leukemia/lymphoma (ATL/ATLL) (Hinuma et al., 1981, Uchiyama et al., 1977). Adult ATL/ATLL is an aggressive lymphoid neoplasm associated with human T-cell leukemia virus type 1 (HTLV-1) (Hinuma et al, 1982). ATL, the first human disease found to be associated with retroviral infection, usually occurs in native individuals from HTLV-1 endemic regions, i.e. southern Japan, the Caribbean, intertropical Africa, and Brazil (Kaplan et al., 1993, Gessain 1996). The HTLV-1 provirus is clonally integrated in $CD4^+$, $CD25^+$ activated T lymphocytes, which are leukemic cells characteristic of ATL. The exact mechanism of HTLV-1-induced tumorigenesis has not been fully elucidated, although HTLV-1 infection appears to represent the first event in a multi-step oncogenic process. (Franchini 1995). Diversity in the clinical features of ATL has been noted and four clinical subtypes of ATL have been defined: the acute form, the chronic form, the smoldering form, and the ATL lymphoma type (Shimoyama 1991). The acute and lymphoma types of ATL have a poor prognosis with a median survival of about six months (Shimoyama 1991). This extremely bad outcome is mainly due to an intrinsic resistance of the leukemic cells to conventional or even high doses of chemotherapy and to a severe immuno-suppression (Hermine et al., 1998, Bozarbachi & Hermine, 2001) reported, but a high toxicity and transplant-related mortality were observed in immuno-compromised patients (Borg et al., 1996, Ljungman et al., 1994, Sobue et al., 1987, Rio et al., 1980). A more effective therapy is therefore needed. Vitamin A and its analogs (retinoid) influence the growth and differentiation of normal and malignant cells, and have been shown to possess anticarcinogenic and antitumor activities in vitro and in vivo (Lotan 1980, Smith et al., 1992). Retinoic acid (RA) influences the clonal growth of normal human myeloid cells and induces the differentiation of both HL-60 cells (classified as a celll from a myeloblastic leukemia) and fresh human acute promyelocytic leukemia cells into normal granulocytes (Tobler et al., 1986, Breitman et al., 1980, Koeffler 1983). It has been reported that RA inhibits the growth of some tumor cells (Lotan 1979, Marth et al., 1986, Jetten et al., 1998)). Tax is a specific gene of ATL that immortalizes human T-cells (Tanaka et al., 1990). Tax, a 40 kD protein, is a transcription trans-activator of HTLV-1 that interacts with cellular transcriptional factors to activate HTLV-1 gene expression and HTLV-1 transformation of human T lymphocytes

(Tanaka et al., 1990, Feuer & Chen 1992). Tax activates HTLV-1 gene expression by increasing the binding of the cyclic AMP-responsive element-binding protein/activating transcription factor (CREB/ATF) proteins and the coactivator CBP (CREB binding protein) to the three 21-bp repeats in the long terminal repeat of HTLV-1 (Zhao & Giam 1991, Kwoak et al, 1996), and also activates immediate early genes (c-fos, c-jun, egr-1, and egr-2), a receptor gene (IL-2Rα), and cytokine genes (IL-2, IL-6, TGF-β, GM-CSF) (Tanaka et al., 1990, Feuer & Chen 1992). Furthermore, tax interacts with the ankyrin motifs in I-κB and NF-κB p105 and dissociates from or interferes with the complex I-κB/NF-κB, which is involved in the transcriptional activation of NF-κB in the cytoplasm (Hirai et al., 1994). It has also been shown that NF-κB was transported into nuclei and activated to induce the expression of cytokine and receptor genes (Feuer & Chen 1992, Baeuerle 1991). Inhibition of NF-kB activity is related for induction of apoptosis, and thus the Rel/NF-κB family plays important roles in the proliferation and differentiation of various cells in vitro. Already, Mori et al. have reported that NF-κB is constitutively activated in primary ATL cells as well as in the HTLV-1-positive T-cell line TL-Om1 independent of Tax protein (Mori et al., 1999). Furthermore, we have suggested that the target molecule of all-*trans* retinoic acid (ATRA) may be tax or some molecule in the tax- NF-κB signal pathway (Nawata et al., 2001). At the present time, the mechanism of ATRA's effect in ATL cells is not clear. In this article, we showed effects of ATRA in the aspect of 1) growth inhibition and CD25 down-regulation, 2) inhibition of NF-□B transcription, 3) effects of thiol compound, 4) effects for skin involvement, 5) mechanism of ATRA action, 6) clinical application, 7) effects for HIV infection.

2. Growth inhibition and down-regulation IL-2Rα/CD25 by ATRA

We initially assessed the effect of ATRA to HTLV-I positive T cell lines, HUT102 and ATL-2 cells. When those cells were treated with ATRA, cell proliferation was decreased significantly (Miyatake & Maeda, 1997). To assess the effect of ATRA to the cell surface antigen, we observed the expression of IL-2Rα/CD25 by flow cytometry. Incubation of those HTLV-I positive T-cell lines for 48hrs with 10^{-5} M ATRA for 48 h also resulted in down-regulation of CD25 expression (Miyatake & Maeda, 1997). Two peaks were apparent on FACS analysis of those cells, treated with ATRA, suggesting the existence of sensitive and resistant clones to ATRA. HTLVI negative cell lines, Jurkat and MOLT-4, were incubated with ATRA for 48hrs and assayed for cell proliferation. However, no growth inhibition was observed on both T cell lines (Miyatake & Maeda, 1997). The mechanism responsible for the difference in sensitivity of HUT102 cell clones to RA with regard to down-regulation of CD25 is not clear. However, this difference may be attributable to: (i) Differences in the expression of retinoic acid receptors (RARs) (Petkovich et al., 1987, Giguere et al., 1987), or retinoid X receptors (RXRs) (Heyman et al., 1992, Zhang et al., 1992). These receptors expression may be associated with the sensitivity to RA. (ii) Differences in the expression of cytosolic retinoic acid binding proteins (CRABPs), which binds RA before its transfer to the nucleus and acts as an intracellular antagonist of RA action (Maden et al., 1981, Eller et al., 1992, Siegenthaler et al., 1992, Wei et al., 1989). The extent of CRABP expression would be expected to correlate with RA resistance. And (iii) differences in the expression of anti-oxidant including ATL-derived factor (ADF). Indeed, our study showed that incubation with ATRA for 48hrs resulted in inhibition of growth for PBMCs and in induction of apoptosis from some patients with ATL, but not for PBMCs from normal individuals

(Maeda et al., 1996). Thus, there is a possibility that specific target cells of RA may be ATL cells in peripheral blood.

2.1 Inhibition of NF-κB transcription activity

We next investigated NF–κB transcription activity by CAT assay with pCD12-CAT. Spontaneous enhancement of CAT activity for NF–κB was detected. CAT activity determined with percent conversion was decreased after treatment with ATRA (% conversion: 60.8% to 21.0%). These results suggested that growth inhibition and CD25 down-regulation by ATRA occurred via the NF–κB signaling pathway (Nawata et al., 2001).Further, we demonstrated typical apoptosis on PBMCs obtained from ATL patients after treatment with ATRA for 48 hrs (Maeda et al., 1996). CAT-measured NF–κB activity was also significantly decreased on these PBMCs after treatment with ATRA for 24 hrs (Nawata et al., 2001). It has been reported that NF–κB is activated by Tax protein, which induces the degradation of I-κBα, which molecule is known to contribute to constitutive activation of NF–κB in ATL cells for cytokine gene, receptor gene and cell proliferation. We carried out a CAT assay for NF–κB using pCD12-CAT on ATL-2 cells in the presence or absence of ATRA (Nawata et al., 2001). Enhanced CAT activity determined with percent conversion was detected on ATL-2 cells (% conversion: 60.8%). It has been reported that Tax-mediated increases in NF–κB nuclear translocation result from direct interaction of Tax and MEKK1, leading to enhanced Ikkβ phosphorylation of IkBα (Yim et al., 1998, Mori et al., 1992). Furthermore, Arima et al. reported that Tax is capable of inducing nuclear expression of all four NF–κB species (p50, p55, p75 and p85) in primary ATL cells of acute type patients (Arima et al., 1999), and inhibition of apoptosis has been reported to be essential for activation of NF–κB. Our results possible indicate that the enhanced CAT activity for NF–κB may reveal that NF–κB protects against apoptosis. After treatment with ATRA, NF–κB activity decreased significantly (% conversion: 21.0%) on ATL-2 cells. Furthermore, we also transfected the *tax* gene in the expression vector (pCMV-Tax-neo) into the HTLV-I negative T cell line Jurkat (Nawata et al., 2001), and examined the effects of ATRA on cell growth. Interestingly, ATRA inhibited the growth of these transient transformants, but had no effect on the growth of control cells transformed with neomycin-resistance gene alone (Nawata et al., 2001). Taken together, these results indicate that the difference in the sensitivity to ATRA may be dependent on the expression of Tax. However, Mori et al. have reported that NF–κB constitutively activates in primary ATL cells as well as HTLV-I positive T cell line TL-Om1 independent of Tax protein (Mori et al., 1992). In summary, we have shown that ATRA could inhibit growth of the ATL cells and induce their apoptosis with suppressed NF-κB transcriptional activity. These results suggest that the target molecule of ATRA may be Tax or some molecule in the Tax-NF-κB signaling pathway, and that the existence of Tax would thus enhance the sensitivity to ATRA. Further study will be needed to determine whether ATRA exert its effects directly, or via some intermediary factor. Plans to administer ATRA to ATL patients in a clinical setting were currently undertaken in our laboratory (Maeda et al., 2000, 2004, 2008).

3. Effects of thiol compounds

In ATL, ADF that is homologous to thioredoxin (TRX) (Tagaya et al., 1989) have been reported to be not only a CD25 inducer, but also an active reducing molecule for active oxygen species. It was reported that the activity of thioredoxin reductase (TRX-R) from melanoma tissue was inhibited remarkably by 13-*cis* RA (Shallreuter & Wood 1990). Cellular redox status modulates various aspects of cellular function when oxidative stress occurs. The balance of oxidative/anti-oxidative influences may play an important role in the modulation of cellular function. It has been reported that L-cysteine and L-cystine act as a buffer of the redox potential of the environment in cells or serum (Bannai 1984, Miura et al., 1992). To study the effects of exogenous thiol compounds on the sensitivity to retinoid in a HTLV-I (+) T cell line, ATL-2 cells (Maeda et al., 1985) were cultured with thiol compounds (10^{-5} M L-cystine, 10^{-4} M GSH and 1 μg/ml TRX), following addition of ATRA or 13-*cis* RA. Significant growth inhibition was seen in ATL-2 cells when 10^{-5} M RA was added. Unexpectedly, similar growth inhibition of ATL-2 cells was shown with each thiol compound added to ATL-2 cells (Miyatake et al., 1998, 2000). These unexpected results may be explained by differences in uptake time into the cells between RA and thiol compounds. Next, we preincubated ATL-2 cells with each thiol compound (1 μg/ml recombinant ADF, 1 μg/ml TRX, 10^{-5} M L-cystine and 10^{-4} M GSH) for 24 hrs, and 10^{-5} M ATRA or 13-*cis* was added to ATL-2 cells in thiol-depleted medium. The reduction rate was decreased significantly by preincubation with the thiol compounds. Especially, preincubation of ATL-2 with L-cyctine or GSH resulted in complete restoration of growth despite the inhibitory effects of RA, this phenomenon suggested that it helped to increase the redox potential of the intracellular environment. Intracellular L-cystine is converted to L-cysteine, which is an active thiol compound that is utilized for GSH synthesis (Bannai 1984) and depletion of L-cystine results in a reduction of intracellular GSH content. These processes are antagonized by antioxidants such as cysteine and GSH (Miura et al., 1992). However, no restoration of growth was obtained in thiol-untreated ATL-2 cells. These reports suggested that L-cystine/GSH and ADF/TRX systems cooperate to support the adjustment of intracellular redox states against several oxidants and, thereby, promote the growth and viability of lymphocytes. Our results suggest that the imbalance of intracellular redox potential in HTLV-I (+) T cell lines may be associated strongly with the sensitivity to RA and exogenous thiol compounds may prepare the intracellular environment to become resistant to RA. In other words, cystine/GSH and ADF/TRX redox systems may act against RA, an antioxidant.

4. Effects of skin involvement

ATL is characterized by infiltration of various tissues by circulating ATL cells. Especially, skin lesions occur in 50% of ATL patients. We observed the effects of ATRA on skin involvement in ATL patients. Eight patients with ATL (2 cases acute type, 5 chronic type and 1 smoldering type) were selected (Maeda et al., 2004). Cutaneous lesions included erythematous plaques, papules, nodules, erythroderma, and tumors. Patients were scheduled to receive oral ATRA 45mg/m^2 daily. During treatment with ATRA, there was no chemotherapy or glucocorticoid therapy administered. Patients were monitored for safety and anti-tumor effect by regular physical examination and laboratory studies including complete and differential blood count and standard chemistry performed at the baseline and repeated at weeks 1, 2, 3 and 4. Skin biopsy was carried out before and after treatment with ATRA Complete response required all skin eruptions coming macroscopically negative. ATRA was effective for skin involvement in 6 patients (Maeda et al., 2004). A typical case is shown below; Case: A 42-year-old Japanese woman was referred to our hospital because of skin eruption with chronic ATL. After detection of proviral DNA in the skin by Southern blot analysis, ATRA (60 mg/day) was administered. The skin biopsy exhibited dense lymphoid infiltrates with atypical cytological features in the dermis. The infiltrate was composed mainly of medium to large cells with irregular nuclei. Neoplastic cells showed mild epidermotropism. There was a clinical and histological improvement after ATRA therapy was given for 4 weeks. Furthermore, proviral DNA for HTLV-I by Southern blot analysis in skin became to be negative after treatment with ATRA. These results indicated that ATRA may be a useful agent for skin involvement of ATL. Adverse effects were seen in 6 of 8 patients, these effects were temporally and generally mild (3 cases of headache, 2 cases of dry skin, 1 case of skin pigmentation). This confirms that as it has been reported ATRA only shows toxicities in a few cases. We had 2 cases that did not respond to ATRA, indicative of ATRA resistant cases. Differences between good responders and resistant cases should be investigated, including the mechanism of ATRA action for skin involvement.

5. Mechanism of ATRA action for ATL cells

At the present time, the mechanism of ATRA's effect in ATL cells is not clear. We observed two critical points; 1) whether ATRA suppresses HTLV-1 replication, and 2) whether ATRA decreases RT activity via a direct reaction. To confirm the anti-retroviral effect of ATRA, detection of HTLV-1 proviral DNA load using real time PCR was carried out in five HTLV-1-positive T-cell lines treated with VP-16, AZT, and ATRA for 48 and 72 hours. HTLV-1 proviral DNA load was only decreased by VP-16 in MT-2. HTLV-1 proviral DNA load was significantly suppressed by AZT in the HTLV-1-positive T-cell lines (ATL-2 and MT-2 at 48 hours, and ATL-2, MT-2, MT-4 and ED40515 at 72 hours) (Yamaguchi et al., 2005). Furthermore, HTLV-1 proviral DNA load was also significantly decreased by ATRA in HTLV-1-positive T-cell lines (all five HTLV-1-positive T-cell lines at 48 hours, and ATL-2, HUT102, MT-4 and ED40515 at 72 hours). These results suggested that ATRA might act as a RT inhibitor (Yamaguchi et al., 2005). Moreover, HTLV-1 tax mRNA load was significantly suppressed by ATRA (HUT102 and MT-2 at 48hours). As ATRA reduced HTLV-1 proviral DNA load, we observed whether it degrades the RT that participates in the cycle of retroviral replication (Yamaguchi et al., 2005). HTLV-1-positive T-cell lines (1×10^5/ml: total 20ml) were cultured with 10^{-5} M ATRA, 64 μM AZT or control reagent. Using the RT detection assay, we measured the RT activity of cell lysates. It was observed that ATRA significantly suppressed the activity in HTLV-1-positive T-cell lines (MT-4 and ED40515 at 48 hours, and HUT102, ED40515, MT-2 and MT-4 at 72 hours). In summary, we found that ATRA reduce HTLV-1 proviral DNA at mRNA level and RT activity of HTLV-1. These results suggest that the mechanism of ATRA's action may be dichotomized into inhibition of NF-κB transcriptional activity related to HTLV-1 and inhibition of RT (Yamaguchi et al., 2005). In another aspect on ATRA mechanism, we focused on the role of retinoids in inducing cellular senescence during the treatment of ATL (Maeda et al., 2011). Cellular senescence was detected by staining for senescence-associated β-galactosidase (SA β-Gal). SA β–Gal-positive cells were observed during the spontaneous culture without retinoids (ATRA or Am-80) in HTLV-I (+) T-cell lines (HUT102, MT-2, MT-4, ED40515, and ATL-2), but not in HTLV-I (-) T-cell lines (Jurkat and MOLT-4). On treatment with ATRA or Am-80, the number of SA β-Gal-positive cells significantly increased in the HTLV-I (+) T-cell lines, but not in the HTLV-I (-) ones. $P16^{INK4a}$ expression was enhanced in all the HTLV-I (+) T-cell lines, but not in the HTLV-I (-) T-cell lines. A telomeric repeat amplification protocol (TRAP) assay revealed that telomerase activity was not inhibited in retinoid-treated HTLV-I (+) T-cell lines; this indicated premature senescence (data not shown). We observed cellular senescence in HTLV-I (+) T-cell lines and in fresh primary cells obtained from patients with acute ATL. The grade of cellular senescence was greater for the HUT102, MT-2, MT-4, and ATL-2 cells than the ED40515 cells, which do not express *Tax* mRNA because of a nonsense mutation. This is an additional report pointing to *Tax* as an oncogene, and oncogene induced senescence (OIS) was possibly induced. These cells cannot re-enter the cell cycle or undergo tumorigenesis once senescence is triggered. OIS is caused by the accumulation of DNA damage. This DNA damage is, in turn, caused by oncogene-driven accumulation of reactive oxygen species (ROS) (Maeda et al., 2011). Chemotherapy using antineoplastic agents that decrease OIS and reduce cellular senescence may rejuvenate these cells and finally induce chemotherapy resistance. In conclusion, retinoids may be a reasonable agent for ATL with facilitating cellular senescence (Maeda et al., 2011).

6. Clinical application

We confirmed the clinical effects of ATRA in 20 ATL patients (Maeda et al., 2008). The median age was 56 years (range, 35–73). In total, 7 men and 13 women were enrolled in the study. Of these, 7 patients presented with the acute type; 3, lymphoma; 4, chronic; and 6, smoldering. The performance status (PS) of the patients ranged between 0 and 2, and 10 patients (50%) had skin involvement and 7 (35%), liver dysfunction. The treatment efficacy was as follows: CR, 0% of the patients; PR, 40%; NC, 45%; and PD, 15%. In the 7 acute patients, a PR was achieved in 2 (28.5%); NC, 2 (28.5%); and a PD, 3 (42.8%). In all the 3 lymphoma-type patients, a PR (100%) was achieved. In the 4 chronic-type patients, a PR was achieved in 1 (25%) and NC was observed in the remaining 3 (75%). Among the 6 smoldering-type patients, a PR was achieved in 2 (33.3 %) and NC was observed in 4 (66.6%). Adverse effects were noted in 10 of the 20 patients (50%). These effects were generally mild (headache in 5 patients; liver dysfunction, 2; hyperlipidemia, 2; and anorexia, 1). No hematological toxicity was observed. Considering the results described above, we indicated that ATRA has a therapeutic effect on ATL and should be the first choice for treating ATL. However, in fact, the present study showed no CR, which is not consistent with the results obtained in previous *in vitro* studies (Miyatake & Maeda 1997, Nawata et al., 2001). Interestingly, in the analysis among subtypes, ATL of the lymphoma-type showed a better PR rate than ATL of the acute-type (Maeda et al., 2008). In conclusion, the causes leading to a favorable response for ATRA treatment remain unknown. However, our clinical trial of ATRA for skin involvement demonstrated that ATRA was effective in the treatment of skin involvement in 6 of 8 patients (74%) (Maeda et al., 2004). Taken together, these results show that ATRA may have potential in the treatment of tumor formation with ATL cells than intravascular ATL cells. The present study showed that some patients are sensitive to ATRA while some are resistant. To elucidate the mechanism of resistance to ATRA, we focused on the intracellular redox potential. The imbalance of the intracellular redox potential in HTLV-I (+) T-cell lines may be strongly associated with the sensitivity to RA, and exogenous thiol compounds may cause the intracellular environment to become resistant to ATRA (Miyatake et al., 1998, 2000). In one of our recent studies, the mechanism by which ATRA acts on ATL cells was examined. The results showed that the mechanism could be dichotomized into inhibition of the transcriptional activity of NF-□B related to HTLV-I and inhibition of reverse transcriptase (Yamaguchi et al., 2005). This dichotomy model means multi-target therapy, and indicated that if one pathway is blocked by some factors, the other one will be available. Furthermore, we should recognize the differences between the clinical outcome and experimental results *in vitro*. We examined the differences in several clinical parameters (LDH, AL-P, sIL-2R, and age) between cases of NC and PR. However, no significant difference was observed (data not shown). Other intrinsic factors (i.e., retinoic acid receptor (RAR)-□ expression, cellular retinoic acid binding protein (CRABP expression etc.) need to be investigated carefully. We previously established a myeloid cell line with retinoid resistance. The cells expressed multi drug resistance 1 (MDR-1) mRNA and p-glycoprotein cell surface protein, we assessed whether verapamil and ATRA would induce the differentiation of the cells, however, they did not. An increased expression of cellular retinoic acid-binding protein (CRABP)-α was also detected on the cells compared with that of HL-60. These results suggest that high level of expression of CRABP-α may contribute to be the mechanism of ATRA resistance (Sumimoto et al., 2000). Further, serum concentration of ATRA would be an important factor, especially trough level should be measured in each case. In the present study, the common adverse effects of ATRA were temporal and generally mild (5 patients had headaches, 2 had liver dysfunction, 2 had hyperlipidemia, and 1 had anorexia). Moreover, the adverse effects ranged between CTC grade 1 and 3. As mentioned above, ATRA may be useful in treating some ATL patients and may also be used in combination with other chemical agents. When ATRA used with conventional chemotherapy, we suggested that dose of anti-neoplastic agents could be reduced significantly. Further, the nonmyeloablative chemotherapy will be able to reduce the opportunities of severe infection and hemorrhagic disorder in the clinical course. In conclusion, we firmly believe that treatment with ATRA can provide some benefits to clinicians and ATL patients.

7. Effects of HIV infection

Finally, we concluded that the mechanism of ATRA's action may be dichotomized into the inhibition of NF-κB's transcriptional activity related to HTLV-1 and inhibition of RT (Yamaguchi et al., 2005). It was reported that vitamin A supplementation reduced HIV-associated disease and slowed the progression toward AIDS (Fawzi et al., 2002). Maciaszek et al. reported that ATRA repressed HIV-1 long terminal repeat-directed expression in THP-1 monocytes (Maciaszek et al., 1998). Furthermore, Hanley et al. reported that a synthetic pan-retinoic acid receptor antagonist, BMS-204 493, activated replication of HIV-1 in a dose-dependent manner (Hanley et al., 2004). This phenomenon suggested that ATRA-induced transactivation of cellular gene expression is required for the viral replication (Recio et al., 2000). On the other hand, it was reported that RA stimulates transcription of HIV in human neuronal cells. The HIV-1 proviral DNA load in 8E5 cells (HIV positive T-cell line) was significantly reduced by ATRA as well as AZT. Furthermore, ATRA affected viral replication in the three HIV patients. Further, HIV proviral DNA load on treatment with AZT, 10^{-5} M ATRA or 10^{-7} M ATRA. Interestingly, ATRA could reduce viral replication not only in the 8E5 cell line but in the primary lymphocytes from HIV patients. Regarding ATRA and HIV infection, there are several interesting reports (Calvo et al., 1997, Kudva et al., 2004). Briefly, four patients were diagnosed with HIV infection and APL at the same time. The use of HAART was not reported in three of these cases. All three patients with APL and HIV infection treated with ATRA achieved a complete remission (Calvo et al., 1997, Kudva et al., 2004). Furthermore, the $CD4^+$ cell count decreased during therapy, but increased once the treatment was completed, and the patient did not suffer any HIV-associated complications (Kudva et al., 2004). This phenomenon may explain why ATRA affects both APL and HIV infection. Furthermore, a case of APL and ATL associated with HTLV-I infection treated with ATRA was reported (Tsukasaki et al., 1995). The patient was diagnosed with APL and smoldering ATL simultaneously, and treated with ATRA (60mg/day p.o.). At day 17 of ATRA treatment, the WBC count was normal with less than 1% APL and ATL cells. Monoclonal integration of HTLV-I was undetectable at that time. Hematological findings showed no abnormality on morphological, phenotypical, cytogenetic and molecular biologic analyses at day 50, when ATRA therapy was discontinued. Moreover, we examined the effects of ATRA on RT activity. RT activity decreased significantly on treatment with ATRA as well as AZT. The mechanism by which ATRA inhibited HIV replication may be inhibition of RT activity (data not shown). Taken together, ATRA may be a useful therapeutic tool for HIV infection.

8. Conclusion

We have believed that treatment with ATRA can provide some benefits to clinicians and ATL patients as having based on several evidences. Finally, we hope that ATRA is a useful agent for other HTLV-I-associated disorders, including HAM (HTLV-I-associated myelopathy), HAAP (HTLV-I-associated arthropathy), HAB (HTLV-I- associated bronchopathy) and HAU (HTLV-I-associated uveitis).

9. Acknowledgements

Author thanks to Mrs. K. Furukawa and Mrs. K. Niki for for technical assistance and Ms. S. Yoshida and Ms. S. Nagayama for preparing the manuscript.

10. References

Arima N, Matsushita K, Obata H, Ohtsubo H, Fujiwara H, Arimura K, Kukita T, Suruga Y, Wakamatsu S, Hidaka S, Tei C (1999) NF–κB involvement in the activation of primary adult T-cell leukemia cells and its clinical implications. *Exp Hematol* 27:1168.

Baeuerle PA (1991) The inducible transcription activator NF-κB: regulation by distinct protein subunits. *Biochim Biophys Acta* 1072: 63-80.

Bannai S (1984) Transport of cystine and cysteine in mammalian cells. *Biochim Biophys Acta* 779:289-306.

Beg AA, Sha WC, Bronson RT, Baltimore D (1995) Constitutive NF-κB activation, enhanced granulopoiesis, and neonatal lethality in I-□B□-deficient mice. *Gene Dev* 9: 2736.

Borg A, Yin JA, Johnson PR, Tosswill Saunders M, Morris D (1996) Successful treatment of HTLV-I-associeted acute adult T-cell leukemia lymphoma by allogeneic bone marrow transplantation. *Br J Haematol* 94: 713-715.

Bozarbachi A, Hermine O (2001) Treatment of adult T cell leukemia/lymphoma: current strategy and future perspectives. *Virus Res* 78: 79-92.

Breitman TR, Selonick SE, Collins SJ (1980) Induction of differentiation of the human promyelocytic leukemia cell line (HL-60) by retinoic acid. *Proc Natl Acad Sci USA* 77: 2936-2940.

Calvo R, Ribera JM, Battle M, Sancho JM, Granada I, Flores A, Milla F, Feliu E (1997) Acute promyelocytic leukemia in a HIV seropositive patient. Leuk Lymphoma. 26:621-624.

Eller MS, Oleksiak MF, Mcquaid TJ, Mcaffe SG, Glichrest BA (1992)) The molecular cloning and expression of two CRABP cDNAs from human skin. *Exp Cell Res* 1992;199: 328-336 .

Fawzi WW, Msamanga GI, Hunter D, Renjifo B, Antelman G, Bang H, Manji K, Kapiga S, Mwakagile D, Essex M, Spiegelman D (2002) Randomized trial of vitamin supplements in relation to transmission of HIV-1 through breastfeeding and early child mortality. *AIDS*. 16:1935-1944.

Feuer G, Chen IS (1992) Mechanism of human T-cell leukemia virus-induced leukemogenesis. *Biochim Biophys Acta* 1114: 223-233.

Franchini G. (1995) Molecular mechanisms of human T-cell leukemia/lymphotropicvirus type 1 infection. *Blood* 86: 3619-3639.

Gessain A. (1996) Epidemiology of HTLV-I and associated diseases. P Hollsberg and DA

Giguere V, Ong ES, Segui P, Evans RM (1987) Identification of a receptor for the morphogen retinoic acid. *Nature* 330: 624-629 .

Hanley TM, Kiefer HLB, Schnitzler AC, Marcello JE, Viglianti GA (2004) Retinoid-dependent restriction of human immunodeficiency virus type 1 replication in monocytes/macrophages. 78:2819-2830.*Hematopathology and Molecular Hematology* 11: 89-99

Hermine O, Wattel E, Gessain A, Bazarbachi A (1998) Adult T-cell leukemia: a review of established and new treatments. *Bio Drugs* 10: 447-462.

Heyman RA, Mangelsdorf DJ, Dyck JA, Stein RB, Eichele G, Evans RM, Thaller C (1992) 9-cis retinoic acid is high affinity ligand for the retinoid X receptor. *Cell* 68: 397-406. Hinuma Y, Komoda H, Chosa T, Kondo T, Kohakura M, Takenaka T, Kikuchi M, Ichimaru

M, Yunoki K, Sato I, Matsuo R, Takiuchi Y, Uchino H, Hanaoka M. (1982) Antibodies to adult T-cell leukemia-virus-associated antigen (ATLA) in sera from patients with ATL and controls in Japan; A nation-wide sero epidemiologic study. *Int J Cancer* 1982; 29: 631-635.

Hinuma Y, Nagata K, Hanaoka M, Nakai M, Matsumoto T, Kinoshita K, Shirakawa S, Hirai H, Suzuki T, Fujisawa J, Inoue J, Yoshida M (1994) Tax protein of human T cell leukemia virus type I binds to the ankyrin motifs inhibitory factor κB and induces nuclear translocation of transcription factor NF-κB proteins for transcriptional activation. *Proc Natl Acad Sci USA* 91: 584-3588.

Jetten AM, Kim JS, Sacks PG, Rearick JI, Lotan D, Hong WK, Lotan R (1998) Inhibition of growth and squamous cell differentiation markers in cultured human head and neck squamous carcinoma cells by β-all-trans retinoic acid. *Int J Cancer* 1990; 45: 195-202.

Kaplan JE, Khabbaz RF (1993) The epideminology of Human T-lymphotropic virus Types I and II. *Med Virol* 3: 137-148.

Koeffler HP (1983) Induction of differentiation of human acute myelogenous leukemia cells: therapeutic implications. *Blood* 62: 709-721.

Kudva GC, Maliekel K, Richart JM, Batanian JR, Grosso LE, Sokol-Anderson M, Petruska PJ. (2004) Acute promyelocytic leukemia and HIV-1 infection: case report and review of the literature. *Am J Hematol.* 77:287-290

Kwoak RP, Lauranca ME, Lundblad Jr, Goldman PS, Shih H, Conor LM, Marriott SJ, Goodman RH (1996) Control of camp-regulated enhancers by the viral transcription Tax through CREB and co-activator CBP. *Nature* 380: 642-646.

Ljungman P, Lawler M, Asjo B, Bogdanovic G, Karlsson K, Malm C, McCann SR, Ringdén O, Gahrton G. (1994) Infection of donor lymphocytes with human T-lymphotrophic virus type I (HTLV-I) following allogeneic bone marrow transplantation for HTLV-I positive adult T-cell leukaemia. *Br J Haematol* 88: 403-405.

Lotan (1980) Effects of vitamin A and its analogs (retinoids) on normal and neoplastic cells. *Biochem Biophys Acta* 605: 33-91.

Lotan R (1979) Different susceptibilities of human melanoma and breast carcinoma cell lines to retinoic acid-induced growth inhibition. *Cancer Res* 39: 1014-1019.

Maciaszek JW, Coniglio SJ, Talmage DA, Viglianti GA (1998) Retinoid-induced repression of human immunodeficiency virus type 1 core promoter activity inhibits virus replication. *J Virol.* 72:5862-5869.

Maden M, Ong DE, Summerbell D, Chytil F (1988) Spatial distribution of cellular protein binding to retinoic acid in the chick limb bud. *Nature* 335: 733-735 .

Maeda M, Shimizu A, Ikuta K, Okamoto H, Kasahara M, Uchiyama T, Honjo T, Yodoi J (1985) Origin of human T-lymphotropic virus-positive T cell line in adult T cell leukemia; analysis of T cell gene rearrangement. *J Exp Med* 162:2169-2174

Maeda Y, Miyatake J-I, Sono H, Matsuda M, Tatsumi Y, Horiuchi F, Irimajiri K, Horiuchi A (1996) 13-cis retinoic acid inhibits growth of adult T cell leuekmia cells and causes apoptosis; possible new indication for retinoid therapy. *Int. Med.* 35:180-184.

Maeda Y, Miyatake J-I, Sono H, Sumimoto Y, Matsuda M, Horiuchi F, Tatsumi Y, Irimajiri K, Horiuchi A (1996) New therapeutic effects of retinoid for adult T cell leukemia. *Blood* 88:4726-4727

Maeda Y, Naiki Y, Sono H, Miyatake J-I, Sumimoto Y, Sakaguchi M, Matsuda M, Kanamaru A (2000) Clinical applications of all-*trans* retinoic acid (Tretinoin) for adult T cell leukemia. *Br J Haematol* 109:677.

Maeda Y, Yamaguchi T, Ueda S, Miyazato H, Matsuda M, Kanamaru A (2004) All-trans retinoic acid reduced skin involvement of adult T-cell leukemia. Leukemia 18: 1159–1160. Maeda Y, Yamaguchi T, Hijikata Y, Tanaka M, Hirase C, Takai S, Morita Y, Sano T,

Miyatake J, Tatsumi Y, Kanamaru A (2008) Clinical efficacy of all-*trans* retinoic acid for treating adult T-cell leukemia. *Journal of Cancer Reseaech of Clinical Oncology* 134:673-677.

Maeda Y, Sasakawa A, Hirase C, Yamaguchi T, Morita Y, Miyatake J, Urase F, Nomura S, Matsumura I (2011) Senescence induction therapy for the treatment of adult T-cell leukemia. *Leukemia & Lymphoma* 52:150-152.

Marth C, Daxenbichler G, Dapunt O (1986) Synergistic antiproliferative effect of human recombinant interferons and retinoic acid in cultured breast cancer cells. *J Natl Cancer Inst* 77: 1197-1202.

Miura K, Ishii T, Sugita Y, Bannai S (1992) Cystine uptake and glutathione level in endothelial cells exposed to oxidative stress. *Am J Physiol* 262, C50-C58.

Miyatake J-I, Maeda Y (1997) Inhibition of proliferation and CD25 down-regulation by retinoic acid in human adult T cell leukemia cells. *Leukemia* 11: 401–407.

Miyatake J-I, Maeda Y, Nawata H, Naiki Y, Sumimoto Y, Matsuda M, Kanamaru A (2000) Important role of thiol compounds to protect oxidative stress on HTLV-I (+) T lymphocytes. *Leukemia Res* 24:265.

Miyatake J-I, Maeda Y, Nawata H, Sumimoto Y, Sono H, Sakaguchi M, Mastuda M, Tastumi Y, Urase F, Horiuchi F, Irimajiri K, Horiuchi A (1998) Thiol compounds rescue growth inhibition by retinoic acid on HTLV- I (+) T lymphocytes; Possible mechanism of retinoic acid-induced growth inhibition of adult T-cell leukemia cells. *Hematopathol Mol Hematol* 11: 89.

Miyoshi I (1981) Adult T-cell leukemia: Antigen in an ATL cell line and detection of antibodies to the antigen in human sera. *Proc Natl Acad Sci USA* 78: 6476.

Mori N, Fujii M, Yamada Y, Tomonaga M, Ballard DW, Yamamoto N (1999) Constitutive activation of NF-κB in primary adult T-cell leukemia cells. *Blood* 93: 2360-2368.

Mori N, Fujii M, Yamada Y, Tomonaga M, Ballard DW, Yamamoto N (1992) Constitutive activation of NF-□B in primary adult T-cell leukemia cells. *Blood* 93: 2360. Nawata apoptosis induced by all-trans retinoic acid on adult T-cell leukemia cells: a possible involvement of the Tax/NF-κB signaling pathway. *Leuk Res* 25: 323-331.

Nawata H, Maeda Y, Sumimoto Y, Miyatake J-I, Kanamaru A (2001) A mechanism of apoptosis induced by all-trans retinoic acid on adult T-cell leukemia cells: A possible involvement of the Tax/NF-kappaB signaling pathway. *Leuk Res* 25: 323–331.

Petkovich M, Brand NJ, Krust A, Chambon P (1987) A human retinoic acid receptor which belongs to the family of nuclear receptors. *Nature* 330: 444-450.

Recio JA, Martinez de la Mata J, Martin-Nieto J, Aranda A (2000) Retinoic acid stimulates HIV-1 transcription in human neuroblastoma SH-SY5Y cells. *FEBS Lett.* 469:118-122.

Rio B, Louvet C, Gessain A, Dormont D, Gisselbrecht C, Matoia R, Auzanneau G, Miclea JM, Baumelou E, Dombret H (1980) Adult T-cell leukemia and non-malignant adenopahties associated with HTLV-I virus. Apropos of 17 patients born in the Caribbean region and Africa. *Presse Med* 1990; 19: 746-751.

Schallreuter KU, Wood JM (1990) The stereospecific suicide inhibition of human melanoma thioredoxin reductase by 13-*cis* retinoic acid. *Biochem Biophys Res Commun* 160:573-579

Shimoyama and members of the Lymphoma study group (1991) Diagnostic criteria and classify-cation of clinical subtypes of adult T-cell leukemia-lymphoma. *Br J Hemato*l 79: 428-437.

Siegenthaler G, Tomatis I, Chatellard GD, Jaconi S, Eriksson U, Saura JH (1992) Expression of CRABP-I and -II in human epidermal cells. *Biochem J* 287: 383-389 .

Smith MA, Parkinson DR, Cheson BD, Friedman MA (1992) Retinoids in cancer therapy. *J Clin Oncol* 10: 839-864.

Sobue R, Yamauchim T, Miyamura K, Sao H, Tahara T, Yoshikawa H, Morishima Y, Kodera Y. (1987) Treatment of adult T cell leukemia with mega-dose cyclophosphamide and total body irradiation followed by allogeneic bone marrow transplantation. *Bone Marrow Transplant* 2: 441-444.

Sumimoto Y, Maeda Y, Naiki Y, Sono H, Miyatake J-I, Sakaguchi M, Matsuda M, Kanamaru A (2000) Establishment of a myeloid cell line, YM711, characterized by retinoid resistance. *Leuk Lymph* 39:373-383.

Tagaya Y, Maeda Y, Mitsui A, Kondo N, Matsui ., Hamuro ., Brown N, Arai K, Yokota T, Wakasugi H, Yodoi J (1989) ATL-derived factor (ADF), an IL-2R/Tac inducer homologous to thioredoxin: possible involvement of dithiol-reduction in the IL-2-receptor induction. *EMBO J* 8:757-764.

Tanaka A, Takahashi C, Yamaoka S, Nosaka T, Maki M, Hatanaka M (1990) Oncogenic transformation by the tax gene of human T-cell leukemia virus type I in vitro. *Proc Natl Acad Sci USA* 87: 1071-1075.

Tolbler A, Dawsaon M, Koeffler HP (1986) Retinoid. Structure-function relationship in normal and leukemic hematopoiesis in vitro. *J Clin Invest* 78: 303-309.

Tsukasaki K, Fujimoto T, Hata Y, Yamada Y, Kamihira S, Tomonaga M (1995) Concomitant complete remission of APL and smoldering ATL following ATRA therapy in a paient with the two diseases simultaneously. *Leukemia.* 9:1797-1798

Uafler (eds). Human T-cell lymphotropic virus type I. John Wiley Sons Lid, pp: 633-664. Uchiyama T, Yodoi J, Sagawa K, Takatsuki K, Uchino H (1977) Adult T cell leukemia: Clinical and hematologic features of 16 cases. *Blood* 50: 481.

Wei LN, Blaner WS, Goodman DS, Nguyen-Huu MC (1989) Regulation of the cellular retinoid binding proteins and their messenger ribonucleic acids during P19 embryonal carcinoma cell differentiation induced by retinoic acid. *Mol Endol* 3: 454-463 .

Yamaguchi T, Maeda Y, Ueda S, Hijikata Y, Morita Y, Miyatake JI, Matsuda M, Kanamaru A (2005) Dichotomy of all-trans retinoic acid inducing signals for adult T-cell leukemia. *Leukemia* 19: 1010–1017.

Yin M-J, Christerson LB, Yamamoto Y, Kwak Y-T, Xu S, Mercurio F, Barbosa M, Cobb MH, Gaynor RB (1998) HTLV-I Tax protein binds MEKK1 to stimulate I□B kinase activity and NF-□B activation. *Cell* 93:875.

Zhang XK, Lehmann J, Hoffmann B, Dawson MI, Cameron J, Graupner G, Hermann T, Tran P, Pfahl M (1992) Homodimer formation of retinoid X receptor induced by 9-cis retinoic acid. *Nature* 358: 587-591 .

Zhao LJ, Giam CZ (1991) Interaction of human T-cell lymphotropic virus type I (HTLV-I) transcriptional activator Tax with cellular factors that bind specifically to the 21-base pair repeats in the HTLV-I enhancer. *Proc Natl Acad Sci USA* 88: 11445-11449.